P9-CKW-971

APPRAISAL AND DIAGNOSIS OF SPEECH AND LANGUAGE DISORDERS

HAROLD A. PETERSON
University of Tennessee

THOMAS P. MARQUARDT
University of Texas

Prentice-Hall, Inc.,
Englewood Cliffs, New Jersey 07632

Library of Congress Cataloging in Publication Data

Peterson, Harold A 1926-
Appraisal and diagnosis of speech and language disorders.

Bibliography: p.
Includes index.

1. Speech, Disorders of–Diagnosis. 2. Language disorders–Diagnosis. I. Marquardt, Thomas P., joint author. II. Title. [DNLM: 1. Language disorders–Diagnosis. 2. Speech disorders–Diagnosis. WM475 P485a]

RC423.P47 616.85'5075 80-16583

ISBN 0-13-043505-8

Editorial/production supervision and interior design by Dianne Poonarian
Cover design by Jerry Pfeifer
Manufacturing buyer: Edmund W. Leone

Printed in the United States of America

10 9 8 7 6 5 4 3 2 1

Prentice-Hall International, Inc., *London*
Prentice-Hall of Australia Pty. Limited, *Sydney*
Prentice-Hall of Canada, Ltd., *Toronto*
Prentice-Hall of India Private Limited, *New Delhi*
Prentice-Hall of Japan, Inc., *Tokyo*
Prentice-Hall of Southeast Asia Pte. Ltd., *Singapore*
Whitehall Books Limited, *Wellington, New Zealand*

This book is dedicated to our clients, teachers, and students, who taught us and made this book possible; to our colleagues and friends who provided invaluable assistance in clarifying the readability of the innumerable versions the text; and to our wives who put up with the seclusion and separateness that a task of this nature engenders. It is an expected and oft quoted truth in dedication statements such as this that those who aided were too numerous to mention for fear of failure to include a name (and that is true here), but the errors that remain are our sole responsibility (and that too is true here).

HAP
TPM

Contents

PART II 47

PART III 171

Preface

A crucial aspect of any rehabilitation program for communicatively handicapped individuals is the appraisal and diagnosis of speech and language disorders. A large number of tests have been developed for this purpose, especially during the past two decades. Some tests are modifications of existing instruments, while others have been developed from new rationales. The purpose of this book is not to serve as a compendium of existing test instruments nor to review critically all test procedures.

You will not find, in the ensuing pages, a block diagram of flow charts to illustrate our theoretical model of diagnosis. Simply stated, the theoretical base from which we are operating is an admonition to describe and, as far as possible, to quantify communication disorders. Quantification is necessary to allow qualitative comparisons on the effectiveness of the therapeutic interventions. To that end, each of the chapters which follow wll include some rationale for testing and sufficient detail on examples of tests to make both the purpose and the mechanics of the tests apparent.

The introductory chapter and the one on information gathering may be taken as philosophical statements—and are identified as Part I. In them we wish to emphasize the importance of careful selection of your measurement instruments and of careful listening and observing. An applicable bromide to insert here may be "a good carpenter measures twice before he cuts once." Part II follows with chapters on a variety of tests for specific types of communication problems. Part III includes diagnostic definitions on some speech and language disorders where a lesser variety of tests exist—and therefore requires a somewhat broader definition of the disorders being described. Part IV contains a chapter on interpretation of psychological tests. We are not assuming the speech and language clinician is also a psychometrist, but rather that the clinician can profit from an explanation of some of the kinds of information available in that domain. The last chapter, on clinical reporting and record keeping, signifies the pragmatic result of the clinical process. The diagnostic endeavor begins with determination of the proper questions to be asked. The testing and observation that are part of the initial and continuing therapeutic contact provide the data on which the answer is based, and the clinical reporting is the communication of that answer.

This book is intended for graduate students and advanced undergraduate students in speech pathology, special education, clinical psychology, and associated rehabilitation specialities—especially those who are inexperienced in diagnostics, or who are interested in comparing a broad range of speech and language tests. Hopefully our professional colleagues, devoted to the diagnosis and rehabilitation of communicatively handicapped individuals, also will find something of interest and value for their daily work.

PART I

The Philosophy of Diagnosis

I

It is the customary fate of new truths to begin as heresies and end as superstitions.

T. H. Huxley

The appraisal and diagnosis of speech and language disorders is primarily a descriptive task. An adequate description should define the speech and language skills observed, judge the communication ability, determine the relevant variables in the speaker, and make obvious a plan of action for remediation if the pattern presented warrants it. Consequently, before discussing the specifics of speech and language description, it is appropriate that we first concern ourselves with the philosophical basis for testing, test construction, and the concept of "normal." Those three variables are inexorably bound. Your philosophical basis for testing will flavor your test selection, and your definition of normal will be some function of the test content and format you choose. We will comment on the need for nonformalized as well as formalized assessment procedures and briefly discuss ethics and responsibilities bound up with the diagnostician's task.

APPRAISAL AND DIAGNOSIS

Before we continue, we need to define two terms and the way in which we will use them. The terms are *appraisal* and *diagnosis.* Appraisal implies calibrated observation and measurement. Measurement requires obtaining direct quantitative data. Some of these performance data can be compared with published "norms"; some cannot. Diagnosis requires placing measurements and other observational data into context and perspective in order to decide whether a problem exists and to differentiate one problem from others which may have similar performance aspects. The diagnosis is then a function of the descriptions which we have collected, and not all of these descriptions will have been easily quantifiable.

Some of the tests we will discuss in the ensuing chapters are identified as *diagnostic,* and others as *screening.* The purpose we have in testing an individual is one of the determining factors in the type of test selected. If we wish to assess the general adequacy of some communicative function, we use a screening test. If we want a detailed description, we use a diagnostic test.

THE NEED TO BE DESCRIPTIVE

Test constructions change over time just as theories change. A new theory is proposed when, in the mind of the theorist, the previous explanation was incomplete. Tests are constructed to fit theoretical biases and to calibrate specific types of observations. More important than the specific tests we select to use as observational tools is our clear understanding of the behavior we set out to describe. The assignment of terms, such as stuttering, or aphasia, or learning disability, is not a description but an abbreviation for a constellation of behaviors. Terms or categories, such as these, may be helpful for filing purposes, but they do not describe what the person does or what he does not do. Call this the first law of diagnostics: *Describe the behavior.* If you cannot describe it, you do not understand it; or, you cannot expect to understand the behavior if you cannot describe it. Description does not guarantee understanding, but description makes understanding possible.

This emphasis on description is important whether or not we can use "standardized" tests to aid our observation. It becomes increasingly important when, as speech-language clinicians,* we are called upon to evaluate "special" populations such as nonverbal or language-delayed children, or those who are referred to us as learning-disabled. With a great number of these children, test results may be inaccurate or even misleading. Muma (1973) has stressed the point that standardized assessment procedures of themselves will not usually yield an adequate description of language function. In his *Language Handbook* (1978, p. 211) he makes a stronger statement:

> Behavior is relative, conditional, complex, and dynamic. Accordingly, clinical assessment must be relative, contextual, process oriented, and

*The word "clinician" as used here is not in contrast to "therapist" or "pathologist" or similar terms but is a generic term to denote one who works in a clinical setting or is involved in clinical activity.

> dynamic. Contrary to some views, it should not be categorical, quantitative, or normative. These three traditional notions need to be challenged. Clinical assessment should be about an *individual* as he functions in natural contexts (Bronfenbrenner 1977) or deals with systems and processes directly relevant to natural behavior.

Siegel (1975) provided similar advice to clinicians with the following statement:

> In my mind, the best "instrument" available is a clinician who has some knowledge of research and theory in language, some experience in describing and dealing with important communication behaviors, and some reservoir of confidence in his or her own abilities to observe behavior, develop hypotheses, and change ideas and approaches when necessary. (p. 213)

Neither of those quotes deny the applicability of standardized testing—of formalized measures. They *do* remind the clinician of the importance of going beyond restricted, structured assessment techniques. Leonard and others (1978) extended Siegel's philosophy in an article concerned with nonstandardized approaches to assessment which they considered

> ". . . as a necessary supplement to the use of standardized tests for the assessment of language behavior. We adopt the position that the use of nonstandardized measures is essential in gaining sufficient information about the child's linguistic system in order to devise effective intervention strategies. (p. 371)

In other words, we do need observations in addition to the "standardized" quantitative, normative comparisons. Normative comparisons are a function of controlled circumstances and can help us make a judgment of speech and language deviance. That is, we can compare how the patient at hand performed in relation to other patients of the same age with the same or comparable stimuli. They do not necessarily describe the communicative function of this person in his "natural" environment. The behavior we observe, in either a controlled or nonrestrictive circumstance, is only a sample from which inferences are made. It is never a complete description of all behavior under all conditions.

The formalized and nonformalized assessments we make are subject to interpretation and that includes a judgment of communicative effectiveness within a situation. A determination of functional effectiveness requires at least the circumstance, or variety of circumstances, in which the child is attempting to communicate (Menyuk 1963, 1964; Sroufe 1970). What a child does, in other than imitative performance, may be taken as some evidence of linguistic competence, but lack of performance should not routinely be accepted as evidence of lack of competence (Cazden 1967).

Bloom and Lahey (1978) describe three dimensions of language: content, form, and function. The normative data that are available bear primarily on language form. Form is described in terms of the acoustic, phonetic shape of segments of the utterance. In other words, quantitative comparisons are available for phonology, morphology, and syntax. There are no quantitative or normative data for the content and function of language. Bloom and Lahey describe content as the topics or concepts discussed and the interaction between context and information processing; function or use of language depends on the context or circumstances (reason to speak) for a decision on the form of language to be used. These definitions of communication bear on the "relative, conditional, complex and dynamic" behavior in Muma's statement and are part of the "knowledge of research and theory" required by Siegel.

Part of the task we are asked to perform, however, is to answer the question as to whether the behavior presented is normal. For this judgment we need information on expected levels of performance as a basis for a definition of normal.

CONCEPT OF "NORMALCY"

Our clinical task is to define a set of procedures which will help to separate "normal" from "abnormal" performance and to gather sufficient description to suggest what can be done about the problems we determine exist. Normal and abnormal are reciprocal terms and need clarification. For example, in a statistical or probability sense, normal means average. One such average that most of us are familiar with is the measurement of intelligence and the expected or average intelligence quotient (I.Q.) of 100. A "quotient" (proportionate score) of 100 implies that the one tested performed no better and no worse than is expected for his or her age.

Two points should be made relative to an "average" score. One is that the practical interpretation of intelligence and similar scores considers average to be a range rather than a single point on the scale. Moreover, the range of normal may not be defined in the same terms on all tests. The "normal range" on most intelligence tests, for example, Wechsler Adult Intelligence Scale (1955), or Stanford-Binet Tests of Intelligence (1960), is from 90 to 110, or approximately one standard deviation on either side of the mean. The Wechsler and the Stanford-Binet tests have been constructed with one standard deviation equivalent to ten points, and both consider a score between plus and minus two standard deviations (a score of 80 to 120) to be within gross normal limits.

On the other hand, the *Peabody Picture Vocabulary Test* (Dunn 1965) yields a score which is convertible to an I.Q. with a standard deviation of about 12 to 13 points. Consequently, gross normal limits of performance according to the *Peabody Picture Vocabulary Test* are from 75 to 125 for the plus or minus two standard deviation range. The second point to be made concerning average scores is that the people measured should belong to the theroretical population against which they are compared. Again, using intelligence scores as an example, the mean or average I.Q. in a university class of undergraduate seniors would probably be between 115 and 120; the mean I.Q. in a grammar school in a low socioeconomic area may be between 90 and 95, and so forth. In other words, a range of scores rather than a single score should be considered normal, and normal or average depends on the circumstances and the population studied.

It is also important to remember that statistical descriptions in terms of numerical quantifications such as these do not automatically imply a value judgment. Being "above" or "below" or "average" is not necessarily good, bad, or otherwise. That is true whether the statistical comparison we are using is concerned with height, weight, shoe size, words in a vocabulary, speech sounds produced correctly, or any other of the variety of behaviors, talents, or attributes measured. A numerical value may be helpful information as part of our total description, but by itself, it only speaks to a person's one-time measurement and comparison to a specific population on a described task. It has no intrinsic evaluational or judgmental connotation.

Figure 1-1 illustrates the hypothetical distribution of an attribute such as intelligence in a population. This is called a "bell-shaped curve," or a normal distribution (DuBois 1965). Points are marked equidistant along the horizontal

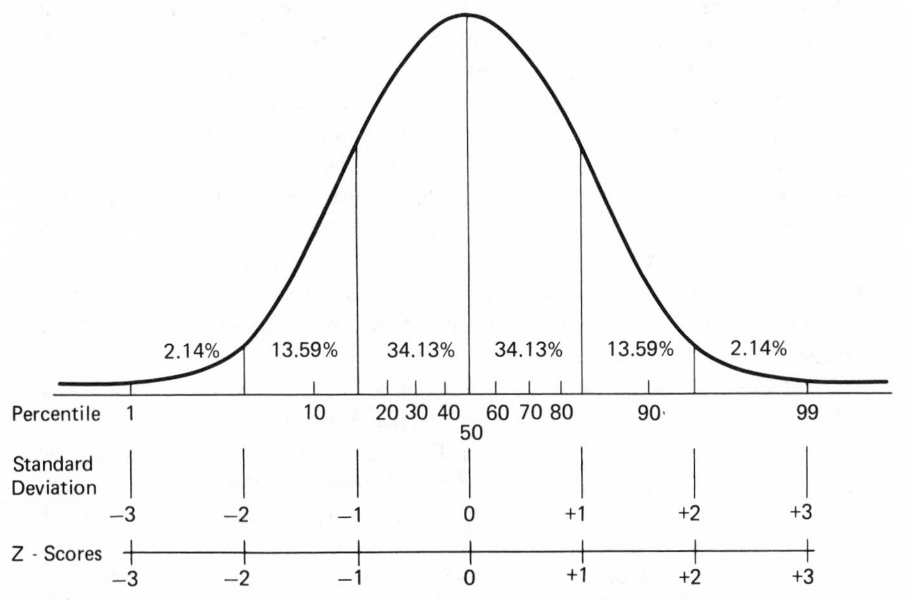

Figure 1-1 Normal distribution curve showing expected proportion of the population within each area of the curve. Also shown with the standard scale divisions are approximate percentile rankings.

axis to indicate standard deviations. Approximate percentile rankings corresponding to those points are also shown. The relative fatness of the curve illustrates the proportion of the total population contained between any two of those points. For example, approximately 34 percent of the population is expected to be between the mean and plus one standard deviation, and another 34 percent, between the mean and minus one standard deviation.* This means that approximately 68 percent of the time, or two times out of three, the individual we test (if we have a large and representative normal sample) is expected to score within plus or minus one standard deviation of the mean for that test. By addition of the proportions shown on Figure 1-1, approximately 95 out of each 100 persons will be expected to score between plus and minus two standard deviations of the mean–the range that was earlier specified as within gross normal limits.

Some of the tests we will discuss specify a normal range of scores in terms of means and standard deviations, some in terms of percentile rankings, and some in neither. These comments on distribution scores will be of no particular value for the tests that use "age scores" and similar interpretative indices, except possibly as a reminder of the "range of normal." However, for a large number of tests which use statistical interpretations, it is pertinent to note that at least part of the decision of "normal" or "abnormal" behavior is based on a statistical or probability judgment. From the percentile rankings and the proportionate distribution in Figure 1-1, it is obvious that if we say the person who scored one standard deviation or less from the mean on our test is "abnormal," we may be wrong in our judgment approximately one time in three. On the other hand, if we reserve our "abnormal" judgment for the individual who is two standard deviations or more from the mean of his population, we would expect to be correct 95 times out of 100, that is, the two standard deviation point is approximately at the 0.05 probability level. Restated, a person may score one standard deviation from the mean by chance alone approximately one time in three but would score two standard deviations or more from the mean by chance alone about one time in twenty. This, of course, also assumes that the test is appropriate to the subject being tested. If the child speaks only Spanish and the test is in English, her score's deviation is not by chance.

One of the judgments we are asked to make from the descriptions of behavior we collect is whether the observed behavior is "normal" or "abnormal." We are on far safer ground in making the "abnormal" judgment when the two standard deviation criterion is used. However, remember that any one test score is only a single number, and more than one measurement is necessary to ade-

*These figures are rounded and approximate values for purposes of discussion. Precise interpretation or the specific proportions of the population within an area differ somewhat with tests. For example, Wechsler (1958, p. 42) included 50 percent of the population within plus and minus one standard deviation. In other words, according to the Wechsler intelligence tests 50 percent of the population will have "average" intelligence (I.Q. scores between 91 and 110).

quately describe a patient. More comments will be made on this point later. For the moment, assume that the score we obtain on any one measure has a probability of error in its prediction.

Figure 1-1 also included percentile numbers corresponding to the standard deviation points. A percentile is a relative ranking of the population on some attribute such as age, height or intelligence. A percentile score is therefore a direct comparison of a particular individual's score with other persons from the population. The mean or average score is obviously at the 50th percentile, with half the population expected to score higher and half the population expected to score lower than this number. One standard deviation below the mean contains 34 percent of the population, therefore the minus one standard deviation point is at approximately the 16th percentile. This in turn means that 84 people out of 100 are expected to obtain a score at this point or higher, and only 16 of each 100 people should score at this point or lower. The minus two standard deviation point is theoretically equivalent to the third percentile above which 97 of 100 people should score and below which only three of 100 people should score. Similar computational comparisons can be made for other points on the scale.

A number of tests utilize percentile scores to separate normal from abnormal performance. For example, some articulation tests use the 16th percentile as the cut-off between "adequate" and "inadequate" articulation skill. Similarly, one language test we will discuss suggests that a score at the 10th percentile or lower represents a significant deviation from normal.

The point to be made with these numbers is that "normal" is a statistical comparison, or a location on a probability curve, and as clinicians we should be aware of the relative value of the scores we use in making our normal and abnormal judgments. In terms of the probability of error in our scoring judgment as mentioned earlier, it would follow that in this case "deviations" may be additive. That is, if the child falls below expected levels of performance on only one measure and related measures place him in a normal range, then two immediate choices present themselves. It may be that our first test result was spurious, and we need a more detailed and alternate measure before making a judgment. It is, of course, also possible that there is a deficiency restricted to that one aspect of behavior, which will be explored with additional testing.

Up to this point, we have been discussing making judgments of "normal" or "abnormal" as if the next patient who walks through the clinic doors is a randomly selected individual from a normally distributed population and that the probability of her performing within the normal range on a test we administer is very high (approximately 97 out of 100 if we use the minus two standard deviation cut-off for "normal"). This is hardly the case. Quite obviously, patients come to clinics because they have a problem, and they come to speech and hearing clinics because they have speech and hearing problems. Therefore, when tests of communicative functioning are administered, we expect that the patient will frequently perform outside the normal range if the tests selected are appropriate to the disorder demonstrated. This observation in no way diminishes the applicability of using statistical concepts to aid in making our decisons, but it is noteworthy because communicatively impaired patients typically represent the lower end of the score distribution when speech and language skills are assessed. Finally, it should be pointed out that some tests use the performance of a sample from a communicatively impaired population to serve as the standardization group for the test. For example, many tests of aphasia provide norms based upon the performance of a group of aphasic subjects. It should be borne in mind then that our interpretation will be based upon the reference group to which the patient is compared, a point we will soon return to.

TESTS: STANDARDIZATION, VALIDITY, AND RELIABILITY

As you no doubt have gathered by now, tests are systematic procedures that yield a score. Two parts of this description are important. The procedures are *systematic* or *standardized* in terms of administration and scoring, and they yield a *score* that allows interpretation of the performance of the individual tested. Tests are important because they aid in making decisions and if they do not aid in making decisions, then they are not worth the time and effort they require to administer and score (Nunnally 1972). On the other hand, many tests are objective and therefore may be of more value than our subjective impressions.

Standardization is the process by which the test or measurement device is administered to a sample from a population with specified physical (age, sex, and so on) and nonphysical (language exposure, socioeconomic status, and so on) characteristics according to specified explicit procedures. Data from the test administration then can be analyzed to determine the mean, standard deviation, and other statistical attributes of the obtained scores. In order to interpret the performance of a new subject by reference to these data, we must assume that the person in question is representative of the population, or at least very similar to the population from which the original sample was drawn and on which the test was standardized. In other words, the subjects within the sampled population must be similar in important respects to the average person in the standardization population. As we have noted, the characteristics of the sampled population utilized to standardize tests which purport to measure a variable may differ considerably. Whether or not you choose to use a particular test because of, or in spite of the standardization population, it is important that you have a defensible rationale for your decision.

Other important considerations in choosing a measurement tool are the validity and reliability of the instrument. Validity typically is described as how well the test does what it purports to do. This is a circular definition analogous to defining a hammer as "something you hammer with" and a horse as "something you horse around with." It is a sufficient definition insofar as it utilizes function to make the meaning known. No test is ever completely valid, and tests are only valid to the extent that they serve their function. The primary functions of tests and the basis on which their validity is determined are prediction, assessment, and trait measurement (Nunnally 1972). These three functions are termed criterion-related validity, content validity, and construct validity.

Criterion-related or "predictive" validity concerns the effectiveness of the test in predicting the individual's behavior in specified situations external to the test (Anastasi 1968). For this purpose, performance on the test is correlated with the behavior to be predicted. One example of a test based on this type of validity is the Predictive Screening Test of Articulation which uses articulatory performance at the first grade to predict whether the child will need therapeutic intervention or whether he will acquire articulatory proficiency without treatment by the third grade. Here performance on a test is used to make a decision regarding treatment. A second example relates to the use of tests to predict improved performance for the patient over time. The Porch Index of Communicative Ability uses the results of testing at one month to predict the performance of the patient at six months post onset of brain damage and therefore performs a prognostic function.

Content validity relates to the assessment function. It involves the careful inspection of the test items to determine if the test covers the behaviors that are to be measured. Rather than being predictive, it involves a sampling of the behaviors that reflect poor or good performance in a particular situation at a particular point in time (Nunnally 1972). It is not important that all possible content be integrated into the test items, only that the important behaviors are examined. For example, in an articulation test, various phonemes are tested, but only in a limited number of contexts. The important behaviors evaluated are the phonemes. The contexts need not all be evaluated, only a representative number. Content validity is sometimes confused with "face" validity. Face validity is the superficial examination of items to assess whether the test items actually cover the behaviors that are to be measured. As such, face validity serves the important function of weeding out items that appear inappropriate, but it is not identical to content validity.

The *construct validity* of a test is the degree to which the test measures psychological traits (constructs). It requires the gradual accumulation of information from many sources. It is broader in scope than the other types of validity we have discussed. Nunnally (1972) has succinctly defined the process of establishing construct validity:

> In essence, construct validation consists of weaving a network of meaningful relations between a new measure and other supposed measures of the same trait. If such relations hold, the new measure then can be trusted in subsequent use. If such relations do not hold, subsequent use of the instrument should be held suspect. (p. 33)

Two primary means used to establish construct validity are factor analysis (major factors and their weightings are used to account for the obtained test scores) and correlations with other tests (concurrent validity). An example of this process might be your development of a new test of aphasia. You select items that appear to measure behaviors typically associated with the disorder, administer the test to a sample of aphasic patients, and analyze the resultant test scores to determine the major factors (traits, constructs) that appear to account for the scores. A second procedure would be to correlate the scores with the scores from a second test of aphasia that is generally agreed to be valid. A high correlation would be indicative of good construct validity for your new test.

The validity of a test then depends upon its purpose; it may be highly valid for one purpose but not for another. This statement points out the fact that many tests serve more than a single function and may need to be validated for each of the purposes.

Reliability means repeatability and talks to the issue of consistency of test scores and the precision of the test. The consistency of test results may be a function of the one being tested, of the test instrument, or of the tester. A test may be reliable without being valid, but a test cannot be valid unless it is reliable. For example, let us say that we want to determine the volume of liquid in a beaker that has been bent out of shape. If we had only a rubber ruler that stretched whenever we made a measurement, it would be neither reliable nor valid. If the ruler were stable, we could determine the height of the beaker in a reliable fashion, but we could not determine the volume of liquid in the beaker. If we now selected a cup, poured the liquid into the cup until filled, and repeated this process until all the liquid has been poured, we would have reliable and valid measures of the volume. This is so because the cup is a valid measure of volume, and the process of measurement could be repeated to demonstrate that we would come out with approximately the same number of cups of liquid every time we did so.

Several procedures are used to establish the reliability of a test, and they all involve correlation. One method is to examine the relationship of scores from two alternate forms of the same test administered to the same subjects. This *alternate-form reliability* is ideal because it examines all the sources of variability that can have an effect on test scores. A second procedure is the *test-retest reliability* method which involves administering the test to the same subjects at two different points in time. A third method, *split-half reliability,* involves for example, the correlating of scores on the odd-numbered items from a test with the scores from the even-numbered items from a test. This method generally overestimates the reliability of the test because there is no instability of the scores over time that would be entailed within alternate-form and test-retest reliability procedures. Consequently, measures of internal consistency, like the Kuder-Richardson formulas are used. The Kuder-Richardson formulas estimate the reliabilities that would be obtained from all possible subdivisions of the test and examines the overlap or correlations between items of the test (Nunnally 1972).

In summary, the results obtained from the variety of tests and observations must be placed in context to interpret their relative importance. Each of the test scores is only a single index and is therefore not the whole picture of the patient. Moreover, the interpretation of results of each of the indices used is dependent on the appropriateness and the quality of the measuring instrument (and the skill of the test administrator). The second law of diagnostics might well be to *interpret each of the quantification numbers with caution.* Or, with data in hand, stand firmly with both feet about three inches off the ground. It is harder to jump to conclusions from that pose.

TESTING NONSTANDARD OR "SPECIAL" POPULATIONS

Earlier, in the section on reliability and validity, we discussed test selection in terms or whether the person to be tested should logically be compared with the population on which the test was standardized. A discrepancy would amount to a test bias. If the discrepancy between test subject and comparative population were not recognized, it could also be termed an examiner bias.

Our biases or our expectations can be a variable in test interpretation. For example, if our task is to screen the speech and language skills of the third grade of the local school, or the entire class of incoming freshman at a college or university, we may well expect to find 95 percent of the subject population to be normal as previously defined. When we, as speech-language clinicians screen those children and adults who are referred to us because someone has been concerned about their speech, the statistics are more likely to be reversed. Our clinical biases tend to be more operative in one situation than in the other. This example is meant to imply a difference between clinical and statistical significance. Where the testing is done, with whom it is done, and the purpose for which it is done may affect our clinical judgment.

Our clinical expectations become an important variable when the population to be tested is culturally different from that which we usually see. Our intent in the speech and language screening is to make a judgment of the efficiency of the communication patterns displayed. Our implicit assumption is that we and the person we are judging share the same communication patterns—the same vocabulary and the same communicative intent. This is a markedly difficult assumption to make when the tester and the testee represent different cultures.

Because of obstacles cultural barriers may raise, there is an expanding array of literature which questions the reliability and validity of test results obtained with culturally different children (for example, Adler 1971, 1973; Cazden 1970; Grimshaw 1969; Severson and Guest 1970). Most of the speech and language measures available have been standardized on middle-class children. Most have used restricted geographic samples. Weiner and Hoock (1973) have discussed the difficulty of standardization assumptions on some frequently used tests when used with the "standard" culture populations. Consider how much more confounded our "standardized" assumptions become with a population which has different culturally generated speech and language patterns.

Adler (1973) has listed some of the linguistic and nonlinguistic factors which may generate a bias against the culturally different child's performance, such as the tested items being outside the cultural experience of the child, or the verbal style being culture specific, or just the fact that the poor, or rural, or ethnic-culture child may be intimidated by the test situation. He reduced the array of specific impediments to two basic problems: motivation and communication. Adler stated that the safest assumption the examiner can make when testing a culturally different child is that it will be difficult to get the child to perform at her potential. Motivation implies a tangible reward but may also include an apparent interest and appreciation on the part of the examiner. Communication barriers may be obvious or may be more subtle. The examiner may not always know which words or syntactic structures used are culture-specific. Because of this uncertainty, Adler urges the examiner to be redundant in the presentation of test instructions, and whenever possible, to utilize a sufficient number of practice items to illustrate to the child what is expected. Put another way, a post-test performance of a child may reflect his better understanding of the task he is to perform as much as it represents his improved performance on the task itself.

Our basic purpose in an evaluation procedure is to measure the tools of communication, and the subject's efficiency in using them. If we have not obtained the person's "best effort," our judgment of capability may be faulty. If the tasks or items we have used for evaluating him are not similar to what is used in his linguistic environment, we may not be measuring his "real" communicative efficiency. And, if the speech and language measures we are using are not appropriate to the population he represents, our judgment of what is expected behavior may be biased. In other words, what we perceive as "language deficiency" may instead be a "language difference." It may be assumed (Wolfram and Fasold 1974; Burling 1973; and others) that the "nonstandard dialect" is an equally well-formed and complex linguistic system. However, unless we understand the phonological structure, the grammar, and the function of the language we are listening to, we cannot judge the efficiency of the speakers' use of it.

TESTING THE COMMUNICATIVE FUNCTION—NONSTANDARDIZED TESTING

Tests for communicative function are almost nonexistent. Most tests of speech and language test grammatical form; function is implied in communication. Our first task, therefore, is to attempt to establish some communicative interchange with the child to be evaluated.

In the previous section we cited Adler's assumption that it may be difficult to get the language-different child to perform to her potential. It would behoove the prudent clinician to approach *all* children in this way. It is a reasonable assumption to make concerning all children, especially preschool-aged children. In the next chapter we define rapport as mutual trust, the ingredient necessary to obtain the kind of personal information requested in the case history interview. We are also asking for a great deal of trust on the part of the child. Even if she is not afraid of whatever unknown lies in your office, the child—and many adults—will at least be shy or uncertain of what is expected by you. The three-, or four-, or five-year-old child who is "completely cooperative" may well be the exception rather than the rule. With this in mind, it may also be logical to expect something less than a full array of completed test results.

ETHICS AND RESPONSIBILITIES

We have been discussing some of the difficulties of testing and test interpretation. There are also some other general comments to be made concerning our responsibilities in an evaluational endeavor. At some time or other we have all heard the exhortation to "treat the whole child." A more realistic statement might be a reminder that "there is a whole child to be treated." Inherent in this paraphrase is the assumption that none of us is adequate to the task of being all things to all people. The Code of Ethics of the American Speech-Language-Hearing Association (1979) reminds all speech and hearing professionals that they must ". . . possess appropriate qualifications" and that they must ". . . use every resource available, including referral to other specialists as needed, to effect as great improvement as possible in the persons served."

Fortunately, that means we are not required to know everything about all problems for all persons. We are neither ethically nor legally required to be right at all times—only to use our best professional judgment and to recognize what we do not know. That means we are allowed to change our minds about the type of treatment, or what we can do to ameliorate problems we have identified—and to seek referral or help when we cannot handle a problem. We are ethically bound to be qualified, certified, capable, and available—but we are not required to "cure" all problems presented.

Dr. Karl Menninger (1958, pp. 19-20) stated it rather succinctly:

> The physician announces (and implies) that he is qualified (trained), authorized (certified), prepared (in equipment and time) and willing to render services to one who needs them. . . . The physician gives the patient his attention and having heard what the patient complains of, makes a decision as to whether or not he—the doctor—can justifiably accept the responsibility of attempting to help this person as a patient . . . He promises to seek the best way to help this patient . . . what the patient pays for is not relief of symptoms but the professional services of the physician . . .

Two points are to be noted from the ASHA Code of Ethics and the quote from Menninger: The clinician must be trained, qualified, and available to do the best he can for the patient, or to find someone better qualified to handle those aspects of the patient's behavior which are not within his (the clinician's) realm of competence. Second you should read in Menninger's "nonguarantee" stipulation that the clinician has no ethical or professional responsibility to be right at all times. Clearly, this means that our best judgment of cause and effect relationships and remediation predictions may not be correct. We should always accept our own as well as other's judgments as being tentative rather than absolute. The judgment we make will be the best and most reasonable we can make according to how we interpret the total problem, but it is changeable. It may be inscribed on parchment, but it should not be treated as if it were chiseled in stone. Don't *expect* to be wrong, but don't commit to a judgment at the expense of the patient.

Diagnostic Law No. Three may be stated as: It is ethically acceptable to be wrong–fallability is forgiveable–*it is legal to change your mind.*

One More Caution

Darley (1964) quoted Beck (1959) in a statement of the basic formulations of science. Briefly stated (and paraphrased) they were:

a. behavior is understandable–deviant as well as normal behavior;
b. cause and effect relationships are expected to maintain some consistency under similar circumstances;
c. the simplest consistent explanation is probably correct;
d. behavioral causes are measureable.

Darley was stressing the need for a scientific approach in speech and language diagnosis. Scientific problem solving is based on the asking of answerable questions. He cautioned the clinician to put more credence in a fact than in a guess or an intuition. "If a fact and a guess are in conflict, the clinician uses the fact. He comes to depend more upon what he can hear, see, feel and verify than upon his intuition. He concentrates upon behavior that can be observed, measured, classified, and manipulated" (p. 4).

In agreement with Darley, our emphasis is on measurement and direct observation, wherever possible. At the present state of the art–or science–we cannot determine and measure all the cause and effect relationships in speech and language disorders. It is still pertinent to assume that behavior is quantifiable. Further, it is imperative that we separate our inferences from our quantifications. We can measure performance. Competence, or capability, are inferences we make from performance or lack of it.

SUMMARY

This chapter has been concerned with the philosophy of testing. We have included comments on what "normal" means, some definitions of terms such as standardization, reliability, and validity, and a caution that not all children and adults are from the same cultural background or speak the same dialect as we do—nor have the same interest in test performance as we may like. We must recognize the purposes we have in testing, the appropriateness of the measurement devices we are using, and the applicability of the norms of behavior which those tests imply. Further, we must recognize the ramifications of our descriptions and judgments. We must know what value to assign to the obtained scores.

We stated, somewhat facetiously, three Diagnostic Laws: to describe rather than to categorize; not to be too sure of each of the numbers we generate; and to make it possible to change our minds about interpretation or significance of the "facts" we generate. They may have been stated facetiously, but the intent is for the clinician to take them seriously.

We commented about a "whole communication system to be treated"—or tested. An efficient communicative system includes appropriate rules and performance in phonology, morphology, syntax, and semantics. Language is "all of a piece." When we make formal or informal value judgments of a child's communication skill, we also must keep in mind the content of what she says (the concepts discussed) and her goals or functions—the reason to speak.

Weiner (1950) formulated one of the strictly linguistic assumptions for decoding a speech sample as, "in the problem of decoding, the most important information which we can possess is the knowledge that the message we are reading is not gibberish." In other words, our first assumption must be that the child knows what he is talking about, and what he is expressing is at least consistent with his understanding of the rules of his language.

In terms of culture-fair testing, Wechsler (1958) has expressed the opinion that "no test is or can be entirely culture-free." Communication skill, however, should not be considered purely an accident of geography or completely conditioned by local mores. Obviously these factors may intrude to a greater or lesser degree, but our task is to make an evaluation of communication skill and efficiency in the communicative functions presented. As clinicians we are being asked to express a professional opinion as to the nature of the problem, if there is one, the prognosis or probable outcome, and the manner of therapeutic intervention.

REFERENCES

Adler, S., Dialectal differences: Professional and clinical implications. *J. Speech Hearing Dis.*, 36, 90-100 (1971).

Adler, S., Data gathering: The reliability and validity of test data obtained from culturally-different children. *J. Learning Dis.*, 6, 429-434 (1973).

Anastasi, A., *Psychological Testing,* 3rd ed. New York: Macmillan, (1968).

Beck, S. D., *The Simplicity of Science.* New York: Doubleday, (1959).

Bloom, L., and M. Lahey, *Language Development and Language Disorders.* New York: John Wiley, (1978).

Bronfenbrenner, U., Toward an experimental ecology of human development. *American Psychologist,* 32, 513-531 (1977).

Burling, R., *English in Black and White.* New York: Holt, Rinehart & Winston, (1973).

Cazden, C., On individual differences in language competence and performance. *J. Spec. Educ.,* 1, 135-150 (1967).

Cazden, C., The neglected situation in child language research and education. Chap. V, in *Language and Poverty,* ed. F. Williams. Chicago: Markham Press, (1970).

Code of Ethics. *American Speech-Language-Hearing Association 1979 Directory.* Rockville, Md.: The American Speech-Language-Hearing Association, (1979).

Darley, F. L., *Diagnosis and Appraisal of Communication Disorders.* Englewood Cliffs, N. J.: Prentice-Hall, Inc., (1964).

DuBois, P. H., *An Introduction to Psychological Statistics.* New York: Harper & Row, (1965).

Dunn, L. M., *Manual for The Peabody Picture Vocabulary Test.* Circle Pines: Minn. American Guidance Service, Inc., (1965).

Grimshaw, W., Language as an obstacle and as data in sociologic research. *Items, Soc., Sci. Res. Council,* June (1969).

Leonard, L. B. and others, Nonstandardized approaches to the assessment of language behaviors. *Asha,* 20, 371-379 (1978).

Menninger, K., *Theory of Psychoanalytic Technique.* New York: Basic Books, (1958). Permission to reprint from Basic Books, Inc., and The Hogarth Press, Ltd.

Menyuk, P., Syntactic structures in the language of children. *Child Develop.,* 34, 407-422 (1963).

Menyuk, P. Syntactic rules used by children from preschool through first grade. *Child Develop.,* 35, 533-546 (1964).

Muma, J. R., Language assessment: Some underlying assumptions. *Asha* 15, 331-338, (1973).

Muma, J. R., *Language Handbook: Concepts, Assessment, Intervention,* Englewood Cliffs, N.J.: Prentice-Hall, Inc., (1978).

Nunnally, J., *Educational Measurement and Evaluation.* New York: McGraw-Hill, (1972).

Severson, R., and K. Guest, Toward the standardized assessment of the language of disadvantaged children, Chap. XV in *Language and Poverty,* ed. F. Williams. Chicago: Markham Press, (1970).

Siegel, G., The use of language tests. *Lang. Speech Hearing Serv. Schools,* 4, 211-217 (1975).

Sroufe, L., A methodological and philosophical critique of intervention-oriented research. *Develop. Psych.,* 2, 150-155 (1970).

Terman, L. M., and M. A. Merrill, *Stanford-Binet Intelligence Scale: Manual for* *the Third Revision,* Form L-M. Boston: Houghton-Mifflin Company, (1960).

Wechsler, D., *Manual for the Wechsler Adult Intelligence Scale.* New York: The Psychological Corporation, (1955).

Wechsler, D., *The Measurement and Appraisal of Adult Intelligence.* Baltimore: The Williams and Wilkins Co., (1958).

Weiner, N., The human use of human beings, Boston, 1959, as quoted in R. Jakobson, C. G. M. Fant, and M. Halle, *Preliminaries to Speech Analysis.* Cambridge: MIT Press, (1969).

Weiner, P. S., and W. C. Hoock, The standardization of tests: Criteria and criticisms. *J. Speech Hearing Res.,* 16, 616-626 (1973).

Wolfram, W., and R. W. Fasold, *The Study of Social Dialects in American English.* Englewood Cliffs, N.J.: Prentice-Hall, Inc., (1974).

Information Gathering

II

Although it may seem rather obvious, it is worth restating that as clinicians we must listen before we speak.

L. L. Emerick and J. T. Hatten

The first part of this chapter will be concerned with the nature and purpose of information gathering, including some of the barriers between the interviewer and the information. In that respect it is an extension of the previous chapter. We will then discuss some of the mechanics of interviewing—how one goes about setting up and accomplishing the interview. Next we will consider some sample questions which may be on a case history form. Last, we will present some examples of social and early developmental measures which are usually completed by interview.

THE PHILOSOPHY OF INFORMATION GATHERING

Much of the context or background information we need in order to interpret the significance of the behaviors we observe is gathered by interview, and all interview information is subject to bias. The informant's biases are an intervening, and often unmeasureable variable between us and the information we are seeking. Some of the available instruments of child development such as the Vineland Social Maturity Scale will be categorized as "interview" rather than as "measurement" devices in this chapter because the descriptions available to us are second hand rather than direct, and data are interpretive rather than observed. The purpose of our information gathering by either direct or indirect means is to determine the current status of the patient and to determine what (and if) changes are to be desired, the direction of these desired changes, and impedance to change. The amount of distortion in our data that can be attributable to the intervening informant bias will, at least initially, be difficult to calibrate. For this reason it may well be appropriate to take all such indirect information *con grano salis.*

THE TASK AND THE TOOLS

As diagnosticians we have two main tasks. One is to analyze and describe the presenting speech, language, voice, fluency, hearing, or other problems. The second is to distinguish the relevant variables in order to understand the dimensions of the problem. The two tasks can be reduced to questions of *what* and *why. What* is the nature of the problem, and *why* did it come to be?

The first task is what we have labelled *appraisal*, or the measurement of the various abilities, and will occupy the bulk of the ensuing pages. The second task, *diagnosis,* is accomplished by putting the measurement results and observations in context. Determining the context of the problem is the concern of this chapter. The information we gather is to be collated with informaton supplied by other professional workers from their observations. With the integration of the many aspects of the client's behavior, it may be possible to arrive at some tentative cause and effect relationships. This task is termed a differential diagnosis which entails distinguishing the problem from similar problems with which it may be confused. From a tentative understanding of cause and effect, decisions can be made concerning prognosis and treatment.

Basically, the diagnostician has two types of tools: measurements or tests, and interview or background information. A test allows the examiner to make measureable judgments without an intervening reporter to distort the picture. A test allows reasonably exact observations and, if quantification is not possible, the clinician at least can reduce her observations to objective, understandable, agreed-upon statements. When she can measure what she is observing and can reduce observations to a numerical value, it is possible to chart improvement or lack of improvement and to determine if the therapeutic intervention is appropriately directed. If the improvement cannot be quantified, it is difficult to defend the judgment of improvement. Quantification is especially important in this age of accountability. For example, later in this text we will mention a device called an oral manometer. With an oral manometer, oral air pressure produced with the nares open and with nares occluded is compared to determine the ratio of the two measurements. This ratio helps determine the efficiency of the velopharyngeal valving mechanism—the closer the ratio is to 1.00 the more capable the speaker is in his ability to close off the nasal port to generate oral air pressure. An alternative to the ratio of nares open to nares closed is a report that the speaker has "some nasal emission." Obviously the latter term expresses an important observation, but the oral manometer ratio yields a quantification of nonverbal velopharyngeal functioning.

The second major tool of the diagnostician is the history-type interview. The examiner wants to obtain information about antecedent and continuing conditions related to the communication difficulty and whatever predisposing, precipitating, and maintaining factors may be present. The determination of these kinds of variables will help delineate the nature of the problem and what can be done about it. An effective interviewer has to be more than a pleasant "asker of questions." The late Wendell Johnson characterized a good interviewer as a "professional eavesdropper." "Professional" in the sense that he has an ethical obligation to maintain the confidentiality of the information gathered, and "eavesdropper" in the sense that he should not influence or intrude upon the information supplied. This is an important concept because it can seriously affect the amount and nature of the information made available. If we ask a question, or slant a question, in such a way that the client (parent) is aware we expect a particular answer, then it is highly probable that we will get the answer —whether it is true or not. If you think an answer could be embarrassing, ask the question in a straightforward manner, and it is less likely to cause embarrassment. To do this, a special relationship must exist between the interviewer and the one being interviewed—a relationship called rapport. Rapport is not something that one establishes before beginning the interview. It is a process or quality that is necessarily maintained throughout the interview to reduce the impedance to communication and sharing. Rapport means mutual respect. In practical terms that means the informant becomes willing to divulge information of a personal nature because she can respect the professional purpose of the interview, and because the interviewer has shown respect for the informant. In order to fulfill our ethical and professional responsibility to adequately describe the patient, we need as much unfiltered information as is available.

The Purpose and the Pitfalls

The professional purpose of the interview is clear when it is apparent to the one being interviewed that the questions being asked have a point, and the point is both valid and obvious. The questions must not be ambiguous; they must not be random. The nature of the information desired by the interviewer should be apparent. Questions should require a factual answer and not just opinion. They should not require merely agreement or denial. The interviewer may have to supply definitions or examples of the kinds of information desired, but be aware that such prompts may also influence the answers received. Do not be afraid to ask for further explanation when answers are contradictory, or when the tone of the response does not appear consistent with the words.

The Apostolic Function, or Giving Advice

Balint (1957) wrote a fascinating book a few years ago entitled *The Doctor, His Patient, and the Illness.* The book was concerned primarily with the practice of psychotherapy by professionals not specifically trained in psychotherapy. When discussing interviewing, he stated that if you ask a question, all you may get is an answer. He stressed the importance of listening to the tone of the responses as well as the words. Filling in answer blanks on the case history form is easy–listening for information relevant to an understanding of the problem is much more difficult.

By virtue of the role played by the interviewer, the implied role of authority, it is frequently expected that the interviewer will be asked for advice. And what is more natural (although possibly dangerous to the best interests of the client) than giving advice? Balint devotes two chapters to what he terms "The Apostolic Function," which means going out and making the world over in our own image. What we say we would do is not necessarily most appropriate for the patient. Professional advice concerning treatment of communicative disorders is appropriate and expected. When the advice requested or offered is less obviously part of our professional jurisdiction, it may still be accepted as from an authoritarian base. The pharmacology of "therapist" has not been determined. We frequently are not aware of how much of ourselves we prescribe and the effect of that dosage. The philosophy we espouse and the words we use in asking questions or supplying information may be interpreted differently from what we intend.

Guiding Principles in Diagnosis

Darley (1964, pp. 9-14) lists six guiding principles in diagnosis and appraisal:

1. *Beware of a priori conceptions.* Each of us is prone to see what we expect to see and to rationalize behavior in terms of a notion we are fond of. It is an occupational hazard for all of us as clinicians to let our biases and preconceptions do our thinking for us. The scientific method demands that we observe the behavior and translate or define it as carefully as possible, without letting our biases interfere with what we observe.

2. *Stick to first-order facts,* with as few inferences as possible. Describe rather than speculate. A break in fluency in a child's speech should be reported as a revision, a part-word repetition, or whatever else it was without labeling it as "stuttering."

3. *Choose the simplest explanation consistent with the facts.* For example, a child may display a tongue-thrust swallow and distorted sibilant sound productions. This does not necessarily mean the distorted sibilants are caused by the tongue thrust.

4. *Keep your conclusions tentative rather than absolute.* Do not be afraid to change your mind. Remember that your ethical and professional obligation is to seek the best possible solution to the communicative problem presented. You are not ethically bound to be correct. Your statement of conclusions and recommendations are professional opinions; they are not pronouncements. Based on your tentative results, you can chart a tentative course of treatment which will include further sampling of behavior. With new data the picture may become more clear and complete. Diagnosis is not necessarily completed before therapy begins.

5. *Respect the relevance of norms.* Understanding what is deviant depends on understanding what is normal. Only approximately one-third of the population has completely normal dental structure. In this case "normal" is not necessarily average.

6. *Seek the counsel of other professionals.* Other professional workers may be in a better position to supply the necessary information than we are from our vantage point. Do not play at being neurologist, psychologist, social worker, educator, or other specialist that you have not been trained for. The code of ethics of the American Speech-Language-Hearing Association, for example, states that the clinician is to consider the welfare of the patient of paramount importance. Among other mandates, she is to ". . . establish harmonious relations with colleagues and members of other professions." She must refer the patient when her limitations to provide the best available treatment are clear.

The Scientific Method. A similar way of looking at Darley's statements is with the assumption that we are engaged in a scientific endeavor. The method of science, as commonly described, consists of asking answerable questions. The organization of a research project follows an outline such as the following:

1. definition of the problem
2. development of hypotheses to be tested
3. development of a procedure for testing the hypotheses
4. collection of data
5. analysis of data
6. support or rejection of hypotheses

Let us assume that our "research project" is a child referred because someone was concerned about the intelligibility of her speech. The six steps just mentioned are then translated as:

1. *Definition of the problem.* Statements to the effect that the child is hard to understand or that she has an articulation problem are not sufficiently descriptive for us to pose hypotheses to be tested. We must at least give an articulation test or otherwise methodically determine error sounds. We need information on the consonant contexts of the errors. We need to know whether or not the errors are consistent; and whether or not the erred sounds can be produced correctly in imitation (stimulability). We need to know the place and manner of error productions in contrast to the expected place and manner of articulation. In other words we need to know whether there is consistency in the pattern of error. We need to know if there are mechanical reasons which could cause or contribute to the speech pattern we hear. In essence we need whatever information we can get to help us narrow or define the problem.

2. *Development of hypotheses to be tested.* Depending partly on the types of information gathered in our definition, possible hypotheses could be related to hearing loss; dental malocclusion; language patterns related to familial or cultural ethnicity; speech and language patterns as a function of unique linguistic rules; inadequate motor control; or velopharyngeal insufficiency. There may be other possibilities.

3. *Development of a procedure for testing the hypotheses.* Essentially this statement means that we must test in such a way that we may believe our results. An important factor may be the willingness or the ability of the child to cooperate in the testing endeavor. Does she understand what is being asked of her? Are the directions clear? Is she sufficiently interested or motivated to perform? Have we established sufficient rapport? Not the least of the variables is whether we can accept the test as a valid measure.

4. *Collection of data.* Simply stated, this means testing for the possible alternatives we listed as hypotheses. For example, in addition to our articulation testing, we would expect to administer at least a test of hearing acuity, appropriate language tests of morphology and syntax, and a complete evaluation of structure and function of the oral-peripheral mechanism. Case history or early developmental information may alert us to areas of more specific interest.

5. *Analysis of data.* In some cases we can now make relatively clear positive or negative statements. Additional judgments may be reserved for a later time. A summary of our data collection is intended to rule out probable causes of the articulation problem we had earlier described, rather than to determine a single cause. In most cases, it is more realistic to look for interrelationships or coexisting factors than to expect a single cause and effect relationship.

6. The last step in our "project" was *support or rejection of hypotheses.* As indicated earlier, some of our hypotheses will be rejected at this point, and some will remain as possibilities which cannot yet be rejected. We will, at least, have some tentative conclusions. For example, our first decision is whether or not the speech and language behavior we have measured is importantly different from what is expected.

The Content of Science: Resolution of Uncertainty. Schultz (1973) has compared the clinical evaluation procedure to information theory (Shannon and Weaver 1964). According to the formulations of Shannon and Weaver, the amount of information conveyed by a message is equivalent to the amount of uncertainty resolved by receipt of the message. By the Schultz comparison, clinical evaluation is a process of generating hypotheses or tentatively predicting judgments with their relative probabilities, for example the probability of hearing loss in a school-aged population. The examination procedures are then tests of the hypotheses. When the hypotheses are reduced to one by virtue of the observations made, the clinician's uncertainty has been resolved, and the examination is concluded. Schultz (p. 153) posed a variety of possible hypotheses, such as, "designation of current status, diagnostic categorization, (re)habilitative requirements." The type of hypotheses entertained would determine the type of observations made and the discriminant ability of the tests selected. The magnitude of the uncertainty determines the value of the test procedure. If there is no resolution of the clinician's uncertainty, new hypotheses must be raised. We only get answers by asking questions, and a good answer requires asking a good question.

As Schultz (1973) stated the final advantage of the evaluation model:

> The early establishment of a set of hypotheses enhances data gathering and data retention efficiencies. Alternatively, the later in the process the hypotheses are first delineated, the more likely it is that the set will include the "true" hypothesis. The examiner must contend with these antagonistic decision pressures; but she knows that, in the event of an unsuccessful outcome (irresolution), she can reformulate any or all of her hypotheses, reconsider the available data, and attempt economically to secure the increment necessary to her evaluative decision. (p. 153)

The Darley statement of six guiding principles in appraisal and diagnosis, the six step outline of the method of science, and the resolution-of-uncertainty evaluation model described by Schultz all speak to the same point. To be effective, our procedures of appraisal must be organized around the specific questions which will be most productive for our diagnostic-descriptive purposes.

The Four Languages for Describing Henry

Although we have mentioned contributing factors which may bear on the problem presented, most of the preceding discussion has been on verbal behaviors. Our concern must be broader. Johnson (1946, p. 411-413) talked about four partial descriptions or "languages"—four general kinds of observations that can be made of Henry, or any other patient. Each of the four factors is incomplete in itself, and all are interactive and interrelated. It is not enough to describe a person merely in anatomical or organic terms, or only in terms of physiology and behavior, or any other single aspect. The four languages which Johnson described are the semantic environment, evaluative reactions, overt and physiological behavior, and the organism. All four are needed to meaningfully talk about Henry. What might be said of one of them depends upon what there is to say of the others.[1]

Semantic environment is defined as the individual's environment of attitudes, beliefs, assumptions, values, ideals, standards, customs, knowledge, interests, conventions, institutions, and so on. Beyond a person's immediate semantic environment is that more extensive environment we call his culture, or the larger social order in which he lives. The individual's semantic environment changes from time to time as people and events exert changing and varying influences on him. The person in question is also part of his environment. *Evaluation reactions* include the individual's own attitudes, beliefs, assumptions, values, ideals, mores, and so forth. They may be regarded as those pieces of his semantic environment that he has internalized or adopted as his own. The evaluative reactions are primarily expressed as verbal behaviors.

Overt and physiological behaviors include what the person does. Generally these are nonverbal behaviors. As far as Henry is concerned, the behaviors which are available to him are those he has practiced before. The stuttering child who has stereotyped an array of "helpful" behaviors which may include facial tics, tongue protrusions, finger snapping, and the like is not likely to immediately accept your logic that he need not do those things to talk. His logic is more likely to be that if he did not go through those practiced behaviors, he may not talk at all. The fourth special language is the organism. *Organism* refers to the relatively invariant relationships involved in the process of growth and deterioration. Restrictions here are physical. They may include the pubertic voice changes of a 14-year-old boy or the imprecise articulation involved in a progressive dysarthria. In one case time may solve the problem–in the other, exaggerate it.

Henry–our patient–is a function of the variety of influences exerted on him, but he is also an active influence in the total picture. Our diagnostic endeavors are an attempt to develop as complete a description as possible in order to determine what and where the significant deviations are, what changes are desired and/or expected, and what circumstances or restrictions mediate against the desired changes. Diagnostic description without prognosis is a meaningless exercise. We must know where we are and where we are going in order to determine how to get there. That statement is equally true whether you are flying to the moon, driving to Peoria, or planning to attempt remediation of a speech or language disorder.

[1]Adapted from Wendell Johnson, *People in Quandaries* (New York: Harper & Row, Publishers, Inc., 1946), pp. 411-413. Reprinted by permission of the publisher.

THE MECHANICS—HOW TO GO ABOUT THE INTERVIEW

As stated earlier, to be a good interviewer, you cannot be a completely dispassionate "asker of questions." You must be interested, and you must listen. The roles of interviewer and interviewee are not equal. The person being interviewed is assumed to be the one who has come for help, and the interviewer is the professional being asked to supply that help. It is expected that you as the interviewer will ask most of the questions and guide the direction of the interview while most of the information will come from the informant. In your role of authority, however, you must not be authoritarian, or aloof, or critical, or judgmental. As an interviewer you cannot afford to act *superior* and still maintain the trust required to obtain the personal information you seek.

The admonition to listen is to keep you from asking for information that has already been supplied in response to a previous question. Nothing will turn off an informant faster than being asked the same question two or three or more times. That would indicate a lack of interest on your part, and the informant should then likely revert to "answers" rather than to provide information.

Tell the Informant What Information You Want and Why

It is not safe to assume that the informant understands the purpose of the interview or the nature of the information requested. Explain the purpose of the interview, the type of information being sought, and the use to which the information will be put. It may be helpful to remind the informant that you may not ask all of the appropriate questions, but that you are asking for her cooperation in obtaining as much information as possible to better understand the nature of the problem being presented.

Informed Consent

Tell the informant who you are. If you are a student in a training program, say so. If there are observers, say so. Everyone has the right to be fully informed, and informed consent requires that you be honest and that you be explicit and clear in your explanations. Tell the informant with whom the information will be shared and with whom it will not be shared. Anonymity cannot be maintained, but the information will be kept confidential. If a report is to be sent, obtain the patient's (or parent's) agreement on a signed release of information form.

Be Economical of Time—
Make Your Questions Clear

The informant should not get the impression that you are in a rush to complete the interview to go on to more important matters—but don't waste time. Give the patient time to answer the questions you pose, but do not encourage "best" answers. The general atmosphere you establish will go a long way toward expediting the information-gathering process. Your questions will be more efficient sources of information if you ask them straightforwardly and primarily in words of one syllable.

"How old was Johnny when he was toilet trained—when could he stay dry all day?", and then, "During the night?" might be a more efficient question than having to sort through clarifications and restatements of something like, "Was it difficult to get Johnny used to bathroom habits, you know, like . . . did he take a long time to be toilet trained, how old was he?"

Don't ask yes or no questions that must be followed immediately by other questions required to get the rest of the answer. "Has Johnny been sick much?" may be less efficient than questions like "What illnesses has Johnny had?" "How severe were they?"

Take Notes, but Be Brief

The ecnomical use of time requires that the interviewer be thoroughly familiar with the interview outline, with the types of information to be gathered, and with the essence of what is expected. That way the interviewer can move rapidly through the interview without leaving too much time for the informant to frame "best" answers. This also requires that the interviewer takes notes as briefly and as expeditiously as possible. Try not to leave long silences while you record everything word by word. Very seldom would you need an exact quote for an answer. Routine, long silences for transcribing answers will tend to inhibit the information to be gathered, and excessive note taking will interfere with eye contact. The note taking should not be surreptitious. Many informants seem to find it reassuring that you are taking notes which at least implies that their answers are important, but it is preferrable to use a clip-board or pad so the informant is not being invited to read what you have written.

Listen

Listen not only to answers given so that you may keep from asking for information already supplied, but listen also for what appear to be contradictions. If you think there is a contradiction in the answers you have received, ask about it, but avoid forcing the informant into being defensive. When you complete the interview, you will have to summarize the information you have gathered, so it is appropriate that you clarify possible points of confusion. Listen to what the words say—and to the tone of the responses. Listen for the concern which may show between the words. Listen for cues that may tell you whether the answers you have been given are real. Have you been given information as well as answers? Listen for questions which the informant asks or wants to ask.

When the Interview Is Over, Close It Gracefully

When the interview is completed, thank the informant for her cooperation and explain again why you have been asking the questions. It is probably not a good idea to volunteer a summary of your impressions of the informant's concern at this point in time. It may, however, be appropriate to ask if there is anything else that the informant thinks you should know to better understand the problem being presented. This sort of invitation frequently may yield a summary on the part of informants—what they think is of primary importance.

Tell the informant that the information you have gathered will be assembled with the speech, language, and other data by you, or whoever is in charge of the case disposition, and that a summary of the findings and recommendations will be discussed with them. Thank her again, and say goodbye.

CASE HISTORY INTERVIEW

A case history, or case study data, must satisfy four criteria: relevancy, sufficiency, representativeness, and reliability (Wallin 1963). There are many versions of case history forms in use, but there are no standardized forms. Theoretically, a complete case history may be gained by simply asking the patient (or parent, or knowledgeable adult) to "tell me about it," or it may be many pages in length with every conceivable question written in advance, and still it may not adequately cover all areas of concern. The appropriate question is not "how long *should* a case history be," but rather, "how long *must* it be." A case history interview must be as long as a piece of string—long enough to do the job.

In addition to the information necessary for filing and retrieval—such as name, address, birth date, file number, referral source, and similar information of a bookkeeping nature, case history interviews would usually expect to cover such topics as family history, physiological data, early development history, speech history, educational history, personal behavioral characteristics, socio-economic data, and a space for the interviewer's statement of general impressions. It is obvious that communication problems in an adult may elicit different areas of concern than would communication problems in children. For example, if the patient is a recently laryngectomized adult, we would not logically be concerned about early developmental history, or speech history, or areas that were not of concern prior to the removal of the larynx. On the assumption that a wider range of questions may be asked concerning a communication problem in a child, consider the following example as an interview of a parent about a child. An example of a case history form for a child can be found in Figure 2-1 as an illustration of the areas discussed. The questions posed in the discussion sections are meant primarily as questions to the interviewer which may or may not be rephrased and asked of the informant. Questions are to be asked one at a time.

Family History

Information concerning age, education, occupation, prior or current speech and language disorders in parent or relatives may provide cues to other questions which need to be asked. A parent may be concerned about what she perceives as early signs of stuttering in her child because someone in her family had "stuttering problems." On the other hand, she may have a lesser level of concern because "Uncle Charlie stuttered as a child, but he got over it." Similarly, information about siblings, their ages and school performance, may or may not be pertinent to the child in question. How many siblings are there, and what are their ages? Is there a sibling rivalry? To what extent might parental aspirations or levels of expectation for the child be a factor? Our task as "professional eavesdroppers" requires that we not make moral judgments or offer unsolicited advice on childrearing. We must remain nonjudgmental so that we can maintain the interviewee's trust while asking for very personal information. From the parent we are seeking an outline of the child's semantic environment. The child's evaluation reactions will have to come from him. A statement that a child is "a good student" is a value judgment—on the part of someone. A statement that a child receives "As and Bs in English and history and arithmetic" is a factual report. When you pool all your information for a diagnostic description, you can interpret the significance of facts—you cannot interpret the significance of value judgments.

Physiological Data

Height, weight, current health, childhood diseases, injuries, hospitalizations, surgery, medications now or formerly used, may all be examples of the kinds of data collected in this section. A probable question to arise is whether reported injuries or illnesses are relatable to the speech problem. From our previous discussion of the "scientific method" and the "resolution of uncertainty," it may be assumed that we are not looking for *the* cause of a speech and language difficulty but for a number of possible factors which could contribute to the

CASE HISTORY (CHILD)

NAME__________ AGE__________ SEX__________

ADDRESS__________ BIRTHDATE__________

__________ ZIP__________

COMPLETED BY__________ PHONE NO.__________

DATE__________

FAMILY HISTORY

Father:

1. Full Name__________ Age__________
2. If dead, state cause and age at death__________
3. Education__________
4. Present occupation__________
5. Did he ever have a speech defect?__________ Voice defect?__________
   At what age did the defect clear up?__________
   Speech defects among relatives__________

Mother:

1. Full Name__________ Age__________
   If dead, state cause and age at death__________
2. Living at home, divorced, remarried, etc.__________
3. Education__________
4. Present occupation__________
5. Did she ever have a speech defect?__________ Voice defect?__________
   At what age did the defect clear up?__________
   Speech defects among relatives__________

Brothers and Sisters:

Name	Age	Sex	Speech Defect	School Grade & Performance
__________	____	____	____	__________
__________	____	____	____	__________
__________	____	____	____	__________
__________	____	____	____	__________

How many living at home? __________

Figure 2-1 Sample Case History Form

PHYSIOLOGICAL DATA

Height__________ Weight__________ Current Health (good, poor)__________

Physical deformities__________

Date of last physical examination__________ Physician__________

Diseases:	Age	Severity	Change in Speech		Age	Severity	Change in Speech
Chicken Pox	___	___	___	Diptheria	___	___	___
Measles	___	___	___	Encephalitis	___	___	___
Scarlet Fever	___	___	___	Mumps	___	___	___
Rheumatic Fever	___	___	___	Meningitis	___	___	___
Pneumonia	___	___	___	Whooping			
Influenza	___	___	___	Cough	___	___	___
Asthsma	___	___	___	Allergy	___	___	___
Hay Fever	___	___	___	High Fevers			
Other respiratory				(104°)	___	___	___
illnesses	___	___	___	Earaches	___	___	___
Others	___	___	___	Convulsions	___	___	___

Surgery:__________

____

Injuries:__________

____

Injuries or illnesses relatable to speech problems:__________

Hearing:

Parent's evaluation of child's hearing__________

Ear infections__________ Otological care or surgery__________

Comments:__________

SPEECH HISTORY

1. a. Age first words spoken:__________
   b. Age 2-3 word combinations spoken:__________
   c. Age first sentences spoken:__________

2. a. Rate of speech development: Fast___ Average_____ Slow_________

   Clearness of child's speech before age 6: below average__________
   average__________ above average__________

3. Verbal output - Evaluation:

	more than average	average	less than average
a. amount of babbling	___	___	___
b. amount of talking when first began	___	___	___
c. amount of talking at present			
d. present rate or speed of talking (fast, slow)	___	___	___

Figure 2-1 Sample Case History Form (continued)

4. Description of child's conversation at home: none________brief responses_______
speaks easily__________gestures with words_______________

Child's speech with peers: none_________brief responses___________
speaks easily_________gestures with words______________

Child's speech with strangers: none _______brief responses_____________
speaks easily__________gestures with words____________

5. Intelligibility of child's speech: easily understood_____understood if listener knows the topic________words understood now and then______
completely unintelligible___________gestures understood___________

6. Language(s) other than English spoken at home:_____________understands second language____________speaks second language_____________

7. Describe how your child gets along with other children/adults__________
____

8. Parents description of speech problem (Now)____________________________

9. When was the problem first noted?_____________Description of speech at that time?____
Who was first concerned (parent, teacher, relative, etc.)_________________
Has any change occurred in speech?____
To what do you attribute this change?_____________________________________

10. Previous speech evaluation?__________Agency_____________________Date_______
Comments____
____

SCHOOL HISTORY

1. Present grade ____________________School___________________________________

2. Age and date of first school attendance______________________________________

3. Other schools attended (year and dates)______________________________________

4. Grades failed_______________________grades skipped_________________________

5. Easy subjects____

6. Difficult subjects____

7. Problems in school____

8. Recreational interests and hobbies____

DEVELOPMENTAL HISTORY

Pregnancy:
Mother's health (illnesses, medicines, accidents)___________________________
____
Previous pregnancies___________________________________
Rh factor_________________Toxemias_______________________
Birth:
Home_____________________Hospital____
Physician__________________________City/State______________________________

Figure 2-1 Sample Case History Form (continued)

Delivery:

Normal______Instrument________Breech________Caesarian______________

Condition at birth: Jaundiced___blue___breathing____crying__________

red___purple___Other_______________________________

Length of labor__________anaesthetic_______birth weight_____________

Term_________Physical deformities_________________________________

Feeding:

Breastfed______Bottlefed_______Nutritional disturbances______________

____

Age of

First tooth_______sitting________creeping______crawling____________

walking________self-feeding_________dressing__________Toilet

training_________Comparison with other children___________________

PERSONAL CHARACTERISTICS

Please indicate how often these behaviors occur in the child by circling the letter which most often describes it. 0 indicates that it occurs often; S indicates seldom; N indicates never

Nervousness	0	S	N	Tongue sucking	0	S	N
Sleeplessness	0	S	N	Hurting pets	0	S	N
Nightmares	0	S	N	Setting fires	0	S	N
Bedwetting	0	S	N	Constipation	0	S	N
Playing with sex organ	0	S	N	Thumb sucking	0	S	N
Walking in sleep	0	S	N	Face twitching	0	S	N
Shyness	0	S	N	Fainting	0	S	N
Showing off	0	S	N	Strong fears	0	S	N
Refusal to obey	0	S	N	Strong hates	0	S	N
Rudeness	0	S	N	Queer food habits	0	S	N
Fighting	0	S	N	Temper tantrums	0	S	N
Jealousy	0	S	N	Whining	0	S	N
Selfishness	0	S	N	Stealing	0	S	N
Lying	0	S	N	Running away	0	S	N
Excitability	0	S	N	Destructiveness	0	S	N
Easily discouraged	0	S	N	Preference for			
Convulsive attacks	0	S	N	older children	0	S	N
				Preference for			
				younger children	0	S	N

Your comments:

SOCIOECONOMIC DATA

1. Type of community (city, town, country, etc.)_____________________

2. Home (owned, rented, bedrooms shared, etc.)______________________

3. Economic condition of family (poor, very poor, comfortable, well-to-do)

____

INTERVIEWER'S IMPRESSIONS

Interviewer________________________

Supervisor ________________________

Figure 2-1 Sample Case History Form (continued)

problem. A child may be reported to have begun to stutter just after he had his tonsils removed or just after the family was involved in an automobile accident. This reported coincidence in time does not necessarily imply a cause and effect relationship. Accept the statement, but record it as a value judgment. We need also to know the parent's definition of stuttering–what did the child do? What was the speech like before and after the incident in question? Is it possible that the perceived problem began earlier or later?

An arrest in the development of speech and language skills following prolonged high fevers, or encephalitis, for example, may be a more acceptable cause and effect relationship, but it is not the end of the search. These may be significant factors but are not of themselves sufficient.

Early Developmental History

Our concern with development begins very early. Questions we raise would have to do with mother's health during the pregnancy (prenatal) and go on to perinatal and postnatal, as well as early developmental milestones. Concerning the mother's physical and emotional health, were any complications reported such as severe nausea or vomiting, toxemias, viral infections, anemia, bleeding, X-ray treatments, nutritional or metabolic disturbances? If so, when during the pregnancy did they occur? Is there any history of miscarriages? Is there a blood incompatiblity, such as Rh factor? What was the term of pregnancy? What was the birth weight of the child? How does that compare with other children of the family? Was labor induced? Was the baby in a breech position? Were forceps required for delivery? Was the mother under anaesthesia or analgesia during delivery? Concerning the baby, was there a report of discoloration, of blueness or jaundice at birth? Was there any delay in respiration? Did the infant require incubation? For how long? (If there are complications which could be of a genetic nature, is there a birth-defects facility in your area which can provide genetic study and counseling?)

In terms of early development, was there any indication of hypo- or hypertonicity? Did the infant have any difficulty nursing? Was she breast fed or bottle fed? Was there ever a feeding problem? Was she a "colicky" baby? How old was she when she could sit up? crawl? stand alone? walk? feed herself? How old was she when toilet trained for day–for night? How do these developmental ages compare with other children in the family? (How do these ages compare with published norms, for example, age norms provided by Aldrich and Norval (1946) who cite sitting-up at approximately six months; crawling or creeping at seven months; standing alone at 10 to 11 months; walking at approximately 12 months.) In a later chapter of this text, motor developmental measures will be discussed with more elaboration.

Speech History

Questions concerning the early speech history of the child may serve a sort of double-barreled purpose. It is usual to ask for approximate ages of babbling and cooing, of early attending behavior to speech, age of first word, age when two- and three-word utterances were assembled, and similar questions on amount and intelligibility of the verbal output. There have been a number of early studies which reported on the age of first word and similar milestones, but they reflect differences in definition of first word by the experimenters. "First word" data for normal children range from 10 to approximately 18 months. With this range for first word, two-word utterances are to be expected by 24 months of age.

We said there was a double purpose in these questions. In addition to ages which can be compared to general ages of expectancy, the second purpose is to get a judgment by the parent as to whether these ages are earlier or later than they expected. If an older child said his first words at 10 months, a later age for the child in question may be considered late although still within the normal range. Part of the information we are asking for with these questions is whether the parents are concerned about the child's speed of development.

In *The Onset of Stuttering* studies (Johnson and others 1959), there was a consistent lack of agreement between judgments of "late" and the child being later than the usual age in reaching developmental milestones. In this series of studies a total of 246 children who were judged by their parents to be stutterers and their parents were compared with 246 children who were judged by their parents as nonstutterers and their parents. More experimental (stuttering) than control group mothers rated their children as being much slower than average, but a comparison of the ages when the two groups of children said their first words and when they said their first sentences did not differ. In other words, ages in the speech history may give us data for comparison with children in general, as well as with other siblings in the family. Judgments of early, average, or late may yield information concerning the *parents'* norms, aspirations, and expectations.

In this section we would also ask for a description of the child's functional communication. How easily does he speak with children his own age? with strangers? Is his speech easy to understand? Is it understood only if the topic is known? Is it not understood? Does he rely on gestures with or without accompanying words? Are other languages spoken in the home? Does the child use more than one language? Who was first concerned about the child's speech? How would the parent describe the speech at that time? How would it be described now? Have any changes occurred in the child's speech? To what does the parent attribute the change?

Educational History

As with many of the other sections of our case history interview, the educational history may or may not be significant to the understanding of every child studied. With children of school age, it is sometimes helpful to know what their educational history has been. Have any grades been failed? Any grades skipped? What are the easiest subjects; what are the most difficult? What kinds of marks does he usually obtain? Have there been any drastic changes? Are there any other reported problems in school?

Here again, we are not dictating questions to be asked but reminding the interviewer to construct as complete a picture as possible to determine if there are areas of potential significance which need be explored. For example, questions concerning social interaction or academic performance in school may allow us to determine if the child's performance is consistent with other performance predictions we may have in terms of intellectual potential, social maturity, and other related indices. Is academic performance consistent with parental expectation?

Personal Characteristics

Under this general heading may be a list of behaviors such as nervousness, sleeplessness, nightmares, shyness, showing off, jealousy, excitability, tantrums, strong fears, strong hates, whining, destructiveness, and the like. The kinds of behavioral characteristics questioned may be normal behaviors to some degree in all children. The behaviors you list may occur often, or seldom, or never in the child in question. This section may be considered an attempt to "flesh-out" our description of the child's nonverbal behavior and add one more dimension to the total picture. Are any of the behaviors described relatable to the "cause" of the speech problem? Are any of them likely to have been caused or aggravated by the child's lack of communication skill?

Socioeconomic Data

Socioeconomic classification systems may have a number of variables in their formulae, but most commonly they include source (rather than amount) of income, occupation, and education of the parents. Of these three, one study (Helton 1974) found mother's education to be the factor which best predicted the child's language skill. The purpose in gathering the social, cultural, and economic information is to help you determine cultural influences or opportunities available for the child. Social-cultural exposure may be important in terms of language form and possibly language function. Do not, however, assume that socioeconomic status tells you everything. Only Aristotelian logic assumes that class determines behavior. Non-Aristotelian logic assumes that behavior determines class. The distinction is important for your remedial intervention. In the extreme, if class determines behavior, language intervention would logically include increasing family income and moving the family across town. While that is not necessarily a poor idea in itself, it may be much more productive to the child's language skills to recommend the kind of language stimulation and interaction commonly found in a more "culturally advantaged" environment.

General Impressions

The premise on which we began this chapter is that we wish to gather as much information as possible which is pertinent to our understanding of the child and the problem presented. Our understanding can be no more complete than our data—and the data no better than our interpretation. This section, therefore, is an invitation to put into words those on-the-spot thoughts and impressions that may not be available when we look back over the answers at a later date. For example, statements concerning general ease or mal-ease of the interview situation and interaction may be obvious at the time but may not be equally obvious at a later time.

OBSERVATION AND INDIRECT TESTING

Different clinical settings have functioned with different procedures. It is difficult to assume that there is only one best way to operate. Some clinicians do an interview first and then test the child, on the assumption that they will have more understanding of the behavior they see. Others do the testing first and then the interview because they feel they can better channel interview questions to areas of prime concern. Clinics with more personnel available may split the task with one clinician taking the case history while another tests the child. If the patient concerned is a child, most clinicians agree that, when possible, it is helpful to make observations of the child separated from the parent and interacting with another clinician and also to observe interactions of child and parent. Sometimes these observations can add considerable information.

The following case is not necessarily unique, but consider it as an example. A 4-year-old boy was brought to the Hearing and Speech Center because of the parents' concern with the child's fluency. The subject displayed normal fluency when he was interacting with a clinician. The descriptions of speech given by his mother did not coincide with our observations of his speech. The boy's mother had also brought a 5-year-old son with her to the Center and when the mother was asked to go into the diagnostic room to continue the activities the clinician had initiated, the other son went along. When the two boys communicated with each other, the speech fluency of both sounded normal, but when the two were competing for their mother's attention, the disfluency which the mother had described was now very evident.

This anecdote only points out that our observations or our test results are not complete in themselves and frequently require "outside" information, not always directly available to us. Many children, due to their age or the way in which they view the test situation, may not be willing to separate themselves from their parent or may not be willing to perform for us, whether or not the parent is present. Especially for these children, and as supplemental information for "performing" youngsters, the social and early developmental scales, which will be discussed in the next section, may be looked on as extensions of the case history or interview information. While they are, by our earlier definition, "second-hand" information, one or more of the following measures may be useful.

SOCIAL AND EARLY DEVELOPMENTAL SCALES

The Vineland Social Maturity Scale

Earlier we talked about tools of measurement as being different from case history or interview forms. The distinction is not always easy to make from the names of the tools. *The Vineland Social Maturity Scale* (Doll 1947) is here defined as an extension of a case history interview in that there is an intervening variable—a reporter—between the interviewer who must make the judgment and the child on whom the judgment is made.

The Vineland Scale was designed to be an alternative to the usual intelligence tests as the basis for making social and academic placements. Doll felt that social competence was the ultimate goal of each individual. Intelligence tests concentrate primarily on abstract (dealing with mathematical and verbal symbols) or concrete (dealing with objects) tasks rather than on social intelligence (ability to deal with persons). Social maturation, or social competence, is measured on the Vineland Scale as successive degrees of social independence in six areas of performance: self-help (eating, dressing, and general self-help); locomotion; occupation (ranging, at an early age from simply keeping himself occupied, to being gainfully employed); communication; self-direction; and socialization.

Socialization does not mean that the child is sociable in the usual sense of the word. Doll's picture of a socially mature nursery school child is one who may be active, nonconforming, resistant, disobedient, and emotional—in short, "independent and rather aggressive." The clinical evaluation of particular attributes is designed to assess the variables related to social competence. In other words, these results should be evaluated in terms of the total clinical study of each individual and the clinician "... will not use the results by mere rule-of-thumb statistical interpretation."

The Vineland Scale was designed to be given as an interview and the listed items were meant as probes, rather than standardized wordings for questions. The items need not be administered in the order listed. The groupings as they appear are merely for convenience, and the examiner is free to adjust the order for herself. The Vineland is not a rating scale, and scores are not based on mere opinion. The informant does not make the scoring judgment, and this is an important point. Empirical observations have demonstrated that the informant is an important variable in the performance level attributed to the child. For example if the child's mother, his teacher, and his speech clinician, all of whom know him well, but from a different frame of reference, were all three (separately) to serve as informant, three different scores are likely to be obtained. The child's mother would likely rate him highest; the teacher, next; and his clinician would rate him lowest. In any case, the informant is asked to supply as much detail as is practical, and the examiner then makes the scoring judgment regarding the behavioristic facts which reveal the manner and extent of the subject's actual performance on each item. Successful performance on many of the items may be relatively clear-cut (for example, walks downstairs one step per tread); others are open to more interpretation (washes hands unaided).

In general, items are scored as "full credit" for reported performance; there is no credit for items on which the child has not succeeded or has succeeded only with what may be termed "unusual incentive;" and half-credit is given for behaviors in an emergent state. A fourth option, "no environmental opportunity," is credited according to the surrounding scores. For example, if there are no stairs in the child's home, you may assume he has had no chance to practice this particular skill and therefore give him credit for "walks downstairs with one foot per tread" even though you don't know if he would or not. That is, you would give him full credit if surrounding items were passed, but give him no credit if surrounding items were failed. A more thorough description of the Vineland Scale and its uses may be found in Doll's (1953) *Measurement of Social Competence.*

The manual is not restrictively specific in the administraton of the Vineland Scale, but five or six minuses in a row is usually indicative that the examiner can discontinue the test. The examiner may, at his discretion, further examine one or two main areas. The score for the scale is the total number of items passed (basal score plus additional items credited), and a conversion chart is supplied to give an age value for total correct points. This index number may also be converted to a social quotient by dividing social age by chronological age and multiplying by 100 ($SQ = SA/CA \times 100$). The usual procedure with age-scale tests is to begin testing at approximately one year below where the child is expected to be scored. If the child is not credited with a series of pluses on five or six consecutive items, work backward until you discover a basal level.

The Vineland Social Maturity Scale spans an age range from 0 to 25 years plus. Items are arranged by age level, and there are an unequal number of items per age. There are 17 items on each of the first two-year levels (0-1, 1-2), 10 on the 2-3-year age level, six items on the 3-4 year level, and four to five items on most succeeding age levels. There are a decreasing number of items per year toward the older age ranges. For example, only four items span the age range from 20-25 years. Age scores are credited to items by interpolation. Item 44 credits the child with a social age of four years; item 50 credits her with five years of social maturity, so intervening items between 44 and 50 each credit the child with approximately two months of maturity. There are, however, no data available to verify that items are equally spaced along the age continuum. In fact, there are no recent studies of the validity or reliability of the scale. The 1965 printing of the 1947 manual did not change any of the form or substance of the test. It was merely a more thorough statement of the information originally gathered in the 1920s and 1930s. It is a widely used instrument because (to our knowledge) it is the only one of its kind, but even Doll (1947) admitted that it would have little significance if not accompanied by a battery of other tests and extensive case-history information.

These nondirect instruments are useful, especially with young children who may not be ready to interact sufficiently with a stranger to allow us to obtain first-hand observational data. Our biases, therefore, would suggest using them as part of the case history interview, particularly with preschool children and supplementing the information with as much first-hand testing as is possible.

Verbal Language Development Scale

The *Verbal Language Development Scale* (Mecham 1971) is an extension of the communication portion of the *Vineland Social Maturity Scale.* The 1971 printing did not make any significant changes from the earlier 1958 edition. Four types of communication items are assessed: listening, speaking, reading, and writing. Scoring is much the same as in the Vineland, with the same rationale and with the same pitfalls.

In this scale, as in the Vineland, the informant supplies the information in response to the examiner's questions, and the examiner makes the judgment of pass or fail. The age range for the *Verbal Language Development Scale* is from one month to 16 years. Again, items are arranged on an age scale, and specific age-scale equivalents are given from a conversion chart and are determined by interpolation.

As a rule of thumb, because there would appear to be more precision in the conversion age scale than is appropriate for the measure, we suggest that the resulting score for both the *Vineland* and the *Verbal Language Development Scale* be reported as an age range. Considering the lack of descriptive and diagnostic precision available from this measure, it is suggested that the resultant score be considered a ball-park estimate at best. That is, rather than attributing a score of 2.72 years to a child, it might be more logical, although admittedly less precise, to report that the child scored at approximately the two-and-one-half-year level or "between the two- and three-year level." This is an empirically derived test, and there are no reliability or validity data available. There is a direct-test version of the *Verbal Language Development Scale* (the *Utah Test of Language Development*) which will be discussed in the chapter on language testing.

Preschool Attainment Record

The *Preschool Attainment Record* (PAR) (Doll 1966) is also an expansion of the *Vineland Scale,* and the assessment procedure is much the same. Like the Vineland, it is an interview procedure. The PAR is designed to provide an assessment in eight maturational categories concerned with physical, social, and intellectual functions of young children aged six months through seven years. The eight categories on which a profile of attainment is scored are ambulation, manipulation, rapport, communication, responsibility, information, ideation, and creativity. There are 16 items per year with eight at each half year. Items are scored as full credit (plus), no credit (minus), half-credit (plus-minus), or no opportunity (N.O.). Since there are 16 items per year, the total raw score is divided by 16 to determine the Attainment Age. An Attainment Quotient is then derived by dividing Attainment Age by chronological age multiplied by 100. The PAR is not normatively standardized.

Birth to Three Developmental Scale

One more scale which fits into the operational definition of general developmental information is the *Birth to Three Developmental Scale* designed by Bangs and Dodson (1979). The age range is obvious from the title–from birth to three years. Five areas of early development are charted: language comprehension, language expression, problem solving, social-personal, and motor behavior. Scoring is by plus and minus for full credit and no credit respectively, a plus-minus as a judgment that the performance is approximate and/or transitional, and the item is left blank for a behavior "not observable." The *Birth to Three Scale* is different from most of the early developmental tests in that, although it may be used as an interview instrument, it was designed to be completed from direct observation of young children when possible. With that in mind, the "not observable" category was probably meant as "no environmental opportunity" or similar translation. Bangs and Dodson placed the items at empirically derived age levels from direct observation. The observer or informant for the test administration may be the examiner, the mother, or other knowledgeable adult.

Age separations are by six-month divisions (0-6, 6-12, 12-18, and so on) and a "developmental age" can be obtained for each of the five areas.

Receptive-Expressive Emergent Language Scale

The Bzoch and League (1970) *Receptive-Expressive Emergent Language Scale* (REEL) was also developed for measurement of language skills in infancy and purports to measure language emergence in age periods from zero to 36 months. This test would seem to allow more variation than some of the ones previously discussed. Age-level periods for the first year are by one month separations (0-1, 1-2, 3-4, and so on); for the second year, by two month separations, and for the third year, by three month separations. At each age period there are three receptive and three expressive language statements. If the informant's information or description convinces the examiner that two of the three items are satisfied at any age, the child is credited with that level of performance. Three age scores and age-score quotients are available from the measure: a Receptive Language Age (RLA), and Expressive Language Age (ELA), and a Combined Language Age (CLA = RLA + ELA ÷ 2). Language Age quotients are found by dividing RLA, ELA, or CLA by chronological age and multiplying by 100.

Validity and Reliability of Developmental Scales. The five social and early developmental scales we have discussed* have all been assembled primarily from empirical bases. They all have an inherent face validity or construct validity, but specific-item validity is much more difficult to determine. The question may well be raised as to whether the items included are significant indices to the maturation under study and also whether the respondent's information would be by the same definitions as ours if we were to make the observations. If the examiner observes a behavior being performed, the child can obviously be credited on the appropriate item; it is equally obvious that the child's failure to perform for our observation does not necessarily indicate that he does not perform the behavior in more familiar surroundings. Reliability determination can suffer from the same variables. The possible variability of reporter is an inherent weakness in any instrument which uses second-hand observations as the primary data.

One other note of caution. Do not be overly fascinated by an age score or a developmental quotient. An age score is merely a test score expressed as a year-month value. Basically it differs in no way from any other type of score given in terms of items passed out of a possible total. The value is the same, and that value is no better than the test items used to derive it. By the same reasoning, a quotient or proportionate score is a comparison of that age score with the

*A summary of the scales appears at the end of this section as Table 2-1 with age ranges and areas examined.

Table 2-1 Summary of social and early-developmental scales

Name	*Age Range*	*Areas Examined*
Vineland Social Maturity Scale	0-25 years	Six social competence areas: self-help, locomotion, occupation communication, self-direction, socialization.
Verbal Language Development Scale	1 month to 16 years	Listening, reading, speaking, writing
Preschool Attainment Record	6 months to 7 years	Ambulation, manipulation, rapport, communication, responsibility, information, ideation, creativity
Birth to Three Developmental Scale	0-3 years	Language comprehension, language expression, problem solving, social-personal, motor behavior
Receptive-Expressive Emergent Language Scale	0-36 months	Receptive, expressive language

hypothetical value to be expected for the chronological age. All three scores—number of items passed, year-month scores, and quotients—have the same arithmetical properties, the same possibilities for evaluation, and the same limitations.

REFERENCES

Aldrich, C. A., and M. Norval, A developmental graph for the first year of life. *J. Pediatrics,* 29, 304-308, (1946).

Balint, M., *The Doctor, His Patient and the Illness.* New York: International Universities Press, Inc., (1957).

Bangs, T., and S. Dodson, *Birth to Three Developmental Scale.* Hingham, Mass.: Teaching Resources, (1979).

Bzoch, K. R., and R. League, *Receptive-Expressive Emergent Language Scale,* Gainesville, Fla.: Computer Management Corporation, (1970).

Code of Ethics. *American Speech-Language-Hearing Association 1979 Directory.* Rockville, Md.: American Speech-Language-Hearing Association, (1979).

Darley, F., *Diagnosis and Appraisal of Communication Disorders.* Englewood Cliffs, N.J.: Prentice-Hall, Inc., (1964).

Doll, E. A., *Vineland Social Maturity Scale.* Circle Pines, Minn.: American Guidance Service Inc., (1947, 1965).

Doll, E. A., *Measurement of Social Competence.* Circle Pines, Minn.: American Guidance Service, Inc., (1953).

Doll, E. A., *Preschool Attainment Record,* Circle Pines, Minn.: American Guidance Service, Inc., (1966).

Emerick, L. L., and J. T. Hatten, *Diagnosis and Evaluation in Speech Pathology.* Englewood Cliffs, N.J.: Prentice-Hall, Inc., (1974).

Helton, J., The value of occupation, education, and income in predicting PPVT scores of preschool-aged-children: Some comments on criteria commonly utilized for social class stratification. Unpublished Master's thesis, University of Tennessee, Knoxville (1974).

Johnson, W., *People in Quandaries.* New York: Harper & Row, (1946).

Johnson, W., F. L. Darley, and D. C. Spriestersbach, *Diagnostic Methods in Speech Pathology.* New York: Harper & Row, (1963).

Johnson, W., and others, *The Onset of Stuttering.* Minneapolis: University of Minnesota Press, (1959).

Mecham, M. J., *The Verbal Language Development Scale.* Circle Pines, Minn.: American Guidance Service, Inc., (1958, 1971).

Schultz, M. C., The bases of speech pathology and audiology: Evaluation as the resolution of uncertainty. *J. Speech Hearing Dis.,* 38, 147-155, (1973).

Shannon, C. E., and W. Weaver, *The Mathematical Theory of Communication.* Urbana: University of Illinois Press, (1964).

Wallin, P., The predicting of individual behavior from case studies, as cited in W. Johnson, F. L. Darley, and D. C. Spriestersbach, *Diagnostic Method in Speech Pathology.* New York: Harper & Row, (1963).

PART II

Articulation Testing

There is no point in giving a test except for a definite purpose.

Wendell Johnson
in *People in Quandries*

There are probably more tests for the measurement of articulation skills than any other single aspect of speech. However, articulation tests, like children, are not all created equal. We will not discuss all of the tests here, but we will explore a sufficient variety for comparison of the rationales for their use. The choice of which test to use will be based on both your purpose in testing and your biases.

One logical division of articulation tests is into screening and diagnostic categories. Some comment was made earlier about this categorization. In general, if you wish merely to separate adequate from inadequate articulation skill, you would use a screening test. If you wish a more detailed description of the subject's ability to produce a wide range of speech sounds in a variety of positions and phonetic contexts, use a diagnostic test. Your choice from this categorization is a function of your purpose in testing.

Not all of the tests we will discuss are labelled in this fashion, however, so a more operational division would be between those articulation tests which are primarily single-phoneme tests compared to those which provide more phonetic detail. A choice between these two categories is largely a function of the clinician's biases. If you believe that a single-phoneme test (or a phonetic inventory) is an adequate description of articulation skill, then you have implicitly assumed that context is not a significant variable in your testing of articulation. If you believe that phonetic context will have an effect on the production of the sound, on the other hand, you will use a more detailed test to sample these effects.

Further, if you agree that speech sounds may represent morphological entities, you will assign a different interpretation to, for example, an omission of an /s/ sound to represent plurality than the omission of the /s/ which is meant to imply possession. For this and other reasons you may make different judgments of articulation skill in connected speech samples than in single-word articulation tests.

Articulation tests vary considerably in their procedures and interpretation. Key issues related to the administration and analysis of the results of any of the tests are the method of eliciting responses, scoring procedures, the effects of stimulation, and interpretation of test results based on age of acquisition.

SPONTANEOUS AND IMITATIVE RESPONSES

In the administration of a test with picture stimuli, the examiner has a choice of showing the subject the picture and asking him to name it or providing the word and asking him to repeat it. The first method is called spontaneous, and the second is imitative. There is some difference of opinion expressed in the literature as to whether the two methods of administration yield comparable results.

The earliest reported study concerned with this issue was by Morrison (1914), who concluded that the two methods yielded similar results. Her subjects were kindergarten and primary school children with "marked" articulatory inaccuracies. Templin (1947a) reported a slight, but not statistically significant, increment from spontaneous to imitative test method with a group of preschool and kindergarten children. Snow and Milisen (1954) used both an imitative and a spontaneous method to test first- and second-, and seventh- and eighth-grade children. Their results showed a consistently higher level of performance for the imitative method, especially among the older children.

Anthony and others (1971) tested three- to five-year-old children and reported no statistically significant difference in the results from the two methods. They indicated, however, that the children probably concentrated more on the pronunciation than the recognition of the picture and therefore gave a less self-conscious articulation example in the spontaneous method. Paynter and Bumpas (1977) found no significant difference between scores for the two methods with 3-0 to 3-6 children. Siegel and others (1973) reported a statistically significant difference between the imitative and spontaneous testing methods for eight of the forty sounds tested with 100 kindergarten children. The differences found were significantly in favor of the imitative method although they were small in magnitude. From inspection of their tabulated data, some of the difference in production may have been related to the familarity of the words and the ease with which the words could be pictured. In view of these diverse findings, an equitable compromise on test procedures may be that the spontaneous method is preferable as a means of eliciting a representative sample from older children, but equivalent results may be expected from the two methods with younger children—probably through kindergarten and first grade.

These findings also indicate the importance of the picture stimuli utilized to elicit responses. For example, it is difficult to draw a picture which has a high probability of eliciting the words "there" or "smooth" to test the production of a voiced /ð/ sound. In general, and in the interest of saving time, it is probably more efficient to ask young children to repeat the words after the examiner. With older children and adults, a sentence test is more likely to yield valid results. If the person being tested does not read fluently enough to provide "spontaneous-sounding" speech, a picture "word" test may be used to elicit spontaneous responses.

STIMULABILITY

Our discussion of methods for eliciting responses suggested that articulation-test procedures attempt to sample the subject's typical performance. A second procedure as part of the testing is to determine if the subject can correct error sounds following the presentation of the correct sounds at several levels of complexity, for example, in isolation, in syllables, and in words. This procedure is called stimulability testing and involves asking the subject to "watch and listen carefully" as the clinician produces the stimulus sound two or three times and then to repeat the stimulus that was presented. The errors observed during the articulation-test procedure and stimulability testing are recorded the same way; the examiner records correct production, a substitution, a distortion, or an omitted phoneme. The results of the stimulability testing are recorded with the level of complexity at which the stimulation was attempted. Stimulation of the error sound, and then testing to determine correct production, would usually be carried out for the sound in isolation, syllables, words, and phrases or sentences.

Stimulability data is obtained because of its prognostic value. On the basis of data obtained from 100 kindergarten-aged children, 50 classified as having mild articulation problems and 50 with severe articulation problems, Farquhar (1961) concluded that children with mild articulation problems are more likely to make the error sound correctly following stimulation. Furthermore she found that when the subjects were retested seven months later, there was greater spontaneous improvement in articulation for the mild group than for the severe group of children. When the results of this study are applied to the spontaneous versus imitative method of administration of articulation testing, it can be concluded that an imitative method is apparently less likely to affect the test results if the child has a "severe" articulation problem.

Milisen (1957) suggested that the error phonemes and the stimulability data be listed in adjacent columns. The first column would list error phonemes in order, so that those errors most distracting to an audience would be at the top of the list. The same sounds in the second column would be listed with the most stimulable at the top. The sounds that are near the top on both lists would be worked with first in therapy to effect a rapid and noticeable change.

SCORING

Articulation test items usually are scored as correct or incorrect. If the tested speech sound is in error, the type of error (substitution, omission, distortion) is recorded. A distortion may be further qualified by a numerical representation of its approximation to the intended phoneme. For example, if "distortions were classified as "1," "2," or "3" to indicate the severity, a "1" rating might be defined as a close approximation to the correct sound while "3" would be a more distant approximation to that phoneme. In practical terms, the qualification of the errors recorded is probably a function of the fine transcription ability of the clinician administering the test. Since our purpose in testing articulation is to gather as much information as possible as to how the error sounds are deviant, it is important to describe the error sounds as completely and as reliably as possible. It has been suggested by Van Riper and Irwin (1958) that the severity of the articulation disorder is closely related to the similarity or dissimilarity of the error sound to the intended target sound. Consequently, large variations between the tested phoneme and the approximation of the speaker to that phoneme will be most disruptive to the communication process.

NUMBER AND TYPE OF ERRORS

There is no universal interpretation among articulation-test makers regarding the importance of total number of errors on their tests. This lack of interpretation is based on the fact that many articulation tests are interpreted on the basis of age of acquisition of speech sounds. Consequently, the specific speech sounds in error are more important than total number of errors. We will discuss age of acquisition of speech sounds in the following section, but for the moment, let us review several studies related to the total number and types of articulation errors and their relationship to judgments of defectiveness.

Historically, the total number of speech-sound errors has been considered the primary factor in judgments of defectiveness. However, there have been few studies which have explored this relationship. Perrin (1954) correlated judgments of trained and untrained listeners with the number of defective sounds, and Barker (1960) derived a numerical value for defectiveness of articulation, but both of these studies used small samples. The Perrin study used only seven subjects while Barker included 45 children. A more complete attempt at determining which factors of misarticulation contribute to defectiveness judgments was completed by Jordan (1960). His study included 150 children who evidenced mild to severe articulation deviations. The correlations within this study were made between judgments of defectiveness of tape-recorded samples of conversational speech and results from the *Templin-Darley Diagnostic Test of Articulation.* He found a statistically significant correlation of 0.72 between number of defective items on the Templin-Darley Test and judged severity. It would seem a generally safe assumption that total number of articulation errors is related to the defectiveness of articulation.

There is a frequently stated assumption (for example, McDonald 1965a) that children develop correct articulation by progressing through several stages of production. In general, as language skills develop, speech sounds first are omitted, substituted, distorted, and then produced correctly. Support for this assumption is implied from data such as that collected by Templin (1957) although her data were cross-sectional rather than longitudinal. Templin's data for all age groups combined showed that the most frequent errors were those of substitution (74 percent), followed by those of distortion (16 percent) and omission (10 percent). As the total number of errors decreased with age, substitutions maintained a relatively constant proportion over the three-to-eight-year age groups, but the proportion of distorted sounds fluctuated with no clear trend from the youngest to the oldest age. The proportion of errors of omission declined with increasing age. In other words, the number of articulation errors of all types was reduced with age, with the most dramatic reduction in errors of omission.

The review of data related to the type and number of articulation errors suggests that both these factors may be related to the judged severity of the disorder. This relationship was explored by Jordan (1960). He found that the variable which most highly correlated with a judgment of defectiveness was the number of single phoneme errors. Second in order of importance to a judgment of defectiveness was the proportion of misarticulations which were omissions, and the variable third in magnitude was the consistency of the misarticulated sounds. As separately contributing variables, errors of distortion and of substitution were of relatively little importance.

In summary, both the number and type of errors are important considerations in analyzing articulation skills. The variables most indicative of defective articulation appear to be the number of omission errors, the total number of single consonants misarticulated, and the consistency of misarticulations. Some inconsistency of articulation should be expected, however, in the child's development of speech production skills.

AGE OF ACQUISITION

Another important consideration in the measurement of articulation skills is the type of test items used to measure these skills. There are approximately 43 phonemes in English; 25 are classified as consonants, and 18 are vowels or diphthongs. Some tests, which we have designated as single-phoneme tests, are constructed on the premise that a representative sample of speech must include all of the consonants and vowels and usually test the consonants in "initial," "medial," and "final" word positions. The assumption implicit in a single-phoneme test is that the articulation of the test sound will be consistent and not significantly affected by context. Since context does make a difference, they cannot be construed as diagnostic as we have defined that term. Since most single-phoneme tests are interpreted according to age of acquisition, this information must be discussed before we review individual articulatory measures.

There are at least five sets of data reported on age of acquisition with a general agreement as to the order of sounds but with discrepancies as to the age at which children have acquired the production of the phonemes of English. The idea of "produced" compared to "acquired" may need some explanation. Several investigators, for example, Irwin (1947) and Miller (1951), suggest that by the time the child has reached approximately 18 months of age he has produced all the sounds his oral mechanism is capable of making. This includes a variety of non-English sounds, but it does not suggest that the sounds have been used meaningfully or correctly in intended words. Consequently "produced" as defined here means that the sounds have been used but not necessarily for intended expressions while "acquired" suggests that they are customarily and purposefully utilized a large percentage of the time.

Phonemes are minimal and nonmeaningful elements in all languages. They are defined by contrast and substitution and are concomitant bundles of features. Features, in the simplest definition, are partial acoustic, perceptual, and articulatory descriptions. For example, we have already divided the phonemes of English into vowels or consonants. By definition vowels have no obstruction of the airstream anterior to the vocal folds and have no narrowing of the vocal tract higher than the tongue position for the high front vowel /i/ or the high back vowel /u/. All vowels are voiced and continuant. Consonants are voiced or voiceless and may have a secondary obstruction anterior to the vocal folds which obstructs or constricts the outgoing airstream through the oral cavity or which diverts the airstream through the nasal cavity. Oral versus nasal, stop versus continuant, and similar descriptions are defined as "manner" of articulation, and the point of major obstruction in the vocal tract is defined as "place" of articulation. These descriptions will be covered in more detail in the chapter on speech-sound discrimination, but the concept was introduced here to give credence or logic to the idea of an order of difficulty of speech-sound production. In an order of acquisition, the sounds with the least number of difficult features are expected to be mastered early while those sounds most complicated in their production will be the last to be mastered. It is not surprising then that Locke (1972) reported a positive correlation between adults' estimates of muscular ease of articulation and children's order of acquisition of speech sounds.

Some other data relative to both ease of articulation and type of error productions were reported by Singh and Frank (1972). Their data are in terms of sound features correctly maintained in children's articulation. The relative stability of each feature is given in the following listing as a percentage of correct production:

Feature	*Percentage Correct*
stop	99.69
nasal	98.75
voiceless	98.04
labial	97.26
voiced	96.92
alveolar	92.42
back	81.82
interdental	78.26

One generalization that Singh and Frank made from these data is that the earlier a feature is acquired, the more stable it is; and that the more stable features are likely to replace less stable features in articulation. In other words, we may assume that the speech sounds most frequently produced correctly are those phonemes which embody features at the top of this list, and that production errors would most often occur on more difficult, less stable, features.

As usually defined, acquisition or mastery is the age when a proportion of children correctly produce a given sound in all appropriate positions in a word. Usually the percentage is 75 percent to 100 percent at a given age level. All the children in the studies to be reviewed had normal hearing and at least normal intelligence.

The first of the five sets of data we wish to compare is by Wellman and others (1931) who tested 204 children ranging in age from two through six years. Test stimuli were pictured on 16 cards plus questions to which the children were asked to respond. The articulation test measured 133 sound units: 66 consonant elements (initial, medial, and final positions, where applicable), 48 consonant blends, 15 vowels, and 4 diphthongs. A sound was considered mastered when 75 percent of the children correctly produced the sound in applicable word positions.

Poole (1934) reported longitudinal data on 140 children over a period of three years with regard to their ability to articulate 23 consonant sounds in initial, medial, and final positions, Each child was tested at four-month intervals with single-word responses elicited by objects, pictures, and questions. Word-position data were pooled, and mastery was defined as approximately 100 percent correct production. That is, "sounds were considered established in the articulation habits of children at the age when the mean frequency of errors approached zero." One other difference in the data reporting of these first two studies is pertinent to mention: Wellman and others designated children under 2-6 as two years of age, children from 2-6 to 3-6 as three years of age, and so forth. Poole classified her 3-0 to 4-0 children as 3-6, the children from 4-0 to 5-0 years age as 4-6, and so forth.

Templin (1957) administered a 176-item articulation test which included vowels, dipthongs, and single-phoneme consonants in initial, medial, and final word positions to 480 children ranging in age from three to eight years. The sample included thirty boys and thirty girls at each half-year level from three through five years and each year level from five through eight years (3, 3½, 4, 4½, 5, 6, 7, 8). Mastery was defined as the age at which 75 percent of the subjects correctly produced the specific consonant elements in all applicable positions in a word.

Sander (1972) criticized the definition of "mastery" as it had been utilized because he thought it was overly stringent. He argued instead for what he termed "customary production" because of varying difficulty of production of a sound according to word-position. For example, /t/ in the initial position of a word is produced correctly at a much earlier age than the medial /t/ in a word such as "biting" or "city." He suggested that a more logical age placement for the consonant sounds would be the age at which 51 percent of the children tested correctly articulated the sound in at least two of three word-positions. Not all sounds occur in all three word-positions, however, so his first suggestion would provide for unequal treatment among the consonants. In order to standardize the treatment of consonants, he placed each sound at an age level where more than 50 percent correct production was achieved at an average of the combined word-positions. For example, Templin (1957) placed the sound of /dʒ/ (the initial sound in "judge") at the seven-year level. The percentages of correct responses for the three positions for 3½-year-old children are 58 percent, 43 percent, and 22 percent for the initial, medial, and final positions respectively. The average of these three is 41 percent. Four-year-old children produced an average correct percentage of 69 percent for the three positions tested, and Sander would therefore place the /dʒ/ sound at the four-year level since it exceeds the 51 percent criterion. Sander did not collect new data from children;

he resummarized the Wellman and others (1931) and Templin (1957) data with the 51 percent criterion as described.

Prather and others (1975) used a 75 percent correct criterion in testing the articulation skills of 147 children aged 24 to 48 months. The sample included groups of 21 children each at four month separations: 24, 48, 32 months and so on. In this study, as in the Wellman and others and Templin studies, children were selected to represent different social classes. Test stimuli were 44 pictures selected from the *Photo Articulation Test* (Pendergast and others 1969) to represent only initial and final position single-phoneme consonants.

Table 3-1 summarizes the data from the five studies discussed. Note that the Sander data derived from the Wellman and Templin studies are quite similar to that collected by Prather and show earlier mastery ages than Poole. It should be remembered that Sander utilized a less stringent criterion judgment than Poole, and Prather tested only initial and final word-positions.

We indicated earlier that single-phoneme tests may be called inventories since they sample speech sounds in a limited number of contexts. There are probably significant effects from even these limited contexts, however, and the data displayed in Table 3-1 can only be used to determine the general level of speech sound development from the age of acquisition data.

The clinician may expect reasonably large variations in the speech-sound mastery of even a limited sample. In general, most children master speech sounds at a relatively early age. For example, Templin (1957) found that approximately 92 percent of the five-year-old children produced more than 75 percent of the tested sounds correctly in the initial position of words, and 85 percent produced these sounds correctly in the final position. Only the final position voiced /ð/, final /ʒ/, and unvoiced /hw/ in initial and medial positions were correct less than 50 percent of the time. In a later report on a five-year longitudinal study Templin (in Smith and Miller 1966) commented:

> Probably the most important observation that I have made up to this time is that the children with many misarticulations in kindergarten continue to have a considerable number of them when they are in the second grade. Because of the consistent findings from the cross sectional studies that mature articulation was achieved by seven- to eight-year-old children, it was originally planned to terminate the identification and longitudinal studies when the children at grade for their age had finished the second grade. This was not possible, however, because a larger number of children than anticipated had not yet achieved adequate production of the phonemes of English. The children who had poor articulation in kindergarten, while they improved considerably as a group, still had far from adequate articulation scores in second grade. (pp. 176-177)

If a single-phoneme articulation test is used, we should probably expect relative mastery of the speech-sound inventory by the age of five years in children of normal intelligence, normal hearing, and normal exposure to a linguistic

Table 3-1 Comparison of the ages at which subjects produced specific consonant sounds

Sound	*Prather*	*Sander*	*Templin*	*Wellman*	*Poole*
m	2	−2	3	3	3-6
n	2	−2	3	3	4-6
h	2	−2	3	3	3-6
p	2	−2	3	4	3-6
ng	2	2	3	*	4-6
f	2-4	2-6	3	3	5-6
j	2-4	2-6	3-6	4	4-6
k	2-4	2	4	4	4-6
d	2-4	2	4	5	4-6
w	2-8	−2	3	3	3-6
b	2-8	−2	4	3	3-6
t	2-8	2	6	5	4-6
g	3	2	4	4	4-6
s	3	3	4-6	5	7-6
r	3-4	3	4	5	7-6
l	3-4	3	6	4	6-6
sh	3-8	3-6	4-6	**	6-6
ch	3-8	3-6	4-6	5	**
th	4	5	7	**	6-6
zh	4	6	7	6	6-6
dzh	4+*	4	7	6	**
th	4+*	4-6	6	*	7-6
v	4+*	4	6	5	6-6
z	4+*	3-6	7	5	7-6
hw	4+*	*	*	*	7-6

*Sound tested but not produced correctly by 75% of subjects at the oldest age level.
**Sound not tested or not reported.

Data are from Wellman and others (1931), Poole (1934), Templin (1957), Sander (1972), and Prather and others (1975). Poole used a 100% criterion level, Wellman and others and Templin used 75%. Poole, Wellman and others, and Templin used initial, medial, and final word positions in their tabulations. Sander used Wellman and others and Templin data, averaged the percent correct, and used a 51% criterion. Prather used the average of only initial and final word positions and a 75% criterion. Ages expressed are in years and months; −2 indicates less than two years. Table adapted from Prather and others (1975).

environment. Children with deficient articulation development at age five can be expected, in most cases, to need help in mastering their phoneme inventory.

ARTICULATION TEST RESULTS AND INTELLIGIBILITY

The reliability of articulation testing and of specific articulation tests is more difficult to discuss than test responses which require a relatively more gross judgment of yes or no, right or wrong. Assessing articulation and intelligibility is basically a perceptual judgment on the part of a listener (Moll 1968). The potential sources of variability which may affect the reliability (repeatability) of articulation test results, according to Winitz (1969), can be attributed to the subjects, to the examiner, and to the test instrument, as well as to the interaction of the subject with the examiner.

Articulation testing usually includes the implicit assumption that the test result will somehow reflect the intelligibility and communicative ability of the one being tested. To a degree this assumption has validity, but it must be viewed cautiously. The ability of a speaker to communicate his intentions to a listener is obviously variable, and less related to the listerner's processing of the acoustic elements of speech than it is to the listener's understanding of the total context. Noll (1970) expressed the proposition this way:

> Since the concept of good speech really can be defined or determined only by the biases and standards of a human listener, articulation testing by the perceptual process of listening is the primary and basic means of assessment. (p. 284)

and further

> To communicate with a listener, a speaker must be able to use intelligible speech. If he has defective articulation, his intelligibility may well be reduced. One way, therefore, to measure articulatory skill is to assess how well the listener understands the message: the degree to which the speaker is intelligible. (p. 291)

A judgment of articulation skill would not be complete with only a reporting of test results; it must also include a statement of judged intelligibility. Probably the most frequently used definitions of intelligibility are from a choice of (1) easily intelligible, (2) understandable if the topic is known, (3) word intelligible now and then, and (4) unintelligible.

"Articulation" and "intelligibility" are related, but they are not identical. If a speaker distorts the sound elements but does so in a consistent manner, her speech may be easily intelligible because of the predictability of the errors. The consistency of the sound errors thus has an effect on intelligibility. As mentioned earlier, the number and type of errors will also influence a judgment of intelligibility, but there is at least one more factor in our judgment. According to Faircloth and Faircloth (1973) syllabic integrity is more critical to intelligibility than is phonetic integrity. They reported that speakers who closely approximate the appropriate number of syllables in a polysyllabic utterance and maintain the correct stress patterns, rhythm, and intonation are more intelligible than those who disrupt syllable integrity, regardless of whether the individual phones are correctly articulated.

The point to be made is that articulation testing is really done in the examiner's ear, and the specific test formats or test stimuli are only the vehicles for the examiner's judgment. Regardless of the test instrument or the means for making the evaluation, the examiner must bear in mind that intelligibility and articulation integrity are not necessarily the same thing and must decide whether he wishes to judge functional communication ability or phonetic accuracy, or both.

The articulation tests to be discussed in the rest of this chapter are therefore assumed to be examples from which—according to her biases and purposes—an examiner may choose the phonetic or phonemic stimuli. The important judgments of functional adequacy and/or accuracy must still be made in the ear (and mind) of the beholder.

SINGLE PHONEME ARTICULATION TESTS

The classification of a test as "single-phoneme" is an approximation. It is perhaps more accurate to call them primarily single phoneme because most of these tests have several blends among the stimulus items. Several single-phoneme tests have no validity or reliability data reported. These include the *Bryngelson and Glaspey Articulation Test* (1951), the *Developmental Articulation Test* (Hejna 1955), and the *Photo Articulation Test* (Pendergast and others, 1969).

The *Bryngelson and Glaspey Test* utilizes picture cards to elicit 51 responses representing 17 single phonemes in various word positions plus three /s/ blends, four /r/ blends, and three /l/ blends. Not all consonants are included. Rather, the authors reportedly included only the "most commonly misarticulated sounds."

The *Developmental Articulation Test* provides picture stimuli for single consonants in all word-positions and some two-consonant blends in the initial position of words. An adaptation of this test by Sanders (1970) utilized format designs from the *Developmental Articulation Test* and the *Photo Articulation Test* with each phoneme identified by the age at which 90 percent of the test subjects of Templin (1957) had correctly produced the phoneme in the word position tested.

The *Photo Articulation Test* uses photographs of isolated objects, rather than pictures, as stimulus materials. On the score sheet for the test, the stimuli are divided into "tongue sounds" (including both front and back tongue positions), "lip sounds," and vowels to allow the examiner to more easily examine the influence of place of articulation on misarticulations. The test stimuli include 24 single phonemes in initial, medial, and final positions where applicable, three blends (/s/, /l/, /r/), and 18 vowels and diphthongs. Sixty-nine of the test items are pictures; the other seven are designed to be elicited by questions or by imitation.

The *Denver Articulation Screening Exam* (Drumwright 1971) was designed to test "culturally disadvantaged" children. The 30 sounds tested represent 22 single-phoneme consonants (primarily in initial and final word positions), one vowel (/ɝ/), one glide plus vowel (/ju/), and six two-element combinations. The sounds tested were taken from the norms established by Templin (1957) as correctly produced by 85 percent of six-year-old children. The published version of the test contains the 30 sounds which were produced by 70 percent of the Drumwright six-year-old sample of economically disadvantaged white, black, and Mexican-American children. The test result is the number of correct sounds converted to a percentile rank for children from 2-6 to 6-0 years of age by half-year separations (that is, 2½, 3, 3½, 4, 4½, 5, 5½, 6). It was designed to be used as an imitiative test, with the examiner saying the word containing the test sound(s) and the child repeating the word. Pictures are included for the hard-to-test child. It is assumed that the presentation mode with the cards will entail both auditory and visual presentation. It was developed as a screening test which could be used by aides and other nonprofessionals to separate economically disadvantaged children who need speech remediation from those whose articulation skill was adequate for their socioeconomic background. The cut-off score was set at approximately the 15th percentile. In other words, the children's articulation skill is considered adequate if they correctly produce as many of the test sounds as 85 out of 100 other children in this lower socioeconomic category. The authors of the test claim validity is demonstrated by comparison of the test results with results from the *Developmental Articulation Test.* However, no validity studies have been reported on the *Developmental Articulation Test.*

Another single-phoneme test, entitled the *Arizona Articulation Proficiency Scale* (AAPS), was published by Barker (1960). She reasoned that speech sounds should be assigned a relative value according to the frequency of their occurrence in the language since an error on a frequently occurring sound should have more effect on a listener's judgment of speech adequacy or intelligibility than an error on an infrequently occurring sound. Barker used the frequency of occurrence data collected by French, Carter, and Koenig (1930) for the Bell Laboratories. The details of the French, Carter, and Koenig study are not important for our purposes except to note that they tabulated the most commonly heard nouns, verbs, adverbs, and adjectives in 500 telephone conversations. From these words they tabulated the frequency of occurrence of individual sounds. Barker (1960) computed the relative occurrence of each sound to the second decimal point. In spite of differences in frequency of occurrence in word position, she assigned equal weight to an occurrence of the sound in initial, medial and final word positions. A picture articulation test was then assembled which sampled 24 single-phoneme consonants and three (/s/, /l/, and /r/) blends, as well as 16 vowels and diphthongs, and four vowel plus /ɚ/ combinations (as in *hair, car, horse,* and *ear*). (The latest version of the AAPS also includes sentences to test older children or adults.) The test values were rounded off to the nearest half point in a modification of the test published in 1962. A later copyrighted publication (Janet Barker Fudala 1963, 1970) tested and assigned values only for initial and final word-position consonants. Vowels and diphthongs were tested in the same stimulus words. The most frequently occurring phonemes, according to the Bell Laboratories data, were assigned more weight than less frequently occurring phonemes. Total values for each word then depend on the assigned weight or value of the sound, the consistency of correct or incorrect production, and the word positions tested. No differential was made for type of error—omissions are scored the same as distortions or substitutions. The total value of all the consonants was set to equal 55 points, the total value for the vowels and dipthongs was 45 points, and the child's score was interpreted as a percentage of intelligibility. Therefore, if the subject's consonant and vowel error values totaled 13 points, he was assumed to be 87 percent intelligible. The 1970 version contains suggestions for interpreting these percentage ranges as well as "norms" of performance for children three to eleven years of age. No data are given to support the interpretations.

We have gone into considerable detail in the description of this test because a mathematically derived score to represent a child's intelligibility would seem to be a very worthwhile endeavor. It would be very helpful to have a quantification of this sort to measure the progress of a child in therapy. Unfortunately, the AAPS quantification does not appear to be a valid measure. One reason may be the lack of distinction for types of errors. Two children could conceivably err on the same phonemes and thus achieve the same score, but because of type or consistency of errors be quite different in intelligibility.

The original subject sample for this test consisted of 45 children from six to twelve years of age. These data were apparently the basis for the 1960 statements of validity. All 45 children were referred by classroom teachers for the test procedure. Nine of the children were receiving speech therapy, two of the children reportedly made no errors in the evaluation, and no description was provided for the articulation skill of the other 34 subjects. The articulation score obtained for each child was correlated with judgments of intelligibility made by speech pathology students from ten-second tape-recorded samples of the subjects' speech. The relatively small number of children over this wide age range with no cell divisions makes the study suspect from a statistical standpoint. The manual for the 1970 revision indicates that current comparisons for age scores were based on a minimum of 25 boys and 25 girls at each half-year age level from 3-0 to 5-6 years and at one year intervals from six to eleven years. It is not clear from the (1970) test manual whether the cited validity data were obtained from any subjects other than the original 45.

In an unpublished study, Peterson (1968) found that AAPS results did not reflect differences in articulation skill, and articulation scores were not in judged agreement with severity. In that study the test sample consisted of 241 children six, seven, and eight years of age. The six-year-old group included 76 children between 5-7 and 6-6; the seven-year-old group included 92 children from 6-7 to 7-6; and the 73 children in the eight-year-old group ranged in age from 7-7 to 8-6. The children were from nine schools in the Northern and Central part of Illinois and were located in communities which represented a range of socio-economic strata. All the children were receiving speech therapy and were judged as having mild, moderate, or severe articulation disorders. Judgments of severity were made by experienced speech pathologists employed in those schools. The severity judgment was on an eight point scale with 7 as very severe, 1 as very mild, and 0 as no problem. The articulation testing was done by experienced graduate and undergraduate students who also rated intelligibility according to ease of understanding of the subjects' speech.

Without going into the rest of the details, data shown on Table 3-2 illustrate the correlations between the test measures listed and judged severity of the articulation problem. Since we would expect a change in proficiency with age (improved skill and reduced variability), it is also pertinent to note the performance of the three age groups on Table 3-3. Table 3-3 lists the means and standard deviations for the *Templin-Darley Screening Test,* the AAPS, the number of distortions, substitutions, and omissions on the 43 single-phoneme items of the Templin-Darley test, and the number of single-phoneme errors which were corrected following stimulation for the error items.

In reference to the mean numbers shown on Table 3-3, the most appropriate comparisons would be between Templin-Darley and AAPS numbers. In terms of the other data shown on Table 3-3, the number of omissions, substitutions, and distortions are obviously proportionate numbers, and the accumulation of the three would be related to total number of errors. The meaningfulness of those numbers would be their relative proportions across the three age groups (and their relative agreement with severity judgments as shown on Table 3-2). The most stable of the three type-of-error means on Table 3-3 is the number of distortions. It is also obvious that the number of stimulable sounds would be related to the number of error sounds—that is, as more errors are made in the production of the single phonemes, more items would be tested for stimulability. Because of the reciprocal nature of these numbers, mean stimulability for groups of children would not be as meaningful as a description of the stimulability change for an individual child.

Table 3-2 Correlations of articulation test measures with judged severity of speech deficiency for six- to eight-year-old children

Measure	*Six Years (N=76)*	*Seven Years (N=92)*	*Eight Years (N=73)*
Templin-Darley Screening Test	.770*	.595*	.611*
Arizona Articulation Proficiency Scale	.468*	.171	.207
Number of distortions (single phonemes)	.165	.201	.334*
Number of substitutions (single phonemes)	.681*	.598*	.669*
Number of omissions (single phonemes)	.587*	.330*	.429*
Intelligibility (0-3)**	.670*	.607*	.539*
Number of stimulable sounds (single phoneme errors)	.421*	.427*	.623*

*Significant beyond the 0.01 level of confidence; df = 72; $r = .23 < .01$.

**Intelligibility judged by the test administrator: 0 = easily intelligible, 1 = understood if topic known, 2 = word understood now and then, and 3 = unintelligible.

Severity judgments were made by speech pathologists who were familiar with the children. Testing and intelligibility judgments were done by student clinicians familiar with the tests but not with the children.

From Peterson (1968).

While the data in Table 3-2 and 3-3 are not comprehensive in that all the varieties of articulation tests are not compared, they do at least indicate that the AAPS was not related to the severity judgments of experienced clinicians as closely as types of errors (omissions and substitutions), and the AAPS score did not reflect an improvement in articulation skill with age as did the Templin-Darley. Numbers can validly represent severity of articulation disorders but apparently not weighted values derived from frequency of occurrence of speech sounds.

The *Goldman-Fristoe Test of Articulation* (1969) was designed to include three levels of complexity. Twenty-three single phonemes and 12 blends (for /s/, /l/, and /r/ combinations) are tested in words in response to pictures. Nine pictures and two stories are used to test the same series of phonemes in what the authors identify as a "sentence" test, for the second level of complexity, and the third level of complexity is a test for the production of the error sounds in single-syllable imitation. Norms are provided for boys and girls separately from ages six to sixteen years by half-year divisions. Norms are expressed in

Table 3-3 Means and standard deviations for articulation measures listed (Ages are shown separately)

Measure	Six Years $\bar{x}$	Six Years sd	Seven Years $\bar{x}$	Seven Years sd	Eight Years $\bar{x}$	Eight Years sd
Templin-Darley Screening Test (number correct of 50)	27.46	13.33	32.97	12.88	37.10	9.76
Arizona Articulation Proficiency Scale	85.27	12.97	83.87	22.62	83.70	25.03
Number of distortions (on single phonemes)	2.92	3.32	2.20	2.10	2.21	2.29
Number of substitutions (on single phonemes)	9.25	6.31	6.78	5.60	4.46	3.99
Number of omissions (on single phonemes)	3.23	6.47	1.79	4.44	1.23	3.50
Intelligibility (0-3)	.53	.72	.43	.71	.31	.68
Number of stimulable sounds (from single phoneme errors)	6.44	5.52	4.03	4.13	3.93	5.39

Intelligibility judged by the test administrator: 0 = easily intelligible, 1 = understood if topic known, 2 = word understood now and then, 3 = unintelligible.

From Peterson (1968).

terms of percentile rankings and are based on a sample of 38,884 children comprising the National Speech and Hearing Survey (1971). The response sheet is designed to allow easy comparison of sound-in-words and sound-in-sentences subtests. The sentence subtest was designed to counter the frequently heard argument that a single-word response does not adequately represent a child's articulation habits. In this subtest, the examiner tells the child a story while showing a series of pictures. The child is asked to retell the story from the same series of pictures. There is a lack of research concerning inter- and intrajudge reliability of this procedure, and we are unaware of any specific validity studies, but at least the sound-in-sentences subtest should have high face validity.

The *Fisher-Logemann Test of Articulation Competence* (1971) differs from other single-phoneme tests in the way that the error sounds are analysed. The response sheet for the 25 single-phoneme consonants tested is separated according to voicing, manner, and place of articulation of the error sound. The test, therefore, is designed to record the feature classification of error sounds, rather than just occurrence of an error. For example, if a /t/ sound were substituted for an /f/, the response sheet matrix would indicate the difference in features of the two sounds as an intruded stop for the intended fricative, and tongue-tip alveolar position intruded for the intended labiodental position.

The sounds are alike in voicing. The error productions would thus be described in terms of the features in error.

Instead of the usual initial, medial, and final word-position description, the three positions are described as prevocalic, intervocalic, and postvocalic. The stimulus words also are chosen to represent standard dialects. For example, the final (postvocalic) sound in the word "garage" is counted correct either with /dʒ/ or /ʒ/ and the voiced /w/ would be accepted as a correct alternative for voiceless /hw/ in a word such as "whistle." The test includes single phonemes, /s/, /l/, and /r/ blends, and vowels and diphthongs. Sentences are included with the *Fisher-Logemann Test* which sample "all the consonants and vowels of English."

There are no separate norms for interpretation of this test. The developmental ages of the single-phoneme consonants according to Templin (1957) are listed as information for the examiner, but as stated earlier, the primary intent of the *Fisher-Logemann Test* is to describe the feature differences in the error sounds.

DIAGNOSTIC ARTICULATION TESTS

We began this chapter with a division of articulation tests into single-phoneme (inventory) and phonetically detailed (diagnostic) tests. It should be borne in mind, however, that the best representation of the tests as a whole would be on a continuum from inventories to phonetically detailed. We have described several single-phoneme tests and have considered their rationales and interpretations. Now we will turn our attention to phonetically detailed, or diagnostic, tests. Two representative diagnostic tests are the *Templin-Darley Tests of Articulation* (1969) and the *Edinburgh Articulation Test* (Anthony and others 1971).

An earlier version of the *Templin-Darley Tests of Articulation* (1960) included a 176-item diagnostic test which contained within it 50 items identified as a screening test. The second edition (1969) has been shortened to a 141-item test while maintaining the 50 screening items. The reduction was accomplished primarily by eliminating the testing of many single-phoneme consonants in the medial position of words and by removing some infrequently occurring consonant clusters. The manual provides means and standard deviations for the 141-item diagnostic test for boys and girls separately, for both sexes combined, and for upper and lower socioeconomic separations for ages three to eight years. The age means are separated by half-year levels from three to five years (3, 3½, 4, 4½, 5) and by one-year levels from five to eight years (5, 6, 7, 8). Eight years is considered adult performance, so an older child's or adult's performance would be compared with the means for eight-year-old children.

To facilitate description of the articulation of the subject, overlays are provided to assist with the analysis of special groups of sounds. For example, overlays are provided to view the 50 screening items separately, 42 consonant singles, 22 initial position consonant singles, 43 Iowa Pressure Test items, 31 /r/ and /ɚ/ clusters, 18 consonant and syllabic /l/ clusters, 17 /s/ clusters, 9 miscellaneous sound clusters, 11 vowel groups, and 6 diphthongs. The manual has means and standard deviations by age groups tabled for each of the above clusters.

The 50 screening test items consist of one vowel (/ɝ/), one consonant glide plus vowel (/ju/), twenty-two single consonants (ten in the initial, eight in the medial, and four in the final position), twenty-two two-consonant clusters, and four three-consonant clusters. The 50 items are those which have been identified as best discriminating between good and poor articulation in preschool and kindergarten children. Templin (1947b) studied the production of 113 speech-sound elements contained in the 176 item diagnostic test by 100 preschool and kindergarten children. From the total test results, the 27 percent of the children with the highest number of correct responses were classified as the "good articulation group," and the 27 percent with the fewest number of correct productions were classified as "poor articulators." Through the use of the Lawshe Nomograph technique of item analysis (Lawshe 1942), a discrimination value (D-value) was determined to identify those sounds which best separated between the two groups of children. The D-value indicates the separation between mean percentages of correct production by the good and the poor articulating groups. None of the 50 sounds had a D-value of less than two. In other words, the sample averages were separated by at least two standard deviations on each of the 50 items constituting the screening test.

In addition to means and standard deviations which are available with the screening test, a cut-off score is included. The cut-off score can be used to separate adequate and inadequate articulation skill by age. These cut-off scores happen to be approximately one standard deviation below the mean for boys and girls combined at each of the age levels. Remember that the adequate-inadequate cut-off score and the mean score for the fifty items were determined by two different statistical treatments, so an exact correspondence is not expected. Recall from the discussion in Chapter I that one standard deviation on either side of the mean usually defines the limits of "normalcy." Insofar as the normal curve model is appropriate, the cut-off score on the test and the minus-one standard deviation point should be expected to approximate.

A response form to illustrate a young client's performance on the Templin-Darley Articulation screening and consonant-singles subtest items is shown as Figure 3-1. She was identified as T.G., and was 4-2 years of age when tested. She was referred because of a concern about articulation skill. T.G.'s mother could understand her, but she was unintelligible to other listeners if the topic was not known. Her mother's description of the problem was that T.G. omitted medial-

Screening Test			
1. ɝ	3	26. br-	bw
2. ju	✓	27. tr-	stw
3. r(i)	w	28. dr-	g
4. r(m)	w	29. kr-	kw
5. l(i)	j	30. gr-	gw
6. v(i)	b	31. fr-	f
7. θ(i)	f	32. θr-	fr
8. θ(m)	–	33. ʃr-	sw
9. θ(f)	–	34. pl-	p–
10. ð(i)	✓	35. kl-	k–
11. ð(m)	✓	36. gl-	gw
12. ð(f)	–	37. fl-	f
13. z(i)	–	38. sm-	m
14. ʃ(i)	s	39. sn-	n
15. ʃ(m)	–	40. sp-	p
16. ʃ(f)	–	41. st-	f
17. ʒ(m)	–	42. sk-	k
18. j(i)	–	43. sl-	sw
19. j(m)	–	44. sw-	fw
20. tʃ(i)	ts	45. tw-	sw
21. tʃ(m)	–	46. kw-	xw
22. tʃ(f)	X	47. spl-	pw
23. dʒ(i)	–	48. spr-	pw
24. dʒ(m)	s	49. str-	zw
25. pr-	p–	50. skr-	kw

Consonant Singles			
Initial		Final	
51. m	✓	52. m	✓
53. n	✓	54. n	✓
		55. ŋ	✓
56. p	✓	57. p	–
58. b	✓	59. b	–
60. t	✓	61. t	–
62. d	✓	63. d	–
64. k	✓	65. k	–
66. g	✓	67. g	–
		68. l	w
69. f	✓	70. f	–
		71. v	–
72. s	✓	73. s	–
		74. z	–
		75. ʒ	–
76. h	✓		
77. w	✓		
		78. dʒ	–

Screening test No. correct	3	Consonant singles no. correct	16
Expected for age: Mean	34.2	Expected for age: Mean	31.7
Standard deviation	10.6	Standard deviation	5.5
Cut-off score (adequate)	23		

Figure 3-1 Templin-Darley Articulation screening and consonant singles subtest scores for T.G. (C.A. 4-2). (✓ = correct production, X = distortion, the phonetic symbol is inserted for substitutions, — = omission).

(Adapted from Templin-Darley Tests of Articulation, Articulation Test Form. Copyright 1968 by The University of Iowa. Used by permission.)

and final-position consonant sounds from her speech. As is shown on Figure 3-1, T.G. correctly produced three of the 50 screening items. Mean performance for a girl of this age is 34.2 with a standard deviation of 10.6. The cut-off separating adequate from inadequate performance for this age is 23 correct productions. She correctly produced 16 of the 42 initial- and final-position single-phoneme consonants included in this test, as compared to an expected 31.7 correct of 42. T.G. was also given the *McDonald Screening Deep Test* and that result will be shown later in this chapter.

The *Edinburgh Articulation Test* is similar to the *Templin-Darley Test* and consists primarily of two- and three-element blends. The rationale for the selection of test stimuli was to represent a "balanced and comprehensive picture of the consonants and consonantal clusters occurring in English at various positions in the word structure in monosyllabic, disyllabic and a few polysyllabic words." Picture stimuli are utilized to elicit 41 words containing 30 blends and 38 single-phoneme consonants. The test utilized item analyses from 371 normal and 153 speech-retarded children ranging in age from 2.5 to 6.0 years of age to establish norms. A conversion table is used for interpretation of test results interpolated with three-month divisions; that is, age groups of 3.75 years but less than 4.0, 4.0 but less than 4.25, and so on. Analysis of the data indicated that 5.5 to 6.0 years of age was the terminal level of the test, or approximately adult level. The standardization sample was reported to be proportionately representative of the boys and girls, social class, and familial status of the population of the Edinburgh, Scotland area. Tabled values from the standardization of the test indicate slight differences for sex, social class, and family standing, but the differences were not statistically significant and the norms do not distinguish among these variables.

The child's responses are scored correct or incorrect for the quantitative portion of the test. The number of correct productions is then converted to a standard score according to age quartile. The standard score is set at 100 with a standard deviation of 15. Fifteen points of this standard scale represents approximately one year, and a standard score of 85 or less at any age is considered "danger level." The examiner is encouraged to look at the error responses in phonetic detail to determine if the child shows speech retardation which calls for therapy.

The test manual also contains a qualitative interpretation of the error responses to each test item. Relative values are implied as a degree of closeness to the correct production by the listing of examples of type of error expected. The test was constructed to allow interpretation of normal performance which would consider local dialectal variants. Since the local dialects used were Scot, the variants accepted are not necessarily acceptable in American English. For example, nine of the 68 test items were voiceless, medial- and final-position plosives for which a glottal stop was considered a local (and acceptable) variant. The idea of local variant is valid, for example, a /d/ for /t/ sound as the medial position stop in the word "bottle," or a schwa vowel for a final position /ɚ/ in many parts of the country, but some revision of the norms may be necessary for use with the bulk of American English populations. No validation studies have been reported. The authors of the test state that the validity of the test is demonstrated by the quantitative test agreement with the "qualitative assessment of the skilled phoneticians [who administered it]" (Anthony and others 1971, p. 23), and by quantitative comparison of results from this (published) version with results generated by a preliminary form of the test (pp. 27-29).

SPECIAL PURPOSE TESTS

The three tests reviewed in this section are set apart because of the different purposes for which they were designed. The *Iowa Pressure Test* consists of 43 items from the 176-item *Templin-Darley Diagnostic Tests of Articulation* which were determined (Morris, Spriestersbach, and Darley 1961) to best separate between adequate and inadequate velopharyngeal closure for cleft-palate speakers. The test items include eight single-phoneme consonants and two- and three-element blends consisting primarily of fricative and plosive consonants. There are means and standard deviations for ages 3 to 8 published with the *Templin-Darley* (1969) test manual, but these "norms" in and of themselves do not indicate adequacy or inadequacy of the velopharyngeal mechanism. That judgment can only be made in terms of the nasality *perceived* with the error production of the intended consonant.

The *Predictive Screening Test of Articulation* (Van Riper and Erickson 1968) was constructed, as the name implies, as a predictor of future performance. The authors indicate that the basic purpose is to

> . . . differentiate children who will master their misarticulations without speech therapy from those who, without therapy, may persist in their errors. More specifically, the PSTA may be used to identify, among primary school aged children who have functional misarticulations at the first grade level, those children who will—and those who will not—have acquired normal mature articulation by the time they reach the third grade level.

The test was designed for school clinicians who have a large percentage of their caseload in the primary grades. The contention of the authors of the test was that a great number of children are scheduled for articulation therapy when maturation would solve their articulation problem. Consequently, it would be inefficient use of therapy time to work with children who would outgrow their errors; and it would also be inefficient not to schedule for therapy those children who would still have clinically significant misarticulations by the time they entered third grade.

A total of 111 experimental items were selected from a larger pool of suggested items assembled from the literature and from practicing clinicians. The 111 experimental items were administered to 167 beginning first grade children in Southwestern Michigan. Each of the children had been judged to have clinically significant misarticulations. At the end of a two-year period when the children were entering third grade, the 134 still available children were retested. Van Riper and Erickson (1968, p. 2) reported that 47 percent of the identified children no longer demonstrated misarticulations, and 53 percent continued to exhibit articulation errors. Item analysis reduced the 111 items to the current 47-item test. This reduced-size test was administered to a similar-sized sample of first-grade children and again the approximate 50-50 division of children occurred. Forty-nine percent were free of misarticulations, and 51 percent continued to demonstrate some misarticulations at the third-grade level.

The first 17 items of the 47-item test sample the child's production of 10 single-phoneme consonants; the next 19 items are two element /r/, /s/, and /l/ blends followed by one /spl/ and one /str/ blend. The remaining nine items are not usually found in an articulation test. They consist of a sentence to be repeated; the continuation of an /s/ and a voiceless /θ/ consonant in isolation; the production of the syllables /seeseesee/, /zoozoozoo/ and /puhtuhkuh/; the production of the syllables /lalala/ while the child has the tip of his thumb between his teeth to test the child's ability to raise and lower the tongue tip independently of jaw movement; the discrimination of an /ɚ/ vowel from a schwa on the end of a word ("finger" vs. "finguh") and the child's repetition of a clapping rhythm. Specific instructions are given for each portion of the test. All stimuli are elicited by imitation.

There are no norms as such included with the test. Rather, the manual includes tabled data to indicate the predicted adequacy-inadequacy of the child's articulation when she reaches the third grade. The selection of a high cut-off score by the clinician would predict that relatively few children who needed therapy would be falsely identified as adequate, but that a relatively large number of children would be identified as inadequate for whom maturation would solve the problem. That would be termed a "false positive error." If, on the other hand, the cut-off were set low, the proportion misclassified as not needing therapy would be high ("false negative error"), but relatively few children scheduled for therapy would have self-corrected through maturation. Van Riper and Erickson (1968) suggest that school clinicians may wish to select their own cut-off score according to their particular circumstances. If there is more room in their clinic load, they could set the cut-off high and risk working with some children whose misarticulations would be corrected by maturation but better ensure working with all the children who would need their professional help. If they have a full clinic schedule, they may set the cut-off low to reduce the false positive error and risk not identifying some children who would need therapy at the third grade. The *Predictive Screening Test* authors recommend a cut-off of 34 which would balance the false positive and false negative errors at about 30 percent of each population.

Table 3-4 illustrates some mid-range cut-off scores with the proportion of children identified at each of the scores. It is important to remember that the scores generated are for beginning first-grade children as predictions of their success at the beginning of the third grade. At the time of this writing, there are no predictions available for first to second grade, or second to third grade, or any other age-grade circumstance. It should also be remembered that the predictions do not necessarily apply to children with hearing loss or other organic deficits and may not apply beyond the population sample on which they were gathered.

The *McDonald Deep Tests of Articulation* include both a "Deep Test" (1965b) and a "Screening Deep Test" (1968) which will be discussed separately because they are slightly different in format and design. Since the tests are based on a theoretical explanation of articulation, it is first necessary that some of the basic concepts be discussed.

McDonald (1965a) based his articulation testing on four concepts:

Table 3-4 Among first graders with functional misarticulations, total proportion classified as requiring speech therapy; proportion misclassified as requiring speech therapy (false positive errors); and proportion misclassified as requiring no speech therapy (false negative errors)—when classifications are based on PSTA scores

Cut-off Score	*Proportion Classified as Requiring Therapy*	*False Positive Errors*	*False Negative Errors*
39	.72	.59	.15
38	.67	.51	.19
37	.64	.49	.22
36	.61	.44	.23
35	.57	.40	.27
34	.54	.37	.30
33	.48	.34	.39
32	.44	.33	.46
31	.37	.26	.51
30	.31	.21	.61

From Van Riper and Erickson (1968).

1. *Articulation is a process consisting of overlapping ballistic movements.** The overlapping ballistic nature of the articulatory movements places varying degrees of obstruction on the outgoing airstream and also modifies the size, shape, coupling, and resonance of the articulatory cavities.

This means that the production of a phoneme will be influenced by the articulatory positions of the abutting phonemes. Said another way, the sound produced is influenced by the context in which it occurs. The amount and the distance of influence has been called coarticulation. Daniloff and Moll (1968), for example, stated that left to right or retentive coarticulation (the articulatory characteristics of a phone observed in later phones in the string) may extend to as many as four consonants, and right to left or anticipatory coarticulation (an articulatory characteristic of a phone observed during production of preceding phones) may extend to as many as three consonants. An example may help here—consider the word "construe." The only lip-rounded phoneme is the high back vowel /u/, but lip rounding has been observed before or during the production of /n/. A discussion of coarticulation is not appropriate for our purposes here and the comment was made only to lend support to the premise of overlapping movements. A more extensive consideration of this topic is provided by Kent and Minifie (1977).

2. *Audible phenomena produced by a series of ballistic movements are highly variable and influenced by the sequences in which they occur.* This concept is a more concise restatement of the comments concerning coarticulation.
3. *Movements which produce these auditory phenomena (the sounds) develop specificity as a result of the interaction of sensory motor activities in time.* Figure 3-2 illustrates what this statement implies. As the child matures, both sensory and motor skills improve from gross to fine abilities. With maturation, he is progressively more capable in terms of both motor and sensory skills to produce more complex sound combinations.
4. *More gross movements must be developed before the fine movements can be produced.* This is self-explanatory and logical. McDonald uses it to account for the child's expected articulatory progression from omissions, to substitutions, to distortions, to correct production. The data on mastery of speech sounds (for example, Templin 1957) does indicate that young children make more errors of omission than older children.

*You remember from basic physiology that there are three types of movements: (a) fixed—the opposed muscles are in balance, (b) controlled—a slightly more powerful contraction of one set compared to the other results in a relatively slow, purposeful movement, (c) ballistic—characteristic of all skilled movements and consisting of three stages: a deep stroke to begin the movement; a momentum stage; and an arresting motion to stop the movement.

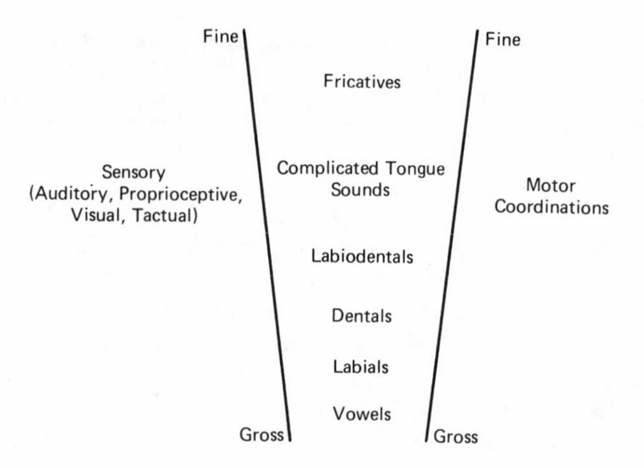

Figure 3-2 Gross to fine development of sensory and motor skills with resultant sound productions.

(Adapted from McDonald, ***Articulation Testing and Treatment—A Sensory-Motor Approach.*** Pittsburgh: Stanwix House, 1965, p. 94.)

We also noted earlier that an error of omission was judged as more important than an error of substitution or distortion in terms of the severity of the judged defectiveness. Although it may be empirically logical, there is no longitudinal data, as such, to suggest that a child would routinely go through this progression.

Two main points in the development or variability of specificity of function may be summarized as the basis for the McDonald test:

1. Articulation is a developmental behavior. There is variability in children, and with maturation the behavior becomes more specific. In practical terms, this means that the mean number of correctly articulated sounds should increase with age, and the variability around the mean should decrease.
2. Some movement sequences are more conducive to correct production of specific sounds. Two implications are contained in this statement. One is that if the articulatory positions for two abutting sounds are close together and do not interfere, those two sounds may be more accurately produced than if the sequential positions are far apart. The other implication is that if we draw a continuum from sound productions being never or randomly correct to always correct, we would expect that the speaker would range on this continuum according to the complexity of the abutting sounds, and probably neither extreme of the continuum is valid.

Percent of correct productions

0%	50%	100%
(never)		(always)

To the degree that the above reasoning is valid the *McDonald Deep Test* results should therefore provide a prediction of spontaneous improvement on the part of the child. For example, if a five-year-old child correctly produced 50 percent (maybe 30 percent or even less) of the /s/ contexts tested on the *Deep Test of Articulation,* it may be logical to expect her to correct her misarticulations as well *without* therapy as with therapy. For a child placed in therapy the implication would be to practice the child in the production of the sound combinations she already makes correctly. McDonald assumes that her production practice will make the child more aware of how the sound is produced and this knowledge will spread to other combinations and result in an easier carry-over to correct productions.

It is obvious by now that the *Deep Test of Articulation* is designed differently from the other articulation tests we have been discussing. According to McDonald, the usual articulation test, with the initial, medial, and final word-position placement of the phoneme in a single-word stimulus, is not indicative of the typical speaking situation. The initial, medial, or final description would frequently imply an intrasyllabic test. If we assume that a conversational production of a statement such as "This is the house that Jack built" contains only one initial sound (the beginning /ð/ sound in "this") and the only final sound is the /t/ in "built," all other sounds in the sentence are medial and primarily intersyllabic (between syllables rather than within syllables). The *Deep Test of Articulation* does not purport to test every phoneme in every and all possible combinations, but it does place the sound tested in up to 30 intersyllabic positions with both an arresting function (final sound on first of two syllables) and a releasing function (beginning sound on the second of two syllables). The sounds to be "deep tested" are determined by the examiner from conversation with the child or from another articulation test or any other means the examiner chooses. Both a picture test and a sentence test are available. The abutting consonants tested are keyed to the same response sheet in each version. The mechanics of test administration can be illustrated by the examiner's instructions to the child to name the pair of pictures presented to him—to make "one funny big word" out of the names of the two pictures presented rather than naming them separately. As mentioned before, this is an intersyllabic test. In English, for example, we have within-syllable combinations of /p/ plus /t/, as in the pronunciation of "capped" or "kept," but not /t/ plus /p/. In a between-syllable arrangement, as in conversational speech, the /t/ plus /p/ abutting would occur in a phrase such as "that point."

There are no norms for the *Deep Test.* The number of combinations produced correctly is converted to a percentage correct for each phoneme. The primary premise, as stated earlier, is that the sound productions are a function of the phoneme context, and some phoneme combinations will be more conducive to correct productions than other combinations. It should further be expected that there will be a common set of correct combinations, for example, among a five-year-old population. A six-year-old population of children should have that group of sounds plus others in correct combinations; the seven-year-old children should add still further to the common core of correct productions, and so on. Appleton (1969) has shown this to be true. Figure 3-3 shows a graph of the progression of percentage of correct response for five-, six-, and seven-year-old children for the /r/ and /s/ phonemes in the various combinations. The children in Appleton's study were selected as having articulation skills at or above the age level according to the *Templin-Darley Screening Test of Articulation* (1969).

The *Screening Deep Test of Articulation* restricts the testing to nine phonemes which McDonald described as frequently in error, in each of ten contexts. In other words, nine consonants are tested in each of ten contexts. While in the *Deep Test* all of the test sounds were placed in a medial (intersyllabic) position in the stimulus syllables, in the *Screening Deep Test* 30 of the 90 test phonemes are an initial or final (therefore, intrasyllabic) location. The

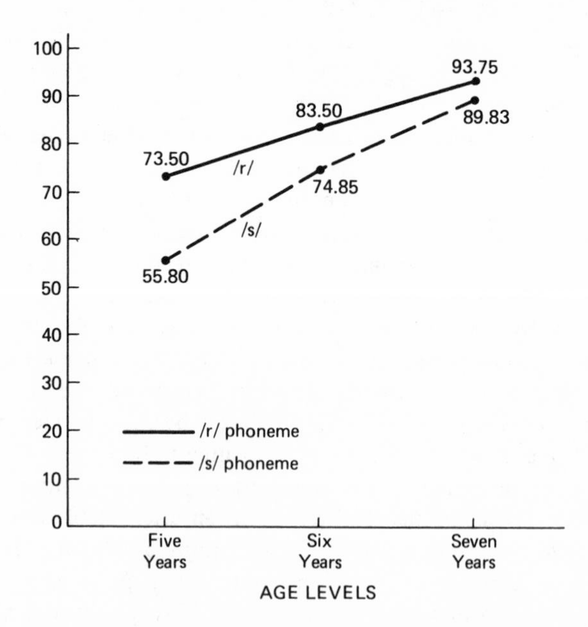

Figure 3-3 Mean percentage articulation scores for five-, six-, and seven-year-old males in the production of the /r/ and /s/ phonemes in 46 phonetic contexts. (From Appleton, 1969)

picture stimuli are paired on a single card, and the instructions to the child are the same: "Make a funny big word" of the two pictures. Originally there were no detailed norms published with the *Screening Deep Test* so interpretation of the results was unclear. However, a later report (McDonald and McDonald 1974) provided longitudinal data on repeated testing of 521 children from beginning kindergarten to beginning third grade. The data reported are in terms of proportion of the children who correctly articulated the nine consonants at each of the six test times (beginning and ending kindergarten and first grade; beginning second and third grade). McDonald and McDonald (1976a,b) reported cross-sectional data on children from prekindergarten to beginning first grade and a comparison of longitudinal and cross-sectional data on the *Screening Deep Test.* The cross-sectional report separates the data for boys and girls and shows a slight advantage for girls over boys in the earliest ages but a similar performance for boys and girls at the beginning of first grade. Table 3-5 shows an example of the type of data reported. Guidelines for interpretation are contained in the reports (1974, 1976a,b), but a general statement such as the following seems reasonable:

> . . . any child who continues to produce fewer than 3 correct productions of any of these sounds from beginning kindergarten to the beginning of first grade should be considered a candidate for therapy at that time. (1974, p. 21)

When discussing the Templin-Darley Tests of Articulation we included (as Figure 3-1), an example of a test result for a young lady identified as T.G. and

Table 3-5 Proportion of 2,125 beginning first-grade children correctly articulating in the indicated number of contexts each of the SDTA tested consonants

Number of contexts correctly articulated	*Consonants Tested on the SDTA*								
	s	l	r	tʃ	θ	ʃ	k	f	t
10	.66	.75	.76	.88	.65	.81	.98	.83	.97
9	.13	.14	.09	.06	.10	.08	.01	.11	.02
8	.07	.07	.04	.02	.05	.03	.001	.05	.004
7	.04	.01	.02	.01	.03	.02	.001	.01	.001
6	.02	.01	.02	.01	.03	.01	.001	.001	.001
5	.01	.004	.01	.002	.02	.01	.002	.00	.00
4	.01	.003	.01	.01	.02	.01	.001	.001	.00
3	.01	.003	.01	.002	.01	.01	.001	.001	.00
2	.01	.01	.01	.001	.01	.003	.00	.001	.00
1	.01	.001	.01	.01	.01	.01	.00	.001	.00
0	.04	.001	.02	.01	.06	.01	.001	.001	.00

From McDonald & McDonald (1976a).

noted that she had been given the McDonald Screening Deep Test as well. That result is shown as Figure 3-4. Most of T.G.'s errors would be described as omissions of medial and final position sounds. Substitution errors were primarily simplification; for example, reducing two-element combinations to a single phoneme, and replacing both /tʃ/ and /ʃ/ with the less marked fricative /s/. The only single phonemes not made correctly in any of the tested combinations or word positions (see Figure 3-4) were /tʃ/, /θ/, and /ʃ/.

The data from the Templin-Darley test and the McDonald Screening test agree that T.G. is significantly below expected performance for a child of her age. Additionally, from both test protocols, she is consistent in her omission of consonants which serve an arresting function (final position) in most stimulus syllables tested. In other words, in planning therapy for T.G., it would be important to note that with few exceptions, the phonemes of English are, at least sometimes, correctly produced. In her case, the position (or function) of the phoneme would appear to be relatively more important than context, per se.

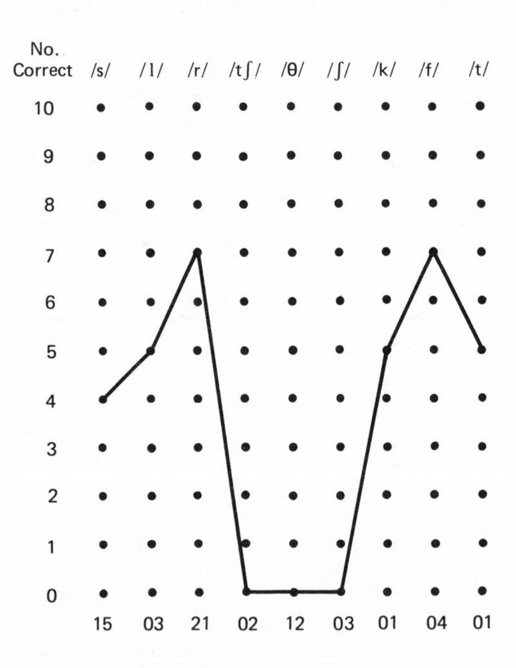

Figure 3-4 T.G.'s phonetic profile on the McDonald Screening Deep Test of Articulation. The graph line represents the number of correct productions of each of the ten phonemes listed. The number at the bottom of each column is the approximate percentile rank that number of correct responses represents as compared to beginning-kindergarten-aged girls according to McDonald and McDonald (1976a).

(Adapted from Teacher's Record Sheet for a Screening Deep Test of Articulation by Eugene T. McDonald. Copyright Stanwix House, Inc., 1976. Used by permission.)

SUMMARY

The articulation tests discussed cannot clearly be separated into categories, but in general, our descriptions were of tests which were either phoneme inventories or phonetically detailed. Although it is a logical division in terms of purpose, very few tests are designated "diagnostic" as opposed to "screening." It is also apparent that some test makers have not considered context an important variable, and they imply consistency of production (an /s/ is an /s/ is an /s/). Other tests' constructions have considered context a highly important variable. Such a diverse display of articulation tests cannot be readily summarized. We are left with a statement which began this chapter; your choice of an articulation test is dependent upon your purpose in testing and your biases.

Once again we wish to repeat a previously expressed caution. Our purpose is not to list all the tests available in articulation or any other phase of speech and language assessment but rather to review some tests and observations that we have designated as representative in order to explore the rationales on which the tests or observations are based.* If you, as a clinician, understand the rationale for a test, then you can decide if you agree with the basic design and whether that particular measurement is valid and appropriate for your purposes in testing. Testing and observation should provide you with information on which to plan a therapy regime, not just to complete a set of forms that you can store in the clinic folder.

Table 3-6 Summary of Articulation Tests

Test	*Age Range*	*Interpretation*
Bryngelson-Glaspey	Usually 3-8 yrs.	Age of acquisition–age range is dependent on whose data you accept.
Developmental Articulation	Usually 3-8 yrs.	Age of acquisition–age range is dependent on whose data you accept.
Photo Articulation Test	3-12 yrs. (½ year separations to 5-11; year separations from 6-0 to 11-11)	Expressed as errors for tongue, lip, and vowel sounds plus total. Boys and girls separately.

*Because of the number of articulation tests discussed, a listing of the tests is included in Table 3-6 with age ranges for which they are applicable and norms or interpretation comments.

Table 3-6 Summary of Articulation Tests (continued)

Test	*Age Range*	*Interpretation*
Denver Articulation Screening Exam	2½-6 yrs.	Percentile rankings—for "culturally disadvantaged" children.
Arizona Articulation Proficiency Scale	3-11 yrs.	Percentage score to give "intelligibility" —based on frequency of occurrence of single phonemes.
Goldman-Fristoe	6-16 yrs.	Percentile scores: boys, girls; words, sentences, stimulability.
Fisher-Logemann	–	Features of sounds in error—interpreted also in terms of age of acquisition of sounds.
Templin-Darley Screening-Diagnostic	3-8 yrs. (½ year separations to age 5)	Means and standard deviations. Screening test has cut-off to designate "adequate."
Edinburgh Articulation Test	2½-6 yrs. (¼ yr. separations)	Raw score correct is converted to standard (scale) score.
Iowa Pressure Test	3-8 yrs.	Means and standard deviations (part of Templin-Darley Tests).
Predictive Screening Test of Articulation	First Grade	Probabilities of normal or defective by third grade. No other norms.
McDonald Deep Tests of Articulation	–	No norms—percentage of correct production for individual sounds tested.
McDonald Screening Deep Test	Beginning kindergarten thru ending third grade	Percentage correct response for 9 sounds in 10 contexts with normative sample comparisons.

REFERENCES

Anthony, A., and others, *The Edinburgh Articulation Test.* Edinburgh and London: E & S Livingstone, (1971).

Appleton, P., A study of the production of the /r/ and /s/ phonemes in forty-six phonetic contexts by five-, six-, and seven-year-old males. Unpublished masters thesis, Univeristy of Tennessee, Knoxville, (1969).

Barker, J. O., A numerical measure of articulation. *J. Speech Hearing Dis.* 25, 79-88 (1960).

Barker, J. O., and G. England, A numerical measure of articulation: Further developments. *J. Speech Hearing Dis.* 27, 23-27 (1962).

Bryngelson, B., and E. Glaspey, *Speech Improvement Cards.* Glenview, Ill.: Scott, Foresman, (1951).

Daniloff, R., and K. Moll, Coarticulation of lip rounding. *J. Speech Hearing Res.* 11, 707-721 (1968).

Drumwright, A., *Denver Articulation Screening Exam.* University of Col. Medical Ctr., Denver, (1971).

Faircloth, S. R., and M. A. Faircloth, *Phonetic Science.* Englewood Cliffs, N.J.: Prentice-Hall, Inc., (1973).

Farquhar, M. S., Prognostic value of imitative and auditory discrimination tests. *J. Speech Hearing Dis.*, 26, 342-347 (1961).

Fisher, H. B., and J. A. Logemann, *Fisher-Logemann Test of Articulation Competence.* Boston: Houghton Mifflin, (1971).

French, N. R., C. W. Carter, and W. Koenig, Jr., The words and sounds of telephone conversations. *Bell Syst. Tech. J.* 9, 290-324 (1930).

Fudala, J. B., *The Arizona Articulation Proficiency Scale: Revised.* Western Psychological Services, (1970).

Goldman, R., and M. Fristoe, *Goldman–Fristoe Test of Articulation.* Circle Pines, Minn.: American Guidance Service, Inc., (1969).

Hejna, R., *Developmental Articulation Test.* Madison, Wis.: College Print and Typing Co., (1955).

Hull, F. M., and others, The national speech and hearing survey: Preliminary results. *Asha,* 13, 501-509 (1971).

Irwin, O. C., Infant speech: Consonantal sounds according to place of articulation. *J. Speech Dis.*, 12, 397-401 (1947).

Jordan, E. P., Articulation test measures and listener ratings of articulation defectiveness. *J. Speech Hearing Res.*, 3, 303-319 (1960).

Kent, R., and F. Minifie, Coarticulation in recent speech production models. *J. Phon.*, 5, 115-133 (1977).

Lawshe, C. H., A monograph for estimating the validity of test items. *J. Appl. Psych.*, 26, 846-849 (1942).

Locke, J. L., Ease of Articulation. *J. Speech Hearing Res.*, 15, 194-200 (1972).

McDonald, E., *Articulation Testing and Treatment, A Sensory-Motor Approach.* Pittsburgh: Stanwix House, (1965a).

McDonald, E., *Deep Test of Articulation.* Pittsburgh: Stanwix House, (1965b).

McDonald, E., *Screening Deep Test of Articulation.* Pittsburgh: Stanwix House, (1968).

McDonald, E. T., and J. M. McDonald, *Norms for the Screening Deep Test of Articulation.* ESEA Title III grant–Project number 73024, (1974).

McDonald, E. T., and J. M. McDonald, *Articulation at Pre-Kindergarten, Beginning Kindergarten, End of Kindergarten and Beginning First Grade on the Screening Deep Test of Articulation.* ESEA Title III grant–Project number 73024H, Report No. 2, (1976a).

McDonald, E. T., and J. M. McDonald, *Comparisons of the Longitudinal and Cross-sectional Norms on the Screening Deep Test of Articulation.* ESEA Title III grant–Project number 73924H, Report No. 3, (1976b).

Milisen, R., Method of evaluation and diagnosis of speech disorders. Chap. 8, in *Handbook of Speech Pathology,* ed. L. E. Travis, Englewood Cliffs, N.J.: Prentice-Hall, Inc., (1957).

Miller, G. A. *Language and Communication.* New York: McGraw-Hill, (1951).

Moll, K. L., Speech characteristics of individuals with cleft lip and palate, in *Cleft Palate and Communication,* eds. D. C. Spriestersbach and D. Sherman. New York: Academic Press, Inc., (1968).

Morris, H. L., D. C. Spriestersbach, and F. L. Darley, An articulation test for assessing competency of velopharyngeal closure. *J. Speech Hearing Res.,* 4, 48-55 (1961).

Morrison, C. E., Speech defects in young children. *Psych. Clinic,* 8, 138-142 (1914).

Noll, J. D., Articulation assessment, in "Speech and the Dentofacial Complex: The State of the Art," ed. R. T. Wertz. *ASHA Reports* #5, (1970).

Paynter, E. T., and T. C. Bumpas, Imitative and spontaneous articulatory assessment of three-year-old children. *J. Speech Hearing Dis.* 42, 119-125 (1977).

Pendergast, K. and others, *Photo Articulation Test.,* Danville: Interstate Printers & Publishers, (1969).

Perrin, E. H., The rating of defective speech by trained and untrained observers. *J. Speech Hearing Dis.,* 19, 48-51 (1954).

Peterson, H. A., SALI: Speech and Language Index. Paper presented to the American Speech and Hearing Association, Denver, Colorado, (1968).

Poole, I., Genetic development of articulation of consonant sounds in speech. *Elem. English Rev.,* 11, 159-161 (1934).

Prather, E. M., E. L. Hedrick, and C. A. Kerin, Articulation development in children aged two to four years. *J. Speech Hearing Dis.,* 40, 179-191 (1975).

Sander, E. K., When are speech sounds learned? *J. Speech Hearing Dis.,* 37, 55-63 (1972).

Sanders, L. J., (modification of Hejna's), *Developmental Articulation Test: D.A.T.* in *Procedure Guides for Evaluation of Speech and Language Disorders in Children.* Urbana, Ill.: Stenographic Bureau, (1970).

Siegel, G. M., H. Winitz, and H. Conkey, The influence of testing instruments on articulatory responses of children. *J. Speech Hearing Dis.,* 28, 67-76 (1963).

Singh, S., and D. C. Frank, A distinctive feature analysis of the consonantal substitution pattern. *Lang. Speech,* 15, 209-218 (1972).

Snow, K., and R. Milisen, The influence of oral vs. pictorial presentation upon articulation testing results. *J. Speech Hearing Dis.,* Monograph Supplement, 4, 30-36 (1954).

Templin, M. C., Spontaneous vs. imitated verbalization in testing articulation in preschool children. *J. Speech Dis.,* 12, 293-300 (1947a).

Templin, M. C., A non-diagnostic articulation test. *J. Speech Dis.,* 12, 392-396 (1947b).

Templin, M. C., *Certain Language Skills in Children.* (Institute of Child Welfare Monograph Series, No. 26), Minneapolis: University of Minnesota Press, (1957).

Templin, M. C., The study of articulation and language development during the early school years, in *The Genesis of Language,* eds. F. Smith and G. A. Miller. Cambridge, Mass.: The M.I.T. Press, (1966).

Templin, M. C., and F. L. Darley, *The Templin-Darley Tests of Articulation.* Iowa City: The University of Iowa, (1960, 2nd ed. 1969).

Van Riper, C., and R. Erickson, *Predictive Screening Test of Articulation.* Kalamazoo: Western Michigan University, (1968).

Van Riper, C., and J. Irwin, *Voice and Articulation.* Englewood Cliffs, N.J.: Prentice-Hall, Inc., (1958).

Wellman, B. I., and others, Speech sounds of young children. Iowa City: *University of Iowa Studies in Child Welfare,* Vol. 5, No. 2 (1931).

Winitz, H., *Articulatory Acquisition and Behavior,* Englewood Cliffs, N.J.: Prentice-Hall, Inc., (1969).

Speech-Sound Discrimination

IV

Are we not constantly surrounded by myth and fashion? Even faced with this there is still a need to understand the prestige of the myth and origin of the fashion.

Maurice Merleau-Ponty
Phenomenology of Perception

Speech-sound discrimination testing is still part of the fashion in the assessment of speech and language disorders. Whether the basis of such testing is also some part myth is not yet decided. Speech pathology has traditionally assumed some cause and effect relationship between speech-sound discrimination and speech-sound production. The relationship, however, has more empirical than statistical basis. Experimental findings for such a relationship have not enjoyed a consensus.

In order to better explore the rationale for speech-sound discrimination testing, our discussion will concern itself with speech-sound discrimination and its relationship to speech production. That discussion, in turn, will lead to a comment on distinctive feature descriptions of speech sounds and lastly to a comparison of dichotic as opposed to diotic identification and discrimination.

DISCRIMINATION TESTS

Speech-sound discrimination, the way we will discuss it here, is not concerned with measurement of hearing acuity, but rather with a relative sophistication or knowledge of the phonemic elements of language. In other words, we will assume essentially normal hearing in our subjects and that the sounds to be discriminated are sufficiently loud (conversational level of loudness) to be easily heard and understood. Specifically, what is being tested is the subject's ability to distinguish between closely related speech sounds.

Travis-Rasmus Speech Sound Discrimination Test

The pioneering work on speech-sound discrimination testing was done by Travis and Rasmus in 1931. That study compared every sound of the English language with every other sound and with itself. This pairing resulted in 366 comparisons which was obviously a monumental task requiring at least 30 to 45 minutes for presentation. The 300 consonant and 66 vowel comparisons were constructed with nonsense syllables. There are no norms per se available for this test and it is mentioned here only because of its historical interest.

Templin Speech-Sound Discrimination Test for Six- to Eight-Year-Old Children

With the Travis-Rasmus paradigm Mildred Templin did a series of studies with nonsense syllable CV (consonant-vowel) and VC (vowel-consonant) combinations. She tested (1943) a group of children in second through sixth grades with 200 items similar to the Travis-Rasmus model. Templin's (1957) *Certain Language Skills in Children* utilized 50 pairs of nonsense syllables which best separated between the good and poor discrimination groups of the earlier study. The 50 pairs of nonsense words (for example, azh - azh, ev - ezh, tha - ta) were presented auditorally, and the child's task was to judge if the two nonsense "words" were the same or different.

Results were reported for boys and girls and for upper and lower socioeconomic groups separately, as well as for the total sample of six-, seven-, and eight-year-olds. The data reflected an increase in discrimination scores with age and a greater number of correct responses for the upper socioeconomic group at all ages. Girls consistently performed better than boys at all three age levels, but the difference was statistically significant only at the eight-year age level. The difference between socioeconomic groups was not significant at the six-year level but was significant at the seven- and eight-year levels.

Templin Speech-Sound Discrimination Test for Three- to Five-Year-Old Children

The use of nonsense syllables with a same or different judgment was obviously too difficult a task for three- to five-year-old children. For these younger age subjects, Templin (1957) chose to use familiar words which could be pictured and which differed by only one phoneme. In this test 59 pairs of words (for example, keys - peas, chairs - stairs, mouse - mouth) are pictured, and the child's task is to point to the picture named. In order to insure that discrimination is being tested rather than vocabulary, it is first necessary to insure that the child knows the objects pictured. With a two-choice test, there is also a possibility that the child can identify the correct picture by chance alone. To control for these two variables, three scoring methods are provided (1957, p. 63):

> Score A. The score is the number of items in which *two out of three* responses are correct and in which no attention is given to whether the test words were identified correctly.
> Score B. The score is the number of items in which *two out of two* responses are correct and in which no attention is given to knowledge of the test word.
> Score C. The score is the number of items in which *two out of either two or three* responses are correct and in which both discrimination words have been correctly identified previously.

In other words, if the child correctly identified all 59 pairs of words in a pretest, scoring method C would be used. If the child failed to name all of the stimulus pictures, the discrimination test must be administered with scoring method A or B. If the child was consistent in the words he pointed to on two consecutive trials, use scoring method B. If the child was not consistent, we must go through the 59 pairs a third time and use scoring method A. It is obvious from the above explanation that progressively less chance behavior is involved as we go from method A to method C. It will come as no surprise that method A derives the highest score and method C the lowest score. Templin reported normative data for boys and girls and for upper and lower socio-economic levels separately as well as total combined samples for ages 3, 3½, 4, 4½, and 5 years. The upper and lower socioeconomic groups differed, but only at the 3- and 4½-year levels did this difference reach the 0.05 level of confidence. In terms of scoring methods, use of method C showed the greatest difference between age levels, and the difference was significant except between the 4½- and 5-year levels.

Auditory Discrimination Test

Wepman (1958) constructed a 40-pair auditory discrimination test which required a judgment on the part of the child that the two words spoken by the examiner were the same or different. Thirty of the 40 pairs of simple words (tub - tug, web - wed) are different, and 10 pairs are the same. The test was designed to yield two types of error scores: X scores and Y scores. An X error score is a judgment that the words were the same when actually they were different (an X score of 30 is possible); a Y error score is a judgment that the two words were different when they actually were the same (a Y score of 10 is possible). If the subject makes more than 15 X errors or more then 3 Y errors, the test is considered invalid. There are no norms on the *Auditory Discrimination Test* as such, but Wepman suggested that "inadequate development" was shown by children of

five years with more than six X errors,
six years with more than five X errors,
seven years with more than four X errors,
eight years with more than three X errors.

There are alternate forms of this test. They are considered equivalent and both are scored in the same way.

Boston University Speech Sound Discrimination Test

The Boston Test (Pronovost and Dumbleton 1953; Pronovost 1974) is slightly different in its design although it too utilizes picture identification. The *Boston Test* is similar in design to a test constructed by Mansur (1950) which utilized four pairs of pictures of two objects on each plate in an a-a, b-b, a-b, b-a arrangement. In the 1974 version there are three pairs of pictures on each plate, and the child's task is to identify which *pair* of pictures was named. For example, the pictures might be a cat and a cat, a cat and a bat, and a bat and a bat. If the examiner's stimulus is "cat-cat" the child should point to the first pair of pictures. The complete test has 36 plates, and by going through the series twice, the long form of the test contains 72 identifications. Twenty-six judgments are requested on a short form of the test.

The test directions suggest that the short form be administered first. If the child has fewer than 16 correct responses, she is considered to have difficulty with the task, and the long form is administered. On a sample of 300 kindergarten children the mean score for the short form was 20.5 with a standard deviation of 3.5. The long form mean score was 65.5 with a standard deviation of 6.55 based on a sample of 700 kindergarten and first-grade children. There are no norms published for younger or older children.

Goldman-Fristoe-Woodcock Test of Auditory Discrimination

The Goldman-Fristoe-Woodcock Test of Auditory Discrimination (Goldman and others 1970) is also a picture-identification task, this time from a choice of four pictures. This test is different in more important ways, however.

A training procedure is included in the Goldman-Fristoe-Woodcock instructions to better insure that the subject understands the word-picture associations. Probably the most important difference is that the stimuli for identification are prerecorded, for both quiet and noisy listening conditions. The "noise" subtest has been recorded with a 9dB signal to noise ratio. That is, the background noise (recorded from a busy school cafeteria) averages 9dB less than the intensity of the stimulus words. In order to maintain the uniqueness of this test, that is, the calibrated difference in quiet and noisy listening conditions, it should be administered through earphones.

There are 30 plates in the quiet subtest and 30 plates in the noise subtest. The manual provides percentile rankings and standard scores for interpretation of error scores. Normative comparisons on these bases are provided for subjects from age three years, eight months to seventy plus years. In agreement with the earlier comment about speech-sound discrimination ability increasing with age, the Goldman-Fristoe-Woodcock test data indicate an increase with age to the 20- to 30-year age range and a subsequent decline with advancing age. Because of the picture stimuli grouping on a plate, it is also possible to compare perceived (confused) consonants with the intended consonants. Most of the sound contrasts differ by only one or two distinctive features. As would be expected, error scores for the noise subtest are generally higher than for the quiet subtest.

Summary of Test Types

The variety of speech-sound discrimination tests discussed as examples may be summarized as nonsense syllables or real words; same or different judgments versus identification of pictures; and choices from among two, three, or four foils.

When the subject's task is to respond that the stimuli are the same or are different, we must assume he knows referents for the two words. With young children, that assumption may need to be tested before we can proceed with the discrimination task. With a two-choice task, the subject has an even chance of making the correct choice if he knows neither of the stimuli. With a two-choice picture test, he could be consistently correct if he knew one of the two choices. With three or four choices from which to choose, the chance probabilities are lowered accordingly. Consequently, a multiple choice test will increase the chances that what is being tested is truly speech-sound discrimination ability.

Relationship of Speech-Sound Discrimination to Speech-Sound Production

We have already made the assumption that the purpose for discrimination testing is to determine the subject's ability to distinguish between closely related speech sounds. Historically, there has also been a common assumption that speech-sound discrimination skill is an important variable in prediction of speech-sound production skill. The available data are not as unambiguous as would be desired for support of this empirical assumption.

The literature concerning correlation between speech-sound discrimination and speech-sound production has not shown a consistent relationship. Many variables appear to have been involved in the correlations which have been reported. For example, one consistent finding in the studies reported is that discrimination scores improved with age. In addition, Templin (1957) commented on the "intellectual development" necessary for children to make discrimination judgments concerning nonsense syllables. Sherman and Geith (1967) reported significantly higher articulation-test scores for kindergarten-aged children with good speech sound discrimination scores than for children with poor discrimination scores. Speech-sound stimuli in that study were the 50 pairs of nonsense syllables constructed by Templin (1957) and discussed earlier in this chapter. The investigators also reported a signficant difference in intelligence test score means for the two groups of children. In other words, they showed a significant agreement between speech-sound discrimination and speech-sound production, but the differences in discrimination-skill scores may well have been a function of intelligence. The correlation of speech-sound discrimination and intelligence test scores is apparently greater for nonsense words, because of the abstract character of the stimuli (Templin 1957), and according to Deutsch (1964) is greater for children of a dull normal range ($r = .52$) than those with average intelligence ($r = .30$). Deutsch also reported a greater relationship between speech-sound discrimination and intelligence scores for first-grade children than for fifth-grade children.

One other variable that has differed in the studies concerning the relationship between speech-sound discrimination and speech-sound production is the definition of articulation skills. For some studies (Mase 1946; Farquhar 1961; Aungst and Frick 1964) the poor articulation group had only one or two sounds in error. For others (Kronvall and Diehl 1954; Cohen and Diehl 1963) four or five sounds in error defined the poor-articulation group. The results of these two extremes have generally indicated that at the low-error end of the continuum, correlations have not been found; and at the high-error end, correlations were more apt to be significant. Between these two extremes, (Carrell 1937; Mase 1946; and Prins 1963) the results have been mixed. Weiner (1967) cited a number of variables such as age, intelligence, and definition of defective articulation which may be responsible for the differing results concerning correlations between speech-sound discrimination and articulation abilities in children. Marquardt and Saxman (1972) reported an agreement between speech-sound discrimination and a test of language comprehension in articulatory-deficient kindergarten children. In summary, it is probable that age, intelligence, and language-comprehension skill all have an effect on speech-sound discrimination abilities, and the results are equivocal for a relationship between speech-sound discrimination and speech-sound production.

DISTINCTIVE FEATURES OF SPEECH SOUNDS AS A VARIABLE

One of the possible variables not discussed by Weiner (1967) or in the comments made above is that some part of that equivocation may be because the minimal differences between speech-sound contrasts may not have been equal. That is, contrasts to be discriminated were usually between single phonemes—but not all phonemes are equally likely to be confused. Phonemes are not minimal entities. Each phoneme is a concurrent bundle of acoustic and/or articulatory features. Features can be thought of as partial descriptions. The descriptions of speech sounds include designations of manner (stop versus continuant, friction versus nonfriction, oral versus nasal); place (bilabial, linguadental, alveolar, velar); and voicing (voiced versus unvoiced). To the degree that two speech sounds have many partial descriptions in common, they would more likely be confused; to the degree that they have few features in common, they would less likely be confused. Vowels and consonants have relatively few contrasts in common. All vowels are voiced, oral, and continuant, and are defined by tongue position and lip rounding. In other words, all are produced in the same manner but differ in place of articulation. In contrast, consonants differ by place and manner.

Order of Feature Acquisition—Discrimination

Crocker (1969) has described an order of acquisition of speech sounds as a function of a hierarchy of acoustic features of sounds. The order of acquisition of distinctive features can be thought of as an order of articulatory and/or perceptual difficulty. Menyuk (1968), Singh and Black (1966), and others have suggested an order of acquisition of features which is similar across differing language groups. Menyuk (1972) listed the rank order of features as nasality, voicing, stridency, continuancy, and place. She stated that production distinctions involving oral versus nasal, labial versus nonlabial, voiced versus nonvoiced, fricative versus stop, and lingual versus velar are accomplished by age three (for English, Russian, and Japanese children). She also noted:

> It is possible that these productive distinctions are made before others because they are probably among the easiest distinctions to hear, but more likely it is because these are the perceptual distinctions that are the easiest ones to translate into articulatory gestures. (1972, p. 27)

Singh and Black (1966) studied the discrimination of consonant sounds by speakers of four language groups. Their results indicated that, across groups, the best discrimination scores were obtained by listeners for their own languages. In other words, these two studies suggest that the listener will best discriminate those features of sounds which are in her productive repertoire, or, that there is some productive base for perceptual distinctions. From the data on order of feature acquisition, Singh and Frank (1972) have listed an order of phoneme acquisition and an order of probable errors in production based on the relative stability of the features involved. Koenigsknecht and Lee (1968) reported a similar order of discrimination difficulty for three-year-old children. From least number of errors to greatest number of errors, the listing ranked: oral - nasal, voiced - unvoiced, stop - continuant, and place. This and many other reports have noted that confusions are more likely between phonemes which differ by only one feature, rather than between phonemes which differ by more than one feature.

Perceptual Distance Between Features

Not only is there an order of discrimination difficulty based on number of features contrasted, but there is a difference in ease of discrimination between phonemes which differ by only one feature. Singh (1971) referred to this phenomenon as perceptual distance and tested the degree of perceptual closeness between stimulus and response consonants differing by one feature. For example, the four consonants /t/, /b/, /f/, and /k/ all differ from /p/ by one feature each. The /p/ (pin) is unvoiced, bilabial, plosive; /t/ (tin) is unvoiced, lingua-alveolar, plosive; /b/ (bin) is voiced, bilabial, plosive; /f/ (fin) is unvoiced, continuant, labiodental (in Singh's classification system both bilabial and labiodental are described as "place 1"); and /k/ (kin) is unvoiced, plosive, and velar. In that study the /p/ sound was recorded six times, and each time it was presented to the listeners a different pair of response choices was available. The subjects were asked to choose which of the pair of response choices sounded most like the stimulus. With this paradigm, perceptual-disparity judgments determined a hierarchy of perceptual distance. With the /p/ phoneme, the order of closeness was /b/, /t/, /k/, and then /f/. The assumption, therefore, is that the pair of "pin-bin" would be a more difficult discrimination task than "pin-tin" or "pin-kin."

From the discussion of Singh's data it is apparent that lack of consistent agreement between speech-sound discrimination and speech-sound production may also be a function of the discrimination choices. The response foils may have differed in degree of difficulty. The historically assumed relationship between children's discrimination and production of speech sounds may be more apparent in a discrimination test which utilizes a balance of feature distinctions and is sufficiently difficult to test perceptual confusions. Such a test was constructed by Miller (1972). She assembled a two-choice picture-discrimination test consisting of 80 items which differed by no more than one feature. An inter-item order of predicted difficulty within the test was assumed by ordering the perceptual distance between choices.

The subjects for this study were six- and seven-year-old males with good and poor articulation as defined by *Templin-Darley Screening Test of Articulation* (1969) scores. Subjects were matched between the good and poor articulation groups in terms of age, intelligence, and socioeconomic status. The purposes of the study were to determine if there were significant differences in feature discrimination ability as a function of age and of articulation skill, and if there were significant agreements between production errors and discrimination errors as a function of the features and the perceptual distance between phoneme pairs. There were slight but nonsignificant (at the 0.05 level) differences between groups in favor of age and in favor of articulation level, but the most important data from this study was the agreement between production errors and discrimination errors—in other words, coincidence of error.

To analyze the coincidence or concordance of errors, only the pairs which occurred both on the discrimination test and in the children's articulation test results were compared. In selecting the concordant pairs, each incorrect discrimination made on the discrimination test by a particular subject was checked on his articulation test to determine if he made the same type of error in production. Each production error in turn was tallied, and a check was made to determine if the same error was made in discrimination.

Table 4-1 lists the eleven pairs of phonemes which were in error in both production and discrimination. The numbers shown in the columns indicate the numbers of errors. For example, the /s/ and /θ/ sounds generated the largest number of errors of production (95); 20 children (of 48) failed to discriminate

Table 4-1 Phoneme pairs, number of errors made (by 48 children) in production of either of the pairs on the articulation test, number of errors in discrimination (of a possible 96), number of concordant errors (of a possible 48), and Singh's (1971) measurement of perceptual distance between the paired phonemes

Phoneme Pairs	*Articulation Errors*	*Discrimination Errors*	*Concordant Errors*	*Perceptual Distance*
s = θ	95	20	3	.75
θ = f	77	38	19	.63
θ = t	73	23	2	.75
ð = z	63	25	4	.82
s = ʃ	63	3	1	.63
ð = v	58	43	11	.63
ʃ = tʃ	47	21	1	.55
ð = d	46	28	9	.75
b = v	18	30	9	.75
g = d	15	7	1	.65
t = k	14	22	4	.75

(From Miller 1972)

between this pair, but only three children failed the discrimination *and* substituted one sound for the other in the articulation-production test. A total of 19 children incorrectly produced /θ/ and/or /f/ and also failed to discriminate between the pair, and so on. Overall there was a relatively small portion of concordant errors in relation to either production errors or discrimination errors. The data reported in this study indicated a nonsignificant correlation between speech-sound production and discrimination ability, and a nonsignificant correlation between discrimination errors and perceptual distance.

Phonemic Versus Phonetic Discrimination

Most research concerning auditory discrimination in children has been done with *phonemic* rather than *phonetic* distinctions as the variable. Tests of phoneme discrimination are what we have discussed until now. As a test of phonetic distinction, the sound is systematically varied along an acoustic continuum. For example, with second formant transitions varying along a continuum, changes should be perceived in quantal steps (/b/, /d/, /g/) and not within those phonetic boundaries (categories) at better than a chance level. Phonetic discrimination is defined as categorical discrimination—how well the sounds of the language are categorized. Thibodeau (1977) studied four groups of young children for their phonemic and phonetic discrimination ability. One group was normal; one, articulation disordered; one, language disordered; and the fourth group was language and articulation disordered. The acoustic parameter varied for the phonetic discrimination was voice onset time (VOT) for the discrimination of /p/ and /b/ sounds. Since the distinction between these two plosives is voicing, the greater the delay in onset of voicing the greater should be the probability of identifying the sound as /p/. Thibodeau found no differences among the groups in terms of mean scores. There were differences among subjects within groups, and the variability among subjects was greater within the disordered groups than within the normal group, but there were no statistically significant differences among means. Phonemic discrimination was tested with the Goldman-Fristoe-Woodcock quiet subtest. All four groups were within the normal range as determined by that test, although the disordered groups performed slightly less well than did the normal group.

SPEECH-SOUND DISCRIMINATION AND SPEECH-SOUND PRODUCTION— THE POSSIBILITY OF A CAUSAL RELATIONSHIP

Investigation of the agreement between speech-sound discrimination and speech-sound production has been inconclusive—possibly for a number of reasons. Some of these possible reasons, or variables, have been mentioned. Most of the studies have reported group data; the Miller (1972) study reported individual child data in an attempt to measure the concordance or coincidence of errors of discrimination and production. Several children in that study showed some evidence of concordance between production and discrimination, but that relationship obviously did not hold for the group as a whole.

The implicit assumption made by many speech pathologists (Berry and Eisenson 1956; Cohen and Diehl 1963; Van Riper 1963; Sherman and Geith 1967; West and Ansberry 1968; Powers 1971) that speech-sound-discrimination training aids and therefore should precede speech-sound-production training may not be a valid assumption.

The alternative to that assumption was investigated by Williams and McReynolds (1975) in a training study. The purpose of their study was to determine if a functional relationship existed between discrimination and production. Specifically, the questions they posed were whether speech-sound-discrimination training had an effect on the production of sounds and whether production training effected discrimination of those targeted phonemes.

Four children between the ages of five and seven years served as subjects for the study. Within a reversal design the experimental tasks included production and discrimination training and production and discrimination probes. The order of presentation was counterbalanced so that two of the subjects received production training followed by a discrimination probe in condition 1, and condition 2 consisted of discrimination training followed by a production probe. The other two subjects had conditions 1 and 2 in the reverse order; condition 1 was discrimination training followed by a production probe, and condition 2 consisted of production training followed by a discrimination probe. The children were trained to 90-percent-response criteria for both discrimination and production tasks for the error sounds selected. The results, most simply stated, indicated that production practice aided both production and discrimination, but discrimination practice aided only discrimination.

Lest we appear to advocate what some may perceive as throwing the baby out with the bathwater, the following quote from Williams and McReynolds should be considered:

> Although the results appear to support a unidirectional position, production training should not be considered single modality training. Rather, it incorporates simultaneous production and discrimination training. When a child responds in production, he receives topographical information from his articulators; he also hears the clinician's production if a model is presented, and, in any event, the acoustic product of his own production. Moreover, the clinician's feedback is directed to the accuracy of both the acoustic and articulatory aspects of a child's response. Consequently production training provides an opportunity for reciprocity between the two modalities. Discrimination training, on the other hand, is limited to one modality. (1975, p. 411)

Summary and Recommendations

It has been noted previously that speech-sound-discrimination abilities tend to increase with age and, especially in younger children, tend to increase with intelligence as measured in the studies reported. As such, speech-sound discrimination would appear to be a maturational behavior and in that way related to language skill. The data do not indicate that speech-sound discrimination results yield a good prediction of speech-sound production. For that reason we would not recommend a routine administration of any speech-sound-discrimination test. On the other hand, it does appear logical that following the administration of an articulation test, the subject be tested on his error sounds for his ability to discriminate between the intended sound and the intruded (substituted) sound. The results may not tell you anything important about articulation per se, but may contribute to your understanding of the child's total language skills. Table 4-2 summarizes the speech-sound discrimination tests discussed.

Table 4-2 Summary of speech sound discrimination tests

Name	*Age and Norms*	*Type*
Templin Picture	3-5 years (half year separations) Means and standard deviation	Two choice picture identification. A,B,C, methods of scoring depending on correct naming of pictures and consistency of discrimination choice.
Templin	6-7-8 years, Means and standard deviation	50 nonsense CV and VC pairs for same or different judgment.
Wepman	Adequate-inadequate for ages 5-8 years	Same-different judgment from real words.
Boston University (Pronovost)	Kindergarten and first grade, Means and standard deviation	Picture identification from choice of three word pairs (for example, cat-cat, cat-bat, bat-bat).
Goldman-Fristoe-Woodcock	3½-70 plus years Percentile rank.	Tape recorded stimuli, picture identification; also tape recorded subtest with calibrated noise background for four-choice picture identification.

DIOTIC VERSUS DICHOTIC DISCRIMINATION

The following discussion concerned with dichotic listening is not an expected example of speech-sound-discrimination testing but is appended here to stress the point that speech-sound indentification really does have relevance to speech and language acquisition.

First, two definitions are needed. The word "diotic" is composed of the Greek prefix "di" meaning two, or double, and "otic" referring to ear; hence diotic means both ears or binaural. "Dichotic" is also derived from a Greek prefix which means to separate into two parts. Dichotic discrimination, therefore, refers to the effect of different or competing signals at the two ears. The usual speech-sound-discrimination task is a diotic testing circumstance, with both ears exposed to essentially the same signal. In a dichotic-listening task, the two ears are exposed to competing signals. A speech signal in one ear and noise in the other would not be competing in this sense of the word. That circumstance may yield a signal-to-noise ratio that is sufficiently poor to make listening difficult and therefore may require more attention to determine *what* signal is being transmitted. The purpose of dichotic-listening tasks is usually to determine *which* of two signals—or which ear—has a preferential perception.

Two well-documented assumptions need to be mentioned. It is generally conceded (Kimura 1961; Berlin 1972; Studdert-Kennedy and Shankweiler 1970; Shankweiler 1971) that within the brain the contralateral (opposite side) pathway from ear to processing brain center is more efficient that the ipsilateral (same side) pathway. The right ear is a preferential pathway to the left hemisphere for processing of speech (linguistically relevant) information, and the left ear is a more efficient route for information processed by the right hemisphere. The second assumption is that for most normal adults the auditory processing areas most important for language are located in the left hemisphere of the brain (Penfield and Roberts 1959). The area on the right hemisphere of the brain analogous to the left hemisphere language area appears to be primarily concerned with making judgments of spatial relationship. The acoustic events most important for communication are consonant sounds, and consonants are apparently handled most efficiently in the left hemisphere (in most persons). It is also assumed that dichotic-listening procedures indicate hemispheric dominance for speech and language functions (Wada and Rasmussen 1960; Berlin and Lowe 1972; Berlin 1972; Berlin and others 1972). In addition, laterality of brain function,* as determined by ear-preference scores, may be considered to be established as early as four years of age (Kimura 1963).

*For clarification, the "laterality of brain function" refers to the relative efficiency of linguistic processing. Based on data collected by Shadden (1979) and others, a left-ear advantage may be expected for a reaction time or a nonlinguistic task. Stimuli that require linguistic processing would generate a right-ear advantage in most linguistically facile subjects.

McDuffie (1975) took these facts one step further. She tested ear preferance for dichotic-speech signals with five- and six-year-old children with varying degrees of speech and language skill to determine what effect, if any, language skill may have on their dichotic-listening performance. Speech signals consisted of the stop consonants /p, b, t, d, k, g/ each paired with the vowel /ɑ/. For the dichotic listening task each of the six consonant-vowel (CV) syllables was paired with each of the other syllables, resulting in a total of 15 stimulus pairs. Each of these 15 competing pairs was randomly presented six times, for a total of 90 dichotic items. She also included a diotic-listening task composed of random-order presentations of each of the six CV stimulus syllables 15 times, for a total of 90 diotic stimulus items. The children indicated their responses by pointing to one of six pictures which represented the perceived stimulus. The data obtained from each of the ten subjects consisted of a discrimination score for the diotic-listening task; and a right ear, left ear, and error score for the dichotic-listening task.

The children were selected for the study according to their relative articulation and language skill. The "good language" group were judged to be syntactically more proficient, and all scored above the cut-off on the *Templin-Darley Screening Test of Articulation* (1969); the "poor language" subjects were judged to be syntactically less proficient and were below the cut-off on the screening articulation test.

Her data indicated that there was not a significant difference in diotic scores for the good versus poor speech-language groups, but there was a significant (beyond 0.01 level) difference between the two groups in the dichotic-discrimination task. Both the good- and poor-language-group children showed a significant right-ear advantage; however, the number of preferred ear responses displayed by the good-language-group children was greater in magnitude than for the poor-language-group children. Of the 90 possible responses, the average number of preferred-ear, nonpreferred-ear, and error responses for the good-language group was approximately 52, 22, and 16 as compared to the poor-language group averages of 37, 22, and 31. Note that the average number of nonpreferred ear responses was approximately the same for both groups. The difference between the two groups was reflected in the preferred-ear scores (for 8 of the 10 children the right ear was the preferred ear) and the error scores. The results of this study suggest that the children with the better language skills were better able to resolve the confusion of the competing messages. The two groups of children were not significantly different in their discrimination of diotically presented syllables but did differ significantly in their ability to handle dichotic presentations.

One other addendum may be pertinent to this discussion of what diotic-dichotic discrimination testing may indicate in children. Minor (1977) utilized the same stimulus materials as McDuffie (1975) with two groups of children similarly defined. The added concern in this study was to determine the trainability of the right-ear preference. Following the test procedure to determine baseline performance, the poor articulation group children were trained for a recognition of the right-ear signals. With the dichotic tape, you will recall, there were six sets of 15 pairs of CV syllables comprising the 90 stimulus presentations. The first set of 15 was used as training in which the children (tested individually) were told which syllables would be presented to the right ear by the examiner pointing to the appropriate picture immediately before each of the dichotic presentations. The second randomized set of 15 was used as a test vehicle (responses recorded but no cues given), the third set was used for training, the fourth for testing, and so on through the six sets on the 90-item tape. By the end of the second complete tape (180 items with six training and six test sections), the poor-articulation children, as a group, performed equally as well as the good-articulation children. As an ad hoc comparison, two of the original 12 poor-articulation group children were retested one month later. Both children performed approximately at their pretraining level. In other words, it is relatively easy to train a right-ear response in children of this age, but what apparently was "trained" was attention to an immediate task. The ear preference as a correlate of linguistic (articulatory) facility was not significantly altered.

In terms of the intended purpose of this chapter, speech-sound discrimination as usually tested (the diotic method) does not appear to consistently predict speech or language skill, but a dichotic-discrimination task may. If we go back to the earlier summary discussion, the historically assumed causal relationship between speech-sound discrimination and speech-sound production is not well supported. This lack of clear prediction may be a function of not testing speech-sound discrimination in a sufficiently difficult circumstance. Or, that speech-sound discrimination is not being tested in the most appropriate mode to determine speech-sound confusions.

REFERENCES

Aungst, L. F., and J. V. Frick, Auditory discrimination ability and consistency of articulation of /r/. *J. Speech Hearing Dis.,* 29, 76-85 (1964).

Berlin, C. L., Critical review of the literature on dichotic effects, 1970. In *1971 Review of Scientific Literature on Hearing.* American Academy of Ophthalmology and Otolaryngology, 80-90 (1972).

Berlin, C. L., and S. S. Lowe, Temporal and dichotic factors in central auditory testing. In *Handbook of Clinical Audiology,* ed. Jack Katz. Baltimore: Williams and Wilkins, (1972).

Berlin, C. L., and others. Central auditory deficits after temporal lobectomy. *Arch. of Otolaryng.,* 96, 4-10 (1972).

Berry, M. F., and J. Eisenson, *Speech Disorders: Principles and Practice of Therapy.* Englewood Cliffs, N.J.: Prentice-Hall, Inc., (1956).

Carrell, J., The etiology of sound substitution deficits. *Speech Monographs,* 4, 17-37 (1937).

Cohen, J. H., and C. F. Diehl, Relation of speech sound discrimination ability to articulation-type defects. *J. Speech Hearing Dis.,* 28, 187-190 (1963).

Crocker, J. R., A phonological model of children's articulation competence. *J. Speech Hearing Dis.,* 34, 203-213 (1969).

Deutsch, C. P., Auditory discrimination and learning: Social factors. *Merrill-Palmer Quarterly,* 10, 277-296 (1964).

Dunn, L. M., *The Peabody Picture Vocabulary Test,* Circle Pines, Minn.: American Guidance Service Inc., (1969).

Farquhar, M. J., Prognostic value of imitative and auditory discrimination tests. *J. Speech Hearing Dis.,* 26, 342-347 (1961).

Goldman, R., M. Fristoe, and R. W. Woodcock, *Goldman-Fristoe-Woodcock Test of Auditory Discrimination.* Circle Pines, Minn.; American Guidance Service, Inc., (1970).

Kimura, D., Cerebral dominance and the perception of verbal stimuli, *Can. J. Psych.,* 15, 166-171 (1961).

Kimura, D., Speech lateralization in young children as determined by an auditory test. *J. Comp. Physio. Psych.,* 56, 899-902 (1963).

Koenigsknecht, R., and L. Lee, Distinctive feature analysis of speech sound discrimination in three-year-old children. Paper presented at American Speech and Hearing Association Convention, Denver, Col., (1968).

Kronvall, E. L., and C. F. Diehl, The relationship of auditory discrimination to articulatory defects of children with no known organic impairment. *J. Speech Hearing Dis.,* 19, 335-338 (1954).

Lee, L., *Northwestern Syntax Screening Test.* Evanston: Northwestern University Press, (1971).

McDuffie, A., Dichotic listening task performance of five- and six-year-old males with different levels of language skill. Unpublished Master's thesis, University of Tennessee, Knoxville, (1975).

Mansur, W., The construction of a picture test for speech sound discrimination. Unpublished Master's thesis, Northwestern University, Evanston, (1950).

Marquardt, T. P., and J. H. Saxman, Language comprehension and auditory discrimination in articulation deficient kindergarten children. *J. Speech Hearing Res.,* 15, 382-389 (1972).

Mase, D. J., Etiology of articulatory speech defects. New York: Teachers College, Columbia University Bureau of Publications, *Contributions to Education,* No. 921 (1946).

Menyuk, P., The role of distinctive features in children's acquisition of phonology, *J. Speech Hearing Res.,* 11, 138-146 (1968).

Menyuk, P., *The Development of Speech.* Indianapolis: Bobbs-Merrill, (1972).

Miller, E. A., A comparison of single feature speech sound discrimination test response in six- and seven-year-old males. Unpublished Master's thesis, University of Tennessee, Knoxville, (1972).

Minor, D., A study concerning the training of dichotic right ear discrimination ability of five- and six-year-old males. Unpublished Master's thesis, University of Tennessee, Knoxville, (1977).

Penfield, W., and L. Roberts, *Speech and Brain Mechanisms.* Princeton: Princeton University Press, (1959).

Powers, M. H., Clinical and educational procedures in functional disorders of articulation. In *Handbook of Speech Pathology and Audiology,* ed. L. E. Travis. Englewood Cliffs, N.J.: Prentice-Hall, Inc., (1971).

Prins, D., Relations among specific articulatory deviations and responses to a clinical measure of speech sound discrimination ability. *J. Speech Hearing Dis.,* 28, 382-388 (1963).

Pronovost, W., *Boston University Speech Sound Discrimination Test.* Cedar Falls, Iowa: Go-mo Products, (1974).

Pronovost, W., and C. Dumbleton, A picture-type speech sound discrimination test. *J. Speech Hearing Dis.,* 18, 258-266 (1953).

Shadden, B. B., Ear differences in reaction time as a function of processing task and mode of stimulation. Unpublished Ph.D. dissertation, University of Tennessee, Knoxville, (1979).

Shankweiler, D., An analysis of laterality effects in speech perception, in *The Perception of Language,* eds. D. L. Morton and J. J. Jenkins. Columbus, Ohio: Chas. E. Merrill, (1971).

Sherman, D., and A. Geith, Speech sound discrimination and articulation skill. *J. Speech Hearing Res.,* 10, 277-280 (1967).

Singh, S., Perceptual similarities and minimum phonemic differences. *J. Speech Hearing Dis.,* 14, 113-124 (1971).

Singh, S., and J. Black, Study of 26 intervocalic consonants as spoken by four language groups. *J. Acous. Soc. Amer.,* 39, 372-387 (1966).

Singh, S., and D. C. Frank, A distinctive feature analysis of the consonantal substitution pattern. *Language and Speech,* 15, 209-218 (1972).

Studdert-Kennedy, M., and D. Shankweiler, Hemispheric specialization for speech. *J. Acous. Soc. Amer.,* 48, 579-594 (1970).

Templin, M. C., A study of sound discrimination ability of elementary school pupils. *J. Speech Dis.,* 8, 127-132 (1943).

Templin, M. C., *Certain Language Skills in Children.* Minneapolis: The University of Minnesota Press, (1957).

Templin, M., and F. L. Darley, *The Templin-Darley Tests of Articulation.* Iowa City: The University of Iowa Bureau of Education Research and Service, (1969).

Thibodeau, L. K., Performance on a test of categorical perception of speech in normal and communication-disordered children. Unpublished Master's thesis, University of Texas, Austin, (1977).

Travis, L. E., and B. Rasmus, The speech sound discrimination ability of cases with functional speech disorders. *Q. J. Speech,* 17, 217-226 (1931).

Van Riper, C., *Speech Correction: Principles and Methods.* Englewood Cliffs, N.J.: Prentice-Hall, Inc., (1963).

Wada, J., and T. Rasmussen, Intracarotid injection of sodium amytol for the lateralization of cerebral speech dominance: Experiments and clinical observation. *J. Neurosurg.,* 17, 166-182 (1960).

Weiner, P. S., Auditory discrimination and articulation. *J. Speech Hearing Dis.,* 33, 19-29 (1967).

Wepman, J. M., *Auditory Discrimination Test.* Chicago: Copyright by J.M. Wepman, (1958).

West, R., and M. Ansberry, *The Rehabilitation of Speech.* New York: Harper & Row, (1968).

Williams, G. C., and L. V. McReynolds, The relationship between discrimination and articulation training in children with misarticulations. *J. Speech Hearing Res.,* 18, 401-412 (1975).

Language Testing

V

'Twas brillig, and the slithy toves
Did gyre and gimble in the wabe;
All mimsy were the borogroves,
And the mome raths outgrabe.[1]

Lewis Carroll
Through the Looking Glass

As listeners we make two assumptions when we hear a language: we assume that the noises or sounds we hear are nonrandom, and that they make sense. In essence that suggests that language is a system. It is the systematic nature of language that allows us to recognize that the jabberwocky lines of Lewis Carroll are grammatical. A definition of being grammatical, in this sense, would include the fact that the lines can be translated. Translation does not mean just that the words can be replaced by more conventional words, but that the syntactic structure, the relationship among the words, is evident. For example, *the slithy toves* is obviously the subject of the second half of the conjoined sentence in the first couplet, and *slithy* is a modifier or qualitative description of whatever a *tove* is; and the predicate (did gyre and gimble–) describes the action of these *toves* and the location.

The study of language, or for our purposes the description of language abilities, is divisible into three areas, defined as semantics, grammar, and phonology. *Semantics* is meaning. It would include the meaning of the words

[1] Lewis Carroll, *Alice's Adventures in Wonderland and Through the Looking Glass.* Copyright © 1962 by Macmillan Publishing Co., Inc. Used by permission.

(approximately what we usually define as vocabulary) but more importantly the meaning of the utterance—the communicative intent. If someone asks, "Can you close the door?" the intent is not usually to determine locomotor and coordination skills of the one addressed. The expected response is not an answer to the question because the intention of the speaker was probably to get the listener to perform an action—close the door. Communicative interactions in this way are frequently defined as an area of language study called *pragmatics* (for example, Bates 1976). There are, at this time, no standard measurements of semantics. There are tests for vocabulary, and we will discuss two such measures.

There is an increasing amount of interest in semantics (for example, Brown 1973; Bloom 1974; Schlesinger 1971; Fillmore 1968; and others) on the assumption that the study of semantics holds more answers to language learning than does syntax. Some comparisons are available between normal-language and language-disordered children in terms of language structures and semantic relations in structured (Leonard and others 1978; Bliss and Allen 1977) and in unstructured language samples (Leonard and others 1976; Miller 1978). These comparisons can more appropriately be terms *descriptions* than *tests* in the way we have been using the terms.

The second area in our tripartite description of the language system is *grammar.* Grammar consists of morphology (a morpheme is the minimal meaningful unit) and syntax (word strings). More completely, syntax is the relationship among the words in a sentence. By analogy, sentences have a structure in the same way that a bridge has a structure. Elements of the sentence, or the bridge, must fit together properly to perform the desired function. Tests specific to morphology and to syntax will be discussed. The third area, *phonology,* or the study of the sound system, is partially assessed through tests of articulation production as were discussed in Chapter III. Assessment of the understanding of the rules of phonology, termed "implicit phonology," has been suggested by Whorf (1956) and utilized by Messer (1967), and Whitacre, Luper, Pollio (1970). The studies reported by Messer and by Whitacre and others (1970) demonstrate that adults and children with better articulation and language-performance skills also have a better understanding of which sounds are combinable in English, that is, which combinations of phonemes are permissable as words.

The language-test examples we will review do not clearly separate into the tripartite structure we have outlined because they are based on a variety of theoretical constructs. To some extent they are separable as receptive versus expressive measures; or as tests for specific descriptive purposes as well as those with more general or broad intent. It will become apparent that no single instrument is sufficient to provide an adequate description of a child's language skills.

Judgments on all three levels of language will be necessary for planning a therapeutic regime if we are to place a child in therapy to correct what we perceive to be a problem. One more caution that bears repeating is that the test score, per se, will give less pertinent information for planning than will the pattern of responses displayed by the child. A test score is useful as a comparison with other populations or as a calibration of progress. In contrast, the pattern of responses can yield a description for our understanding and plan of therapy. This description is what Siegel and Broen (1976, p. 118) term assessment:

> Assessment is a broad concept that includes and goes beyond formal tests. Before an adequate assessment program can be devised, the clinician must have a general notion of what is to be subsumed by language . . . successful assessment always requires that the clinician go beyond the bounds of specific procedures to the basic language dimensions themselves. (and) . . . the most reliable and useful language assessment device is a clinician who has a good grasp of language in its various aspects and a willingness to probe and be inventive in creating new approaches to language assessment.

Of necessity, because of the instruments available, the test responses will yield more description of language *forms* than of language *function.* From our understanding of the language system and the communicative interaction requirements, we can arrive at some judgment of function.

LANGUAGE TEST MEASURES

The array of tests included as examples will begin with measures of verbal output. Following descriptions for length and complexity, we will discuss vocabulary testing, tests specific to grammar (morphology and syntax), and then tests of more generalized format.

Mean Length of Response (MLR)

The idea of length of response as a criterion of a child's progress in speech was suggested at least as early as 1925 by Margaret Morse Nice. She divided speech development into four stages identified as

a. single words,
b. early sentences (an average of more than one but less than three words),
c. short sentences of three to four words, and
d. complete sentences of six to eight words.

She assumed that 30 or more sentences would comprise an adequate sample.

McCarthy (1930) elaborated on this general idea, collected 50 responses per child, and developed mean length of response norms for children at six-month age separations from 18 to 54 months. McCarthy (1954) and later Templin (1957) modified the critical descriptions of what would be considered a word and how responses were to be determined. Templin reported norms for children from age three to eight years of age. Both McCarthy (1930, 1954) and Templin (1957) reported alternatives to the Mean Length of Response, such as Mean of the Five Longest Responses, Number of One-Word Responses, Number of Independent Clauses, and the like. Minifie, Darley and Sherman (1963) reported the Mean Length of Response to be the most reliable of the seven language measures they compared.

A considerable amount of time is required to elicit 50 responses from most youngsters,* and for at least this reason the clinical usefulness of such a measure is offset by its awkwardness. To determine if reliable information could be obtained from fewer than 50 responses, Darley and Moll (1960) collected 50 responses from 150 children and calculated the MLR from 5,10,15,20,25,35, and 50 responses. They determined that 25 responses was adequate for most descriptive purposes, although the highest reliability was obtained from the 50 responses.

Even with 50 responses, MLR is only an approximate measurement. The norms published with 50 responses do not discriminate between age levels. For example, with the Templin (1957) norms, the five-year-old mean is 5.7 words with a standard deviation (SD) of 1.5. One SD spread on each side of this mean (4.2 to 7.2) nearly reaches the mean performance of three-year-old children on one side ($\bar{x}$ 4.1, SD 1.3) and eight-year-old children on the other side ($\bar{x}$ 7.6, SD 1.6). Shriner (1969, p. 66), from a comparison of MLR data, concluded that

> . . . response length does not appear to be a significant indicator of expressive language for children who are approximately five years of age and older, because of increased response variability. . . . Whether or not one sampling of 50 responses is representative of a "true" MLR for children below the age of approximately five years has not been determined.

Mean Length of Response is no longer a frequently used measure, but some of the research done with it is important for an overall consideration. For example, in a study by Hahn (1948), one of her peripherally reported findings was that (p. 365) ". . . the child's response and completeness of his sentence structure depend more extensively on the immediate situation and the topic. Skills, as we measure them here, are high when speaking is fun." In other words, it is important to remember that the child is likely to perform better on whatever speaking task we are observing, if we appreciate his performance and show that

*Wintz (1959) suggested tape recording the responses for greater accuracy and also recommended that at least 60 responses be recorded. The first ten responses are discarded on the assumption that early in the interview the child may be reluctant to talk. The next 50 responses are then analysed.

we are interested in what he is saying. Under pleasant circumstances and before an appreciative audience he is more likely to provide a good sample of what he can do.

The elicitor and the setting of the language sample may also be important variables for consideration. Olswang and Carpenter (1978) compared language samples collected by mother and by clinician for young language-impaired children. They reported that the children's samples generated similar lexical, grammatic, and semantic data for the two elicitors (mother versus unfamiliar female clinician) but that mother generated more utterances within the restricted time period. Both of the samples were collected in the clinic. Scott and Taylor (1978), on the other hand, reported that mother (at home) was likely to generate more complex language structures than was a clinician in the clinical setting. This difference in favor of the home and mother was primarily true of "good-language" children with utterance lengths which averaged three or four or more morphemes. They reported (p. 494) that "Clinical sampling underestimates the frequency of complex utterances, questions, modals, and volitional verb forms and predisposes the child to talk about ongoing or imminent activity and the location of things."

Mean Length of Utterance (MLU)

The distinction between *response* and *utterance* is not in the definition of the word meanings, but in the way the terms are used. A Mean Length of Utterance (or MLU) is counted in morphemes rather than in words. In that sense, MLU is probably a more valid index of linguistic maturity. There are no norms, per se, for MLU by age. Roger Brown (1973) has described the stages of language development with MLU ranges to mark off arbitrary I to V stages. In the early stages—from one to four and five morpheme averages—he stresses that children differ in age of acquisition but show considerable consistency in the morphemic elements used with stages of progression.

To illustrate the difference between the measurement of words and morphemes, the phrase "the deer were running" contains four words but seven morphemes. An MLR procedure would tally only words; a count of morphemes (MLU) would credit *deer* as plural, *were* as past tense, and *running* as progressive and give the child appropriate credit for more linguistic talent.

Structural Complexity Score (SCS)

McCarthy (1930) was probably one of the first to suggest an analysis of children's utterances in terms of linguistic complexity of the response. Williams (1937) used measures comparable but not identical to McCarthy and assigned weights of 0 to 4 according to response complexity. Templin (1957) modified the definitions slightly and assigned a weight of 0 to 4 as:

0. incomplete responses, including those which are functionally complete,
1. a simple sentence with or without phrases,
2. a simple sentence with two or more phrases or a compound subject or predicate with a phrase,
3. a compound sentence, and
4. complex and elaborated sentences.

Templin published norms for three- to eight-year-old children (age, 3, 3.5, 4, 4.5, 5, 5.5, 6, 7, 8) and noted that while the performance increased from age three through age eight, the increments from age to age were not as stable as they were for most language tests. The norms are based on 50 responses, each of which is valued on the 0 to 4 scale, making a possible score of 200. Similar to the MLR example of an expected score for a five-year-old child, on the SCS score with Templin's norms (1957, p. 82) the mean for a child of five years is 56.9 with a standard deviation of 21.5. The three-year-old mean is 34.3 (SD 18.3) and for an eight-year-old child the mean is 77.7 (SD 33.8). It can be seen that one standard deviation on each side of the mean SCS given for a five-year-old clearly is within the range of normal performance for both the three-year-old and the eight-year-old children on this measure.

Darley and Moll (1960) also investigated the reliability of the SCS. Their data showed that while 50 responses was a sufficient sample for the MLR in terms of reliability, 50 responses was not sufficient to give an equally reliable measure of structural complexity.

The advantage of the SCS, over what was then available, was the fact that it supplied a qualitative measure of language complexity–not just sentence length but the linguistic complexity of the utterance. In that sense, both the *Developmental Sentence Scoring* and the *Length Complexity Index* to be described next have some beginning in the SCS.

Developmental Sentence Scoring (DSS)

Developmental Sentence Scoring (Lee and Canter 1971, Lee 1974) was developed to analyse the syntactic growth of children who are at the stage where at least 50 percent of their utterances are complete. If less than 50 percent of the utterances are complete, the Developmental Sentence Types (Lee 1966, 1974) is a more appropriate instrument. In *Developmental Sentence Scoring* fifty consecutive complete utterances are selected for analysis. "Complete" in this sense means a subject and predicate relationship are expressed and not necessarily that the sentence is grammatically complete by adult standards. That is, "Me go" or "Daddy broke car" are both considered complete. A modifier plus a noun such as "red car" would not be complete, but an imperative such as "Go" or "Don't" would be complete because in the adult standard an imperative sentence can omit the implied subject.

As in the MLR procedure, the clinician is advised to discard the first few sentences as "warm-up" and then take fifty consecutive responses beyond that point, preferably selecting that portion of the total discourse which represents the child's highest level of language skill. Repeated utterances are scored only once, so if a child says "I know, I know, I know." the second two repetitions are discarded and not scored. Unintelligible responses are also usually omitted from scoring. An exception to this rule is if an unintelligible word occurs in a sentence but its function is obvious. For example, in "he chased the ___ and the lion" the unintelligible word might reasonably be interpreted as a noun, and the sentence could be included. Exact imitations of the clinician's sentences are also omitted from analysis. As utterances are omitted, further consecutive responses are added to obtain the suggested 50.

Segmenting utterances is logical, but somewhat discretionary. As in the MLR, intonational and inflectional cues are useful in separating utterances, as are pauses in the child's ongoing commentary. Conjunctions, such as *and* occurring as the initial word in a sentence are usually excluded. Initial position conjunctions which introduce dependent clauses are included: "When I grow up, I'll be a fireman." or "If I want to, I can have another cookie." The conjunction *and* may be included any number of times in a series listing: "Sam and Andy and Betty and Jack went to the store," but *and* between series of clauses may be omitted at the clinician's discretion. For example, "And I went to the store and I got some candy and then we went to the zoo and I saw a tiger and . . . ." The first *and* would be omitted, the first sentence would be presumed to have ended with ". . . some candy," the next *and* would be omitted, and the second sentence for analysis would begin with "We went. . ." Conjunctions other than *and* are usually maintained, but other "run-on" sentences as the one illustrated may be separated at the clinician's discretion. Sentence tags are given sentence status: "It's a red car, I think."

Scoring for DSS. The 50 sentences selected for scoring are copied onto a record form. Scores are entered on the record form for each of eight grammatical categories: indefinite pronouns or noun modifiers, personal pronouns, main verbs, secondary verbs, negatives, conjunctions, interrogative reversals, and wh- questions. Words in each of these categories are valued from 1 to 8 points. For example, the conjunction *and* is given three points; *but, so, or,* and *if* are given five points credit, *because* is six points, and so forth. Structures are credited only if they meet the adult standard for correct usage. A sentence point is given if the sentence meets all semantic, syntactic, and morphologic requirements of the adult grammar. Total points for the 50 sentences are summed and divided by 50; the resultant mean score constitutes the DSS. The child's performance can be compared with norms provided for children from two years to six years, eleven months at six month levels. Norms are in terms of percentiles with the 90th, 75th, 50th, 25th, and 10th percentiles charted.

The subjects for the normative data were two hundred normally developing white children between 2-0 and 6-11 years, with five boys and twenty girls between 2-0 and 2-11, 3-0 and 3-11, and so on. All but three of the 200 children were from middle-income families, and all were from monolingual homes where standard English was spoken. The normative data indicates a progressive increase of DSS with increasing age and a statistically signifiant ($p = < .01$) separation between all five one-year age groups.

Developmental Sentence Types (DST)

The DST was proposed by Lee in 1966, then discussed in more detail in 1974 as the classification procedures were refined. When discussing the DSS, you will recall that it was suggested for use when at least 50 percent of the child's utterances contained a subject-predicate relationship. If less than 50 percent of the sentences were complete in that respect, the DST was suggested as an alternate tool. The DST was designed as a measure of the "pre-sentence" stage in language development, by which is meant those sentences which have only partial subject-predicate relationships expressed.

The DST chart for "clinical" children's utterances contains three horizontal levels: (1) single words, (2) two-word combinations, and (3) multiword constructions which are not complete sentences. The vertical dimension has five segments: (1) noun phrases, (2) designative phrases, (3) predicative sentences, (4) subject-verb sentences, and (5) fragments. The *fragment* designation includes all utterances which are mere appendages to the three main sentence types: the designative, the predicative, and the subject-verb sentences.

The DST classification is a linguistic description of the child's utterances but does not generate a score, and as such is not a measurement device in the sense that we have been discussing them. The kinds of data which result from a DST analysis are the proportion of the utterances which were single words, the proportion that were two-word combinations, and the proportion which were elaborated as different sentence types. In other words, the chart is an informational source for tracking a child's progress in the acquisition of syntax but does not provide a calibration or a numerical value.

Length-Complexity Index (LCI)

The *Length-Complexity Index,* as the name implies, is based on both length and complexity. It was developed by Shriner and Sherman (1967) and modified and elaborated by Miner (1969). Using language samples from 200 children ranging in age from 2-6 to 12-0 years, Shriner and Sherman obtained an equation for predicting language development as measured by psychological scale values. The initial battery used *Mean Length of Response* (MLR), *Mean of*

Five Longest Responses (M5L), *Number of One-Word Responses* (N1W), *Standard Deviation of Response Length* (SD-RL), *Number of Different Words* (NDW), and *Structural Complexity Score* (SCS). The measures retained as the best predictors included M5L, N1W, NDW, and SCS. MLR was not maintained in the final equation although it correlated more highly with the dependent variable than did any other single predictor variable. According to Shriner and Sherman (1967, p. 46), its lack of significant prediction in the equation may be because it also correlated highly with each of the retained predictor variables.

From this base, Miner assigned score values to phrases or constructions in terms of their length and complexity. He assigned values of 1-7 and 1-6 respectively to noun phrases and verb phrases according to inclusion of modifiers, morphological endings, use of auxiliary words, and verb tenses. Additional points are scored for negatives, for interrogatives, and for conjunctions.

Segmenting of responses follows the same general rules as the MLR and DSS. There are some arbitrary rules for counting words, such as hyphenated words, compound words, and proper nouns being counted as single words, and not counting prepositions when they appear as the last word in a sentence ("I want to"), but generally these rules are similar to those followed in MLR, SCS, and DSS scoring procedures. From the typescript protocol of a child's responses, slash marks are inserted to mark off responses, and the sentence responses are numbered consecutively and transferred to a scoring sheet. Major sentence components (NP_1 and NP_2, VP_1, and VP_2) plus the extra point categories (conjunctions, negatives, and additional points) are then considered for scoring. An example may help to visualize these categories.

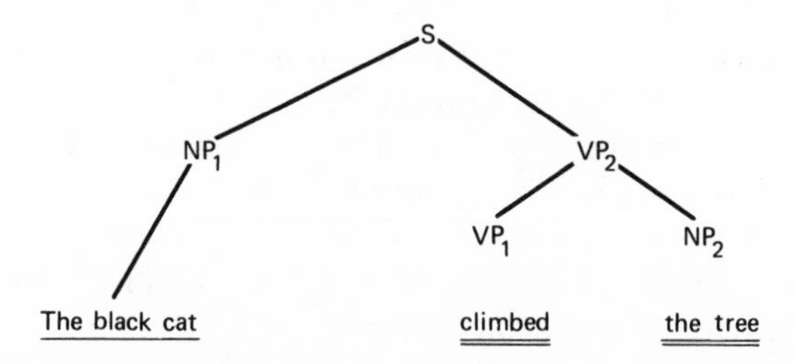

After the sentence has been transferred to the score sheet, the NP_1 (subject of the sentence) is underscored with a single line and the VP_2 (predicate) is underscored with a double line. The number designations illustrate that the marking is from left to right. VP_2 is the predicate which dominates VP_1 and NP_2. In the examples given, NP_1 (the black cat) is an Article plus Modifier plus Noun and is credited with three points; NP_2 is Article plus Noun and is given two points. VP_1 is a past tense verb and is given two points. The total credit for the sentence is then NP = 3 (NP_1 = 3) and VP = 4 (VP_1 = 2 and NP_2 dominated by VP_2 = 2) or 7 points.

Three measures can be computed from these analyses: a noun phrase index (NPI = NP_1 points divided by the total number of NP_1's); a verb phrase index (VPI = VP_1 points divided by the total number of VP_1's) and the length complexity index (LCI = NP_1 points plus VP_2 points plus additional points divided by number of sentences).

In terms of identification of children with delayed language development, the DSS norms provide a numerical comparison which the LCI does not. The LCI on the other hand, like the DST or the DSS, can provide the clinician with a description of the child's language usage which would be essential to therapy planning.

As an example of the types of information generated by a child's language sample, the following examples are inserted from a boy we will identify as L. B. who was five years, six months old at the time of testing. A short sample of 35 utterances were elicited from L. B. in response to pictures and from conversation with the examiner. The Mean Length of Response (MLR) for the 35 responses was 3.87, and the Mean Length of Utterances (MLU) was computed as 4.84. Templin's 1956 norms for a child of 5-0 years show a MLR of 5.7 words with a standard deviation of 1.5. L. B.'s MLR is just outside the −1 SD point by that comparison. The MLU is not normed.

L. B.'s responses were also scored on the LCI and the DSS. For purposes of comparison on those two measures, the 35 responses were reduced to 18 which were grammatically complete. The remainder of L. B.'s responses were functionally complete as answers to questions but were grammatically incomplete and thus eliminated from the analysis. Figure 5-1 lists the 18 scored responses and their value on the LCI. Figure 5-2 identifies the same responses by number and how they were valued according to the DSS. The LCI, as you recall, is not normed so no comparisons can be made against a hypothetical normal group. The DSS computation gave a score of 8.50. Lee's DSS norms show a mean of 9.19 for children of chronological age 5-6. The 25th percentile is 7.89, and the 10th percentile point is 6.72. If we assume the −1 SD point to be approximately the 16th percentile, then the two normed measures of the four utilized are in relative agreement. By most standards of comparison, L. B. would not be considered to have a language problem—or no more than a mild delay in his expressive language or grammatical skills.

VOCABULARY

We earlier defined "semantics" as including word meanings. Vocabulary testing usually includes primarily "referent" (lexical) or pictureable words and must avoid "nonreferent" (nonlexical; function words) items. In practical terms, that means it is more likely to expect a child to recognize a picture of a dog, or a horse, or a chair, or an action such as sitting, eating, and the like, than a picture

Sentence #	NP NP1	NP NP2	VP VP1	VP VP2	Con.	AP Neg.	?
1. He used to be two,	1	1	3	4	1		
now he's one.	1	1	1	2			
2. I don't know.[a]	1	0	2	2		2	
3. Yeah, I got two brothers,	1	3	2	5			
one of them's Eric	3	1	1	2	1		
and one of them's Bobby.	3	1	1	2			
4. Eric's this much (holding up three fingers).	1	2	1	3			
5. Yeah, I'm this many (five fingers).	1	2	1	3			
13. We got animals and tigers and raccoons and I don't know and lions and all the animals.	2	10	1	11	5		
19. I seen this at the store.	1	4	2	6			
25. He's waving 'bye.	1	1	3	4			
26. There's a tweety-bird.	1	2	1	3			
27. Tweety-bird hit on the cat.	1	3	1	4			
28. They like this.[b]	2	1	1	2			
29. He's trying to catch that tweety-bird.	1	2	4	6			
30. It's snowing there.	1	1	3	4			
31. He's trying to catch that tweety-bird again.	1	3	4	7			
32. He's cooking a pie.	1	2	3	5			
33. He's snowing again.	1	1	3	4			
34. He's got his trunk caught and	1	3	4	7	1		
tweety-bird went with her.	1	3	2	5			
35. He's talking.	1	0	3	3			
	28	46	47	93	8	3	--

[a] Do is a modal, part of VP

[b] For example: they (N+P1) like this (V + N)

$$L.C.I. = \frac{NP_1 + VP_2 + AP}{\#\ Sentences} = 7.33$$

Figure 5-1 A short language sample from a five-year-, six-month-old boy scored according to the Length Complexity Index (LCI).*

*We are indebted to Dr. Lynn E. Miner for checking the accuracy of the LCI values.

	Indef Pro	Pers Pro	Main Verb	Secon Verb	Neg	Conj	Inter Rev.	Wh Ques.	Sent Pt.	Total
1	3,3	2,2	2,1	5					a	18
2		1	4		4				1	10
3	3,3,3	1,3,3,	-1,1[b]			3			-	21
4	1,7		1						-	9
5	1,7	1	2						-	11
13	3	3	-[b]		c	3,3,[c] 3,3			-	18
19	1	1	-						-	2
25		2	1						1	4
26			1						1	2
27			1[d]						-	1
28	1	3	1						1	6
29	1	2	1	5					1	10
30	1		1						1	3
31	1	2	1	5					1	10
32		2	1						1	4
33		-[e]	1						-	1
34		2,2,2	7[f],2			3			1	19
35		2	1						1	4
										153

[a] no sentence point because not semantically accurate
[b] got not acceptable for have
[c] and I don't know excluded from scoring
[d] verb hit has no past tense marker
[e] he is wrong pronoun--not credited
[f] has got caught credited as passive

DSS = 8.50

Figure 5-2 The language sample displayed in Figure 5-1 is shown as scored by the Developmental Sentence Scoring (DSS) procedures.* Sentence numbers refer to the listing as on 5-1.

*We are indebted to Professor Emeritus Laura Lee who graciously consented to score this sample for DSS values.

of *the* or a picture of *is.* Vocabulary recognition tests are not "semantic" tests as we have defined them here. That is as good a reason as any why we would not expect to find high correlations between picture vocabulary recognition tests and the other language tests to be discussed.

The Peabody Picture Vocabulary Test (PPVT)

The Peabody Picture Vocabulary Test (Dunn 1965) was designed to provide a standardized estimate of a subject's verbal intelligence. More specifically, this test attempts to determine a subject's ability to recognize common meanings of words through the identification of appropriate pictures. The obtained raw score can be converted to a mental age, intelligence quotient, and percentile equivalent. For our purposes, and in awareness of the fact that intelligence is more than vocabulary recognition, we would suggest that the score be reported as a vocabulary-recognition age score to make it more obvious how the test result should be interpreted.

Test Design. The original 360 PPVT subjects, ranging in age from 2 to 18 years, were asked to respond to more than 2,000 pictures representing what Dunn described as all the pictureable words in a Merriam-Webster New College Dictionary. From those responses, each of the items was placed at an age level where 40 percent to 60 percent of the subjects at an age level correctly identified the picture. From those data, 200 pretest plates were developed with four pictures per plate for a total of 800 pictures. Eight plates were designed for each age level from below 2-6 to above 18-0 years. An additional 16 plates were added for below the 2-6 level to test young retarded subjects, but these plates were not included in the standardization process. The mental age and percentile equivalent norms which are provided below 2-6 are extrapolations derived from extension of curves below that level.

The 200 test plates were developed to provide three forms of the test so that a substitute word could be available on each plate for making up the final two forms (A and B) of the scale. The three forms of the pretest plates were administered to 750 subjects in counterbalanced order. From the responses, the final test plates were drawn or redrawn if decoy substitutions were needed, and new curves of success were drawn to analyse the effectiveness.

The final test battery of 150 plates was developed from these data to provide A and B forms of the test. The plates were arranged in an empirically determined order of difficulty. Selection criteria for the four words to be used on any one plate included the following: (1) all four words were at the same difficulty level; (2) all four words demonstrated the same linear growth curves in terms of percent passing at successive age levels; (3) no sex differences were found to exist; (4) words were singular and collective nouns, some gerunds, a few adjectives and adverbs; and (5) words were omitted which seemed to be culturally, regionally, and racially biased, as were dated words, scientific terms, plurals, double words, and the like.

Standardization was based on 4,012 subjects. All subjects were administered forms A and B of the final battery. The alternate forms were counterbalanced for order of presentation. Dunn listed no other prerequisites for his population except that their intelligence test scores predicted a normal probability curve of I.Q. (Kuhlmann-Finch Intelligence Test) scores.

Administration and Scoring. To administer the PPVT, the examiner provides a stimulus word orally, such as, "show me arrow." The subject then points to, or otherwise indicates, the picture on the plate (of the choice of four pictures) which best illustrates the meaning of the word. The carrier phrase can be varied but should not include articles or other cues which might assist the choice to be made. Therefore, "point to jumping" should be used rather than "point to a girl jumping." The examiner records the subject's response on a score sheet. We suggest that the number of the response be recorded rather than merely a credit or no credit indication for the item. This method does two things. First it does not indicate to the subject any judgment of her response. (If we only mark the score sheet when the subject makes a wrong choice, we may discourage her continuing.) Second, if you mark the number of the response, it may indicate a pattern of guessing which can aid in interpretation of the result. You can keep track of errors by putting a slash mark through the item numbers of error responses.

Each subject is tested from a basal of eight consecutive correct responses to a ceiling of six errors in eight consecutive responses. The manual contains suggested beginning items for ages, but in general it is usual to begin approximately one year below where you expect the subject to score. Remember that there are eight plates per age. If the subject errs within the first eight plates, work backward in order until you have established a basal level. Administration of the test should take from ten to fifteen minutes. The raw score for a subject is the basal score plus the number of items identified correctly up to his ceiling. "Mental age" scores, percentile rankings, and I.Q. scores are provided by locating the raw score and the subject's chronological age in tables provided for the A and B forms of the test. Scoring is accomplished in two or three minutes. According to data quoted in the manual, individual or group administration is equally reliable.

Reports in the PPVT manual are mainly of alternate-form reliability. The reliability coefficients reported (Dunn 1965, p. 30) range from a low of 0.67 to a high of 0.84. Dunn has assumed, with those data, that the two forms yield approximately equivalent results. Nicolosi and Kresheck (1972) disagree. They administered the two forms (A and B) of the PPVT to a group of 36 first-grade children and found differences of 10 months or more in mental age scores for 17 of the 36 subjects. Twenty-seven (75 percent) of the children obtained higher scores on Form A. This difference in result would obviously be important if the two forms of the PPVT were being used in a pre- and post-test measurement. If Form A were utilized as the pretest and Form B as the post-test (or vice versa) for some vocabulary recognition intervention program, differences reflected in a comparison of scores may be attenuated or inflated. It is also important to note that the point of lowest correlation reported by Dunn (0.67) is for the six-year-old population. That is also the age of the Nicolosi and Kresheck population—which means there may be smaller or less consistent differences between the two forms of the PPVT at other age levels.

Validity is more of an arguable point. Weiner and Hoock (1973) point out that since the standardization subjects were all caucasian and all lived in and around Nashville, Tennessee, these vocabulary-recognition norms may not adequately represent "intelligence" for children from different ethnic backgrounds or from different parts of the country.

Validity studies reported in the PPVT manual show significant relationships between PPVT-I.Q. and MA (mental age) scores and results of the Wechsler Intelligence Scale for Children and the Stanford-Binet Intelligence Test. It should also be noted that Wechsler reported a high agreement between Vocabulary subtest scores and the Full Scale Score for both his children's (WISC) and adult's (WAIS) intelligence scales.

In summary, it may be concluded that the PPVT probably provides an adequate measure of vocabulary recognition for most populations. While vocabulary recognition at least relates to intelligence as usually measured, vocabulary is not all of intelligence, and we should be especially cautious in interpreting the PPVT score as "intelligence" with populations other than the ethnic groups on which it was standardized and on populations which may have hearing problems. From the nature of the items included on the PPVT, it is also *not* expected that the PPVT score will correlate with articulation or with tests of grammar (morphology and syntax).

Vocabulary Comprehension Scale (VCS)

The *Vocabulary Comprehension Scale* (Bangs 1975) is a restricted vocabulary test. It assesses the understanding of pronouns and words of position, size, quality, and quantity in children two to six years of age. Objects, rather than pictures, are utilized in the assessment; that is, the child is requested to "push the car around the tree" rather than to identify a picture of "around." Materials utilized include a tea set and two dolls (for pronouns); a "garage set" which includes toys such as ladder, fence, trees, and cars; a sponge and wooden and metal cubes. The child is required to name or point to all the objects used before the scale is administered.

Normative data were collected from 60 children: ten at each six-month age separation from two to six years of age (2-0–2-5, 2-6–2-11, and so on). The children for the standardization population were all from middle-income families of mixed ethnic backgrounds and were enrolled in preschool programs in Houston, Texas. Selection criteria included a judgment by the teacher that the children presented no obvious language deficits, and that each child scored at or above his age level, or no more than six months below his age level, on the *Peabody Picture Vocabulary Test.*

The primary purpose of the *VCS* is not to determine a vocabulary age per se, but to demonstrate to the examiner which specific pronouns and words of position, size, quantity, and quality are understood by the subject. The 61 words on the scale include 17 pronouns (I, my, mine, they, their), 6 quantity words (more, less), 6 words of quality (hard, soft), 6 of size (big, little), and 26 words of position (around, next to, beside). The manual lists each of the stimulus words with the percentage of the standardization sample at each age level which demonstrated understanding of that word. A criterion of 80 percent was selected as "mastery" level.

The test subject's performance is marked on a scoring form (+ for pass, – for fail, and blank for not administered). The scores on this form are then transferred to a summary section which has the stimulus words listed in developmental order. A summary of the results could yield a vocabulary index for classes of words, an overall vocabulary age, and information for planning instructional activities. The manual for the *VCS* does contain suggestions for classroom activities to be utilized in teaching pronouns, positional words, and so on, but it does not contain any statistical data for reliability or validity.

TESTS OF GRAMMAR

In the tripartite description of language which we defined earlier, *grammar* consisted of morphology and syntax. For the tests to be discussed in this section, we will use a rather broad definition of syntax.

Morphology

Morphemes were earlier defined as the smallest units with meaning. Morphology is therefore a study of the rules by which morphological units are applied to indicate the intended meaning function of words. Jean Berko (1958) reasoned that if a child were asked, for example, to give the plural of chair or glass or cat, her correct response of adding a /z/ to chair, /Iz/ to glass, and /s/ to cat could have been because she had been taught those specific responses and may not indicate knowledge of rules to apply in the three instances. These would be examples of known elements in known circumstances. One alternative to this paradigm would be to place unknown items in known circumstances, which is what Berko did. (If we were to place unknown elements in unknown circumstances, the subject would not know what rules to apply, so little knowledge of a rule system would be gained.)

Berko constructed 27 brightly colored picture cards described by elliptical sentences. The sentences contained both real words and nonsense words. For example, the child is shown a picture of a birdlike creature and below it on the same page a picture of two of the creatures. The examiner reports that: "This is a picture of a wug (/wʌg/). Here is another one. Now there are two _______." The child is expected to say "/wʌgz/." On another plate, a man is pictured balancing a plate on his nose, and the captioned stimulus is that "Here is a man who knows how to rick (/rIk/). He is ricking. He did the same thing yesterday. What did he do yesterday? Yesterday he _______." and the child's response should be that the man "/rIkt/."

Sentence-completion tasks, such as these, were generated to test the child's knowledge of plurals, singular and plural possessives, past tense, present progressive, comparative and superlative forms of adjectives (quirky, quirkier, and quirkiest for a dog with spots, more spots, and even more spots), and derived compounds (a wug-house as the name of a house where a wug lives).

Berko administered this test to a control group of 12 college graduates who were native speakers of English. The answers given by 100 percent of the adults were assumed to be the correct responses. In practical terms, that also means that only regular endings would be included on the morphology test.

The *Berko Test of Morphology* was published as the Berry-Talbot Exploratory Test of Grammar (1966). For the Berry-Talbot version, the pictures were redrawn, but no norms were published. The Berko percentages of correct response may be viewed as an approximate order of difficulty among the morphological elements tested, at least for preschool and first-grade children but are not normative.

Validity. Validity for the Berko test paradigm appears to be questionable (or at least equivocal). Templin (1966) followed 435 children from preschool age through the second grade and charted the changes in their morphology scores and related the scores to articulation skill. Sylvester (1969) found significant differences in morphology test scores between good and poor articulation first-grade-age children, but these and other studies using samples of children with normal intelligence apparently cannot be generalized to retarded populations. Newfield and Shlanger (1968) investigated the Berko morphology test responses and a group of meaningful words paralleling Berko's nonsense words with a group of 30 educable mentally retarded children, and a group of 30 normal children. The normal children performed better on both tests of morphology than did the retarded children and, although the retarded children paralleled the normal children's performance in many respects, the retarded children showed a greater inability than the normal children in generalizing rules from familiar to unfamiliar words. Dever (1972) made a stronger statement.

Dever tested the ability of the Berko test paradigm to predict errors made by retarded children while speaking. He found that although many children who scored 100 percent correct on the test also showed 100 percent correct usage in their speech, many other children scored 0 percent correct on the test and 100 percent correct in their speech.

The interpretation of these last two studies would suggest that we may not be able to use the Berko test results as a basis for what is to be taught in a language-intervention program. On the other hand, Ramer and Rees (1973) used a modification of some of the Berko items with black children and reported that the responses were an adequate representation of forms used in black dialect.

Northwestern Syntax Screening Test (NSST)

The *Northwestern Syntax Screening Test* was developed by Lee (1969, 1971) and intended as a screening instrument only. It should not be considered a general language measurement, nor even an "in-depth" evaluation of syntax. Therefore, it should be accompanied by other measures of language development. It was patterned after the Imitation-Comprehension-Production (ICP) paradigm used by Fraser, Bellugi, and Brown (1963). Fraser and others reported an increasing degree of difficulty, in terms of reduced percentage of correct response, when the children were asked to repeat the stimulus sentence (imitation), identify a picture associated with the stimulus sentence (comprehension), or, having been given a choice of descriptions, were asked to produce the sentence (production) which best described the indicated picture.

The NSST contains both receptive and expressive portions with identical syntactic forms on the two parts of the test. The receptive portion contains twenty plates with four pictures per plate, two of which are to be identified on each page. The vocabulary items on each plate are controlled, with minimal distinctions to be made between pictures. For example, plate number one has four pictures with a cat and a chair, and the critical distinction is the preposition denoting the relationship of the two elements. (The cat is in front of, on, under, or behind the chair.) With the plate of four pictures before the child, two of the four pictures are described, but the specific pictures are not identified. For example, the examiner may say that "On one of these pictures the cat is behind the chair, on another, the cat is under the chair. "Show me '*The cat is behind the chair.*'" (Wait for a pointing response.) "Now show me '*The cat is under the chair.*'"

The range of syntactic structures tested includes prepositions; personal pronouns; singular and plural noun-verb agreement; present vs. past tense; singular and plural possessive; present progressive vs. future tense; *who, what, where* contrasts; *this* and *that* designators; active vs. passive constructions; and subject + verb + indirect object + direct object (the mother shows the baby the kitty) vs. subject + verb + direct object + indirect object. The clinician is cautioned not to emphasize the critical distinctions between stimulus items or to give exaggerated intonational patterns for questions. There are demonstration items included to help illustrate for the child what is expected. The NSST is not intended as a measure of speed of comprehension nor as a test of memory, so Lee allows the examiner to repeat the sentence more than once if necessary.

The syntactic structures illustrated on the 20 pages are in an increasing order of difficulty, which means that if the child were to fail on the first ten items, it would be logical to terminate the test. With scattered errors, however, it is probably safest to continue testing. The entire test is not expected to take more than 10 to 15 minutes to administer.

The expressive portion of the test contains the identical structures but with different pictures. There are two pictures on each of the twenty plates for the expressive portion. The two pictures are described, and the child is asked to listen carefully and then to copy the exact words of the examiner. For example, the first plate contains a picture of a baby who is asleep and a picture of a baby who is awake. The clinician would say: "The baby is sleeping. The baby is not sleeping. Now, what's this picture?" (Examiner points to one of the two pictures.) "Now, what's this one?" If the child were to say: "The baby is awake," she would be grammatically and syntactically correct, but her response would not reflect use of the negative. If this type of response were to occur on the first few plates, it might be wise to assume that the child had forgotten the rules of the game. Remind her again that she is to say "exactly what you say," and try the plate a second time. Responses which are different from your stimulus, even though they are grammatically correct, are to be considered errors for the purpose of testing these syntactic constructions.

Scoring. There are two correct identifications of each of the twenty receptive-portion plates, and two correct responses on each of the twenty expressive-portion plates. Each response is credited as correct or incorrect, which yields 40 possible points on each half of the test.

Norms are provided for five age-year levels: 3-0 to 3-11, 4-0 to 4-11, 5-0 to 5-11, 6-0 to 6-11, and 7-0 to 7-11. Tabled norms are expressed in terms of percentile scores (90th, 75th, 50th, 25th, and 10th percentile) and are based on a total of 344 children. Norms are for receptive and expressive scores separately to allow for the expected higher numerical performance on the receptive portion compared to the expressive portion of the test. The means and percentile rankings are also shown on a graph provided in the manual which allows the clinician to find an interpolated point on the graph for evaluation of a child who is at either extreme of the age categories given. For example, if a child were 4-11 or 5-0, it would be more appropriate to compare his score to a point midway between the vertical lines indicating the four-year-old and the five-year-old groups. An additional line on this chart indicates a point two standard deviations below the mean which would be equivalent to the second or third percentile for the age groups.

Validity. Ratusnick and Koenigsknecht (1975, p. 59) reported that the NSST "assessed consistently the syntax and morphology used by children with atypical language development." These authors used tests of internal consistency in evaluating the responses of 20 preschoolers with normal language development, 20 with severe expressive language impairments but normal intelligence, and 20 mentally retarded children. The normal and the language-delayed children did not significantly differ on the receptive portion of the test but did differ on the expressive portion. The retarded children differed from both normal-intelligence groups on both expressive and receptive portions.

Prutting, Gallagher, and Mulac (1975), using a normal-intelligence, language-delayed sample of about the same age, determined that the expressive portion of the NSST did not present an accurate representation of the children's language performance. They indicated that 30 percent of those syntactic structures incorrectly produced on the NSST were correctly produced spontaneously in the language sample gathered for comparison.

Arndt (1977) has criticized the NSST on the basis of what he termed "serious inadequacies" in its meeting psychometric standards. Specifically, the complaints have to do with the small and socially restricted normative population sample, the inability of some items to consistently separate between adequate and inadequate language skill in children, and the relatively small difference in scores expected between ages (especially at the high end of the age range).

Lee (1977) has acknowledged that the norms may be restrictive and that they should not necessarily be used to judge populations which are culturally or ethnically different from the urban, middle-class children primarily used as her normative base. The studies which have been critical of the NSST have generally done so on the basis of false negative findings. That is, children (who may not have been appropriate to the normative base) have been falsely identified as being language-deficient according to the NSST scores. In a rebuttal to Arndt, Lee (1977) reported that she was not aware of any studies in which language-delayed children had been falsely identified as normal.

In light of these critiques, it is probably appropriate to caution the clinician to use the NSST according to its stated purpose, namely as a screening rather than a diagnostic instrument. It would appear to be a more discriminating instrument below the 7-0 to 7-11 age level, and it is probably safe to assume that a false positive finding is less likely than a false negative. That is, it is more likely that a child with normal language skill for his sociocultural environment will be falsely determined to be delayed, than that a child with delayed-language will be judged normal.

Carrow Elicted Language Inventory (CELI)

The CELI (1974) is a sentence repetition task (one phrase plus 51 sentences) with the stimuli ranging in length from two to ten words. Carrow described it as a diagnostic test. It was designed to assess linguistic structures through repetition of sentences rather than eliciting spontaneous language samples from the child for clinician analysis.

Linguistic theories frequently assume that children's imitation of sentence structures is a fair representation of their linguistic skill. Children as young as two years (Slobin and Welsh 1973; Brown and Fraser 1963) and three years (Fraser, Bellugi, and Brown 1963) will frequently imitate nonsense words in a sentence which they do not understand (but which have been assigned a grammatical function by location in the utterance), providing the sequence is short enough. Young children will spontaneously utter sentences which they cannot imitate (Slobin 1968) and will generally repeat sentences from their own production rules rather than from the adult model. Smith (1973) has reported that in repetition tasks with ungrammatical utterances, children frequently err by making the sentences grammatical. Slobin and Welsh (1973, p. 487) also reported that: "Number of words, or number of morphemes is clearly not a relevant measure of how much of a sentence a child can imitate."

From these and other data, there is general agreement in the pscyholinguistic literature that children understand utterances they cannot accurately repeat, and further, that if a child can repeat an utterance, it is probably safe to assume he has those linguistic structures in his repertoire. It is also true, empirically, that some children will repeat (to the limits of their retention span) utterances which they do not understand. Frequently these repetitions will be monotone or mechanical sounding. In that sense, sentence repetition tasks, such as the CELI, will be assumed to have some descriptive value concerning syntactic skill for most children. When there is a qualitative distinction in your mind between the child's spontaneous productions and her repetitions of sentences such as these, it is suggested you treat the CELI data with caution. Norms are provided for children 3-0 to 7-11 years.

Administration and Scoring. None of the 52 stimuli are embedded or coordinated sentences. Of the 51 sentences, 47 are in the active voice, 4 are passive; 37 are affirmative and 14 are negative; 37 are declarative, 12 are interrogative and 2 are imperative. The grammatical categories and features included in the test are articles, adjectives, nouns, noun plurals, pronouns, verbs, negatives, contractions, adverbs, prepositions, demonstratives, and conjunctions. The test is administered by the clinician reading the sentence and asking the child to repeat. Carrow suggested that a high-quality tape recording be made of the child's responses for more accurate scoring. The clinician's task is to mark any errors in production on the score sheet. The average time for administration, transcription, and scoring is approximately 45 minutes. In addition to the total error score, subscores are obtained for each grammatical category and error type (substitution, omission, addition, transposition, or reversal). With few exceptions, only one error per word would be tallied.

Normative comparisons can be made with total error scores, grammatical category scores, and error types on percentile rankings according to age. Carrow attempted to fit the error scores to a year-month score, and those data are reported in an appendix to the manual. It is interesting to note that in the comparison of age-by-month with error scores, errors decrease to about age 6-7 years and then *increase* steadily to the 7-11 limit of the test. According to those data (1974, p. 31) expected number of errors at the 7-11 age are approximately equal to the number expected at 5-3. A curvilinear relationship between age and language score is not to be expected. The percentile rankings do not show these curvilinear relationships, possibly because they are plotted by whole year divisions rather than one month divisions. The clinician should probably pay more attention to the grammatical category descriptions of the child's errors and relatively less attention to the "normative" comparisons, especially for children above the 6-6 year level.

Other Reliability and Validity Data. Carrow reported that the test-retest reliability or stability of the CELI was high. In terms of validity, she assumed that a progression of scores with increasing age demonstrated the validity of the CELI. She also reported a statistically significant agreement between CELI error scores and clinician judgment and a high correlation between CELI error scores and the *Developmental Sentence Scoring* procedure. The reports (1974, p. 9) did not indicate the age or the number of comparison subjects. In summary, the CELI would appear to have good construct validity, at least, and may be a more valid measure of grammatical skill with younger (children 6-6 and younger) than with older children.

Assessment of Children's Language Comprehension (ACLC)

The ACLC (Foster, Giddan, and Stark 1973) is a four-part receptive language test. The four parts include a short vocabulary section and three sections in which the vocabulary pieces are combined into two, three, and four critical-element statements. The vocabulary items (section A) are presented first. There are ten plates with five pictures per plate in this section, for a total of 50 words. Thirty of the pictures identify common nouns; 10 are action verbs; 5 are adjectives; and 5 are prepositions. Sections B, C, and D of the test require two, three, and four critical-element identifications, respectively. In a linguistic description these elements would serve *functions* as agents, actions, objects, relations, and attributes. For example: The boy (agent) is sitting (action) on (relation) the big (attribute) chair (object). The purpose of the ACLC is to assess the child's core vocabulary and his comprehension of the elements in increasing element contexts. The ACLC is described by its authors as "diagnostic" in the sense that it should indicate to the clinician the level of difficulty at which performance breaks down. The authors also state that one consistent problem they have found with language-impaired children is poor auditory memory span (Foster and others 1973, p. 14) and the ACLC is heavily weighted to assess auditory memory span. Specifically, it is "designed for the purpose of identifying individual children who have difficulty processing auditory information" (1973, p. 31).

Administration and Scoring. The ACLC takes approximately 10 minutes to administer. The vocabulary portion (Part A) is administered first, and all 50 items are to be identified as the examiner names them. There is not a specific cut-off for the test, but it would obviously be a futile effort to continue if the child missed a large proportion of the vocabulary items. Part B, two critical elements, has two word combinations such as agent + action (a horse standing, from a choice of a swan flying, a swan standing, a horse standing, and a horse running); attribute + noun (dirty box), or noun + noun (chair and horn). Part C has three elements, for example, attribute + agent + action (happy lady sleeping), or agent + action + object (boy riding the horse); and Part D has four critical elements which allows more complex combinations such as attribute + attribute + agent + action (happy little girl jumping) or agent + action + relation + object (monkey sitting on the fence). In all the pictured stimuli, the vocabulary is balanced. Each of the incorrect choices has only one element in error. For example, with the stimulus *monkey sitting on the fence* the choices in order on the page have a monkey sitting on a chair, a monkey sitting in front of the fence, a monkey sitting on the fence, a monkey standing on the fence, and a boy sitting on the fence. The score sheet allows the examiner to mark if the first, second, third, or fourth element was in error.

Part A has 50 points possible, one for each of the 50 words; Parts B, C, and D have ten points each, one correct answer for each of the ten plates per part. Four scores are determined, one for each of the four parts. Part A score is expressed as a number correct; Parts B, C, and D, as the percent correct for comparison with the norms.

The normative data published with the 1973 (experimental) edition are mean scores only for boys and girls separately at six-month separations from 3-0 to 6-5. There are no percentile rankings or standard deviations provided. A minor revision from the 1972 manual changed some of the pictures which were found to be not effective, and this actuation would be likely to have an effect on the mean scores expected. There are no reliability or validity data published with the 1973 edition, so at least for now, the mean scores provided should be treated as suggestive rather than normative.

Another comparative example may be helpful here. Remember T.G., the little girl (C.A. 4-2) whose articulation test data were used for example in Chapter III? As part of her diagnostic testing, she was also tested in language skills. As reported earlier, she was so difficult to understand that an expressive-language sample was not analyzed. Language comprehension was tested, however. On the Peabody Picture Vocabulary Test she scored beyond her age-level expectations. On the receptive portion of the Northwestern Syntax Screening Test her score was approximately at the 50th percentile for children her age with 22 correct picture identifications of the 40 chances. Errors were in identification of *in-on* prepositions, singular-plural designations, inflected endings, *who-what* and *this-that* designators, present-past tense, and passive constructions. There was also some question of her identification of the correct concept but the wrong picture. For example, for "The deer are running" she correctly pointed to the picture of the two deer; for the singular designation "The deer is running" she pointed to one of the two deer on the same picture. The same type of error occurred in her choices for "The boy sees the cats/the cat." Her understanding of the concept appeared to be correct, but her choice of pictures was in error. As would be expected, more errors occurred on the more complex linguistic structures. As discussed earlier in the section on the NSST, T.G.'s score may be a minimal estimate of her language skill, but there does not appear to be a problem.

As a further example, T.G. was also given the ACLC test. In this receptive measure, she correctly identified 45 of the 50 vocabulary pictures (Part A), erring on three of the five prepositions tested and two present progressive verb forms. It is always at least possible in a picture-identification test that the child's errors may be a function of the pictures, rather than with the concept purportedly represented, but the *in-on* error was in agreement with her NSST responses. In the two-three-four-critical-element sections (B, C, D) she was correct in identification of all the items tested, including those erred on the vocabulary section.

For the record, her hearing was normal according to pure-tone screening responses; oral-peripheral structure and function, pitch, voice quality, and fluency were also judged to be normal.

GENERAL TESTS OF LANGUAGE

Under the rubric of "general" tests will be included a diverse selection. Some, such as the *Michigan Picture Language Inventory* and the *Test for Auditory Comprehension of Language,* cover a similar breadth of language skills, but test the elements differently. The *Illinois Test of Psycholinguistic Abilities* is included because it is unique in the linguistic model after which it was patterned. Also included are a number of scales which are generally developmental, rather than specific to language. To add further to the diversity, the *Basic Concept Inventory* is included.

Michigan Picture Language Inventory (MPLI)

The *Michigan Picture Language Inventory,* constructed by Lerea (1958), was a forerunner in many ways to the kind of language structure tests which became popular in the 1970s. This test evaluates both expression and comprehension of vocabulary and language structure.

The vocabulary section is administered first, and as in the language structure portion, the child is first asked to name the pictured items (primarily nouns). Items named correctly are scored on the expressive scale. For the comprehension test the child is credited with comprehension of an item if she succeeded in the more difficult task of naming it, so only those items are tested on which the child erred in the expressive test. In other words the first time through, the examiner displays the pictures and says: "Let's see how many of these pictures you can name. What's this?" On the receptive portion of the vocabulary section, for those items not named by the child, the examiner says "Let's look at some of these pictures again. This time I'll name the pictures and you point to the ones I name." In scoring this portion, each item has a value of one. Expression and comprehension scores are obtained by totaling the number of correct responses.

The language structure portion of the MPLI is administered in a similar fashion. It consists of 50 cards associated with 60 expression and comprehension responses. There are nine classes of words tested: singular and plural nouns, personal pronouns, possessives, adjectives, demonstratives, articles, adverbs, prepositions, and verbs and auxiliaries. Each section is tested separately. First the examiner describes every card within a section; next the examiner returns to the first card to test the key items for expression; and, third, after completing the cards in that section, the examiner returns to test for comprehension of items not correctly named in the expressive portion. For example, one of the cards concerning personal pronouns has a series of pictures with a boy, a girl, and a rabbit running toward a tree. The examiner describes these pictures in sequence as, "He ran to the tree. She ran to the tree. It ran to the tree." To test expression (the second step in the sequence), the examiner would return to this card, point to the appropriate pictures and say: "In this picture *it* ran to the tree. In this picture *she* ran to the tree, and here _____." The child is expected to reply that "He ran to the tree." If a wrong answer is supplied, or if the child fails to respond when a cue such as "Who ran to the tree?" is given, the examiner returns to that card after other items in that section have been tested and asks the child to "Show me the picture where he ran to the tree."

Scoring. As in the vocabulary section, each correct response receives a score of one. Total expression and comprehension scores are obtained by totaling the scores for the nine subtest sections. Remember that an item credited on expression is also given comprehension credit although it is not tested separately.

Norms. Lerea administered his test to 140 normal children between the ages of three and nine years and reported that both comprehension and expression appeared to be a function of age. Lerea did not separate his population age groups by sex. Wolski (1962) administered Lerea's MPLI to 180 normal children from four to six years of age, 30 boys and 30 girls at each age level. Differences between boys and girls were not significant for the three age groups, and both expression and comprehension showed significant gains with age. It is interesting to note that Wolski's mean scores for vocabulary were higher than those collected by Lerea; the language structure mean scores were lower than Lerea's for the three age groups. Neither Wolski's nor Lerea's criteria for normal included a definition of articulation skill, and this oversight may make both sets of normative comparisons suspect. Wall (1970) investigated the relationship between articulation skill (as defined by the *Templin-Darley Test of Articulation*) and linguistic skills as defined by the MPLI. Her population included 30 five-year-old male children, 10 described as having good articulation, 10 with mildly defective articulation (between 16 and 31 correct responses* to the 50-item screening test), and 10 with severely deficient articulation responses on the screening test. Her data revealed that the MPLI demonstrated a high degree of predictability for the articulation subgroups although not all of the subtests of the MPLI were equally important in separating among the groups of normal and articulation-deficient children.

For comparison, the means and standard deviations reported for five-year-old children by Lerea (boys and girls combined), Wolski (boys and girls separately), and Wall (boys) are shown (Table 5-1) for the MPLI language structure section. What is most apparent from this comparison is that the means do not agree. Lerea's sample population was selected from children "who were normal with regard to language development," but articulation skill was not noted; Wolski's sample was not described in terms of articulation; and Wall's sample was separated in terms of articulation skill. In summary, the MPLI is probably a valid measurement of some aspects of language skill, but we do not have definite norms of performance.

Test for Auditory Comprehension of Language (TACL)

Carrow published her preliminary findings on the *Test for Auditory Comprehension of Language* in 1968, and the fifth revision in 1973. The TACL was designed to serve two functions: measurement of the developmental level of

*This range of scores is approximately 1 to 2 standard deviations below the mean score for children of this age.

Table 5-1 Means and standard deviations for the Language Structure subtests of the Michigan Picture Language Inventory as reported for five-year-old children by Lerea (boys and girls combined), Wolski (boys and girls separately), and Wall (boys)

		Lerea	*Wolski*		*Wall*
		Boys and Girls Combined	Boys	Girls	Normal Articulation Boys
Language Structure Comprehension	mean	80.00	53.83	54.77	66.30
	s.d.	8.39	5.25	5.17	2.16
Language Structure Expression	mean	59.65	43.67	45.90	57.40
	s.d.	11.73	6.50	5.84	4.19

auditory comprehension of language structure; and diagnosis of deficits within specific areas of language comprehension. It was designed to assess oral-language comprehension without requiring language expression. The test consists of 101 plates on which the child is to point to the designated picture—usually from a choice of three. Pictures represent referential categories and contrasts that can be signaled by form classes and function words, morphological constructions, grammatical categories, and syntactic structures. The form classes and function words (mainly the vocabulary section) measured on the TACL are nouns, adjectives, verbs, demonstrative, interrogatives, adverbs, and prepositions. Morphological constructions tested are agentive and comparator suffixes formed by adding "er" and "ist" to free morphs such as nouns, verbs, and adjectives. Grammatical categories evaluated involve contrasts of case, number, gender, tense, status, voice, and mood. Also tested are syntactic structures of predication, modification, and complementation.

Scoring. The entire test should probably not take more than 20 minutes to administer. It is a standardized test in the sense that it is to be given with standardized instructions. Instructions are given in either English or Spanish, and norms are provided for both English-speaking and Spanish-speaking children from ages 3-0 through 6-11. Each of the 101 items is scored as pass or fail. Four subscores are possible: vocabulary (41 points); morphology (9 points); grammar (39 points); and syntax (12 points). Norms are available for comparison only with the total raw score of the TACL. Normative data were collected from 200 middle-class black, Anglo, and Mexican-American children, ages three through six, with 50 children in each age group. Normative comparisons can be made for each six-month age separation either with percentile rankings or with mean and standard deviation data provided in the manual.

Validity. Validity is reported in terms of test results following the developmental trend of children; that is, the scores are expected to increase as the children increase in age. Carrow (1973) also reported studies indicating that the TACL separated normal from language-deficient children (Carrow and Lynch 1973; Weiner 1972) and normal from articulation-deficient children (Marquardt and Saxman 1972).

In a study with 36 normal-intelligence five-year-old children (12 with good articulation, 12 with mildly defective articulation, and 12 defined as having severe articulation deficiencies), Dean (1975) sought to determine which sections of the TACL provided the best prediction of articulation level. A stepwise discriminant function analysis indicated that the most accurate predictor of correct classification was a paired combination of areas testing vocabulary and morphological constructions. This combination was better than the total TACL score as a predictor. All four sections did contribute to the prediction of articulation level in some combination, and the total score separated good and poor articulation groups, but the only section which was a significant predictor by itself was vocabulary. The predictive value of the vocabulary score was not expected, especially since the three groups of children did not differ on their *Peabody Picture Vocabulary Test* scores. The most logical interpretation of this finding is that the vocabulary section of the TACL may test more than what is usually tested on a vocabulary test.

As part of L.B.'s language evaluation (the examples shown as Figures 5-1 and 5-2), the CELI and the TACL were also administered and are included here as Table 5-2 and Figure 5-3 respectively. The CELI performance summary sheet (Table 5-2) credits him with a total error score which is just over the 4th percentile for a child of C.A. 5-6. The numbers of errors are also shown for the Grammar and the Error-type subscores with percentile conversions. Figure 5-3 displays the number of correct responses according to structures tested on the TACL. The total score of 69 (35 Vocabulary + 28 Morphology + 6 Syntax) converts to the 16th percentile according to the TACL Manual. The expected score for the age range of 5-6 to 5-11 is 79.5 with a S.D. of 9.6. In other words, L.B.'s score is about one standard deviation below expected performance on the TACL and approximately two standard deviations below on the CELI. Some relative comparisons can be made within and between categories—for example, his relative mastery of noun class versus verb class morphological endings.

Bankson Language Screening Test (BLST)

Another test with relatively broad coverage is the Bankson Language Screening Test (Bankson 1977). It was designed to be a broad-based screening device. Of the 153 items on the test, 38 have been designated for "quick screen" purposes. Five general areas are assessed within the Bankson test: *semantic knowledge,* which would include vocabulary type items such as nouns and verbs,

Table 5-2 CELI Performance Summary, L.B., C.A. 5-6

	No. Errors	*%ile Rank*		*No. Errors*	*%ile Rank*
Total Raw Score	40	4.2			
Grammar Subscores					
articles	5	7.3	negation	5	3.1
adjective	1	11.5	contraction	0	100.0
noun	0	100.0	adverb	0	100.0
noun plural	2	6.3	preposition	0	100.0
pronoun	7	3.1	demonstrative	0	100.0
verb	18	9.4	conjunction	2	12.5
Error-type Subscores					
substitution	15	14.6	transposition	0	100.0
omission	21	1.0	reversals	1	35.4
addition	3	15.6			

Adapted from Carrow Elicited Language Inventory *by Elizabeth Carrow. Copyright 1974 by Elizabeth Carrow, published by Teaching Resources Corporation, Hingham, Massachusetts. Reproduced by permission.*

prepositions, quantitative opposites (for example, big - small, easy - hard, and so on) and pictured objects to be identified by function. This part comprises nearly half of the entire battery. Part II, or the second area of the test, is designated as testing *morphological rules* and includes pronouns, verb tenses, plurals, and comparatives. *Syntactic rules* (Part III) includes subject-verb agreements, sentence repetition tasks, and the child's judgment as to whether sentences read by the examiner are syntactically correct. Part IV (*visual perception*), with matching, discrimination, association, and sequencing tasks, and Part V (*auditory perception*), with short-term memory and discrimination tasks, complete the battery.

It is a test for expressive language function in the sense that the child's task is to supply the word for the action or picture identified by the examiner or to complete an elliptical sentence begun by the examiner. Bankson also suggests, in the instructional manual, that seven of the eight semantic knowledge tests can be tested receptively. If an item is erred expressively but the correct response is identified receptively, the item is still scored as an error for comparative purposes, but the examiner has some more information on which to plan a remedial program.

Comparisons for the child's test performance are available as means and standard deviations and as percentile rankings for the total raw score according to half-year age separations from 4-1 to 8-0 years. Validity is expressed in terms of correlations with the *Peabody Picture Vocabulary Test* (Dunn 1965), the *Test of Auditory Comprehension of Language* (Carrow 1973), and the *Boehm Test of Basic Concepts* (Boehm 1971). The correlations are moderate at best, ranging from 0.54 to 0.64.

VOCABULARY SUBSCORE Score	41	35
Nouns 1-10, 29, 30	12	11
Adjectives 11-28	18	16
Color 11-13	3	3
Quality 14-20	7	5
Quantity 21-28	8	8
Verbs 31-38	8	6
Adverbs 39-41	3	2
MORPHOLOGY SUBSCORE Score	48	28
Noun, Verb, Adjective, & Derivational Suffix "er" 50-52, 54, 55	5	5
Noun + Derivational Suffix "er" + masculine suffix 53	1	0
Adjective + Derivational Suffix "est" 56	1	1
Noun + Derivational Suffix "ist" 57, 58	2	1
Noun (Number) 66-69	4	2
Pronouns	8	6
Demonstrative (Number) 42,43	2	2
Personal (Number & Gender) 59-63, 65	6	4
Verbs	18	7
Number 70,71	2	1
Tense 64, 72-77	7	3
Voice 78-81	4	2
Status 85-88, 98	5	1
Prepositions 44-49	6	3
Interrogatives 82-84	3	3
SYNTAX SUBSCORE Score	12	6
Simple Imperative Sentence 89, 90	2	1
Noun-Verb (Number Agreement) 91, 92	2	0
Complex Sentence with Independent Clause & Dependent Adjectival Clause 93, 94	2	2
Direct-Indirect Object 95	1	0
Noun Phrase with 2 Adjective Modifiers 96, 97	2	1
Complex Imperative Sentence with Conditional Clause 99	1	1
Complex Imperative Sentence Using neither/nor 100	1	1
Compound Imperative Sentence 101	1	0

Figure 5-3 Analysis Section for TACL for L.B.

(Adapted from ***Test for Auditory Comprehension of Language*** by Elizabeth Carrow. Copyright 1973 by Elizabeth Carrow, published by Teaching Resources Corporation, Hingham, Massachusetts. Reproduced by permission.)

Bankson's interpretation of the test results (1977, p. 4) is that:

> . . . children who score at the 30th percentile and below need further language assessment. Those at the 15th percentile and below are those who are most certain to be enrolled for clinical language instruction, while those from the 16th through 30th percentile are those for whom a classroom enrichment approach, directed to specific linguistic weaknesses, may be appropriate.

Illinois Test of Psycholinguistic Abilities (ITPA)

The *Illinois Test of Psycholinguistic Abilities* was published as an experimental edition in 1961 (McCarthy and Kirk), and in a revised edition in 1968 (Kirk, McCarthy, and Kirk). The ITPA is based on the Osgood (1957) theoretical behavior model. The Osgood two-stage ($S - r_m - s_m - R$) model is similar to language models for aphasia which utilize decoding, association, and encoding components. Aphasia tests such as *The Language Modalities Test of Aphasia* (Wepman and Jones 1961) would fit in this category. Aphasia tests will be discussed in Chapter X.

The ITPA was designed to be a diagnostic tool in the sense that it identifies areas of relative strength and weakness. Paraskevopoulos and Kirk (1969) described the ITPA as a ". . . diagnostic psychoeducational test . . . that assesses specific abilities and achievements of a child in such a way that remediation of defects can logically follow" (p. 4). For this purpose the ITPA subtests represent:

1. Four channels of communication
   a. auditory reception
   b. visual reception
   c. verbal expression
   d. manual (gestural) expression
2. Two levels (hierarchy) of organization
   a. representational
   b. automatic (called automatic-sequential in the 1961 edition)
3. Three psycholinguistic processes
   a. receptive processes
   b. organizing processes (formerly called association)
   c. expressive processes

Norms are provided for children two through ten years of age, and the test takes approximately 30 to 45 minutes to administer. The titles are generally descriptive of the content of those subtests, but the degree to which they are actually separable functions is a theoretical question. Because this test is unique and model-specific, a short description of the subtests will be given.

Test 1. *Auditory Reception.* This is a yes-no type test with simple, short

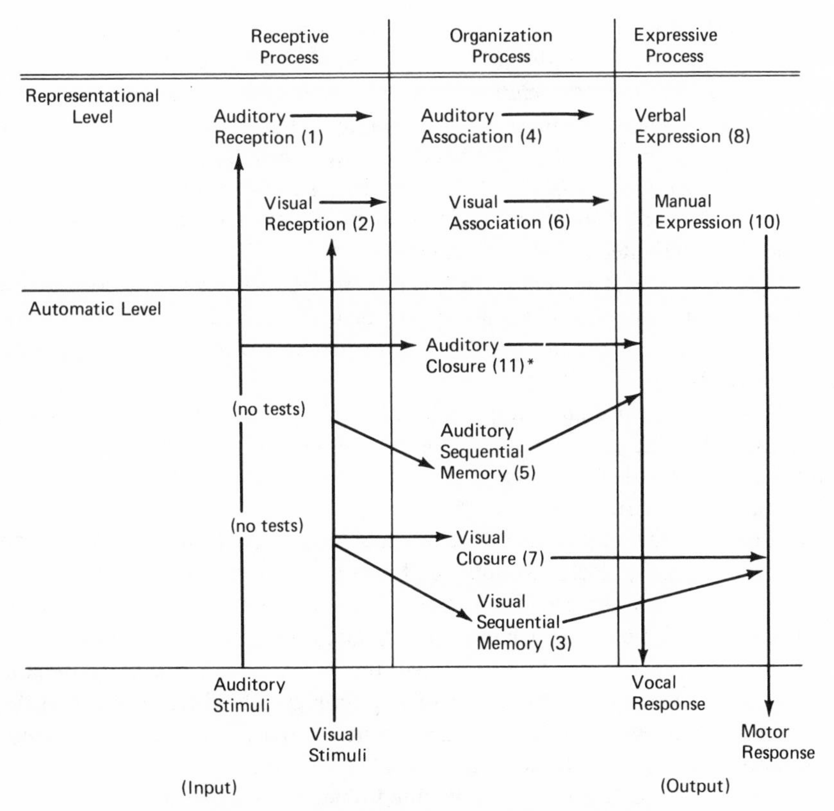

Figure 5-4 Three-dimensional clinical model of the Illinois Test of Psycholinguistic Abilities (ITPA) showing two input and two output channels, two levels and three psycholinguistic processes. The numbers included with the subtest names indicate the order in which the subtests are administered.

(Adapted from Kirk, McCarthy and Kirk, 1968. By permission of The University of Illinois Press)

questions. It is actually a controlled vocabulary test with questions of the type: "Do dogs eat?," "Do airplanes fly?," "Do sidewalks sprinkle?"

Test 2. *Visual Reception.* The child is first presented with a stimulus picture (for about three seconds) and is then asked to find a similar picture from a choice of four pictures. The correct choice is semantically similar but not physically identical. For example a picture of a boy running is to be matched with a choice of four pictures of girls: one reading, one standing, one writing, and one running. In other words, the child must identify the *meaning* of the picture not just the object pictured.

Test 3. *Visual Sequential Memory.* A series of from one to eight chips with geometric designs is illustrated in the test manual. A test pattern is shown to the child, then removed after about five seconds. The child is asked to reproduce the illustrated order of the chips from the available 17 chips.

Test 4. *Auditory Association.* This is an analogy-type test where the child is asked to complete sequences such as "Daddy is big, baby is ____," "Smoke goes up, rain comes ____," and "A bee has a hive, a man has a ____."

Test 5. *Auditory Sequential Memory.* This is a digit-span test which differs from most other digit-span tests (such as in the Binet or Wechsler tests) in that the digits are presented at half-second intervals.

Test 6. *Visual Association.* In this test, the child is asked to associate one centrally located picture with one of four pictures located peripherally on the page. For example, a picture of a bone to be matched with a choice of a pencil, a baby's rattle, a pipe, and a dog.

Test 7. *Visual Closure.* In this subtest the child is shown picture strips with dogs, fish, bottles, and the like. He is first shown the sample picture of the object to be identified and then is asked to find as many of those as he can in the picture strip in 30 seconds.

Test 8. *Verbal Expression.* Five common objects are shown (separately) to the child: nail, ball, block, envelope, and button. His task is to describe the object as completely as he can. The response is credited with points for labels (it is a nail), for descriptions (the nail has a point), and functions (carpenters use it).

Test 9. *Grammatic Closure.* What the ITPA categorizes as grammatic closure, we earlier discussed as a test of morphology. The difference is that the ITPA uses real words with responses which require past tense, plurality, possessive, comparative, and some derived adjective forms.

Test 10. *Manual Expression.* Pictured objects are shown to the child and his task is to *demonstrate* the appropriate actions. For example, objects pictured include a hammer, a telephone, and a toothbrush.

Test 11. *Auditory Closure.* Words with sounds omitted are auditorally presented to the child, and his task is to supply the completed word. For example, a da–y is daddy, and bo–le is bottle.

Test 12. *Sound Blending.* This subtest is approximately the reverse process from what is tested in Auditory Closure. In one of the three sections the child has a plate of pictures as a guide, and the examiner divides the words into two or three parts: d-og, f-oot. The second section divides words with two to seven sounds which the child is to identify without picture cues; and the third section divides nonsense words into three to six sounds for the child's identification.

The subtests all have standardized instructions and specific guidelines for probes to be used in eliciting responses. Some of the subtests have specific basal and ceiling levels depending on the age of the child and the accuracy of his performance.

Scoring the ITPA. Each of the 12 subtests will generate a raw score, and tables in the manual convert these scores to Psycholinguistic Age scores and

Scaled Scores for interpretation. For purposes of scoring, the Auditory Closure and the Sound Blending subtests are considered supplementary tests. A conversion chart also is included in the manual to convert the *total raw score* to a Psycholinguistic Age score. A comparison of the child's Psycholinguistic Age score (PLA) and his chronological age (C.A.) will yield a Psycholinguistic Quotient (PLQ) which the ITPA authors suggest (1968, p. 64) has close correspondence with overall intellectual level. The primary diagnostic purpose of the test, however, is accomplished by use of the Scaled Scores (SSs). These SSs are charted as a profile of abilities for the subtests, and from this profile should come the information as to whether or not the child has important discrepancies in her abilities. The point of reference for comparison is the mean Scaled Score (the sum of the basic Scaled Scores divided by 10). A median rather than a mean SS is used when profile discrepancies are all unidimensional, that is, when discrepancies are either all high or all low. Differences of ± 6 SSs are considered within the average range of variability; ±7, ±8, ±9 are considered borderline discrepancies; and differences of ±10 are considered "substantial" discrepancies. In other words, these would indicate significant strengths or weaknesses in the child's psycholinguistic profile according to the ITPA. The suggested remediation procedure would be to utilize the areas of strength in an attempt to improve areas of weakness.

Reliability and Validity. The ITPA was standardized on approximately 1,000 "average" children from two to ten years of age. That is, the children were selected to be of average intellectual functioning, school achievement, personal-social adjustment, and sensory-motor integrity and were from predominantly English-speaking families (Paraskevopoulos and Kirk 1969). Because the test was designed for the primary purpose of identifying educational deficiencies, the choice of "average" children as a standardizing population seems highly logical. Weiner and Hoock (1973) have expressed some concern about the socioeconomic levels represented and the geographical location of the sample population. They have stated (p. 622): "The published ITPA norms are most adequate for white children who live in small cities in the midwestern U.S." Paraskevopoulos and Kirk (1969) have recognized the geographical restriction and called for the development of normative data for more diverse socioeconomic and geographical groups.

Reliability in terms of both internal consistency of test items and stability (test-retest) is relatively high for all subtests. "Statistical significance" and "psychological significance" are two different constructs, however. The validity of the ITPA would concern its psychological significance. Comparisons have been made primarily with intelligence test results. Data published by Paraskevopoulos and Kirk (1969, p. 162) revealed highly significant ($p = 0.01$) correlations between all 12 subtest scores and chronological age of the subjects in the standardization sample, but these data do not necessarily mean that the subtests or the complete ITPA profile measures *language* skill as it is usually defined in the clinic.

In a review of the ITPA, Carroll (1972) spoke to this point. He felt that the term "psycholinguistic abilities" was a misnomer and suggested instead ". . . (it) might less misleadingly have been named something like the 'Illinois Diagnostic Test of Cognitive Functioning'" (p. 819). Later in the same review he summarized his *cognitive* rather than *linguistic* complaint in these words (p. 821):

> To a degree then, the ITPA may be regarded as just another test of a limited number of intellectual abilities—verbal comprehension and general information, immediate memory span, and perhaps special capacities in the visual and auditory perceptual domains, as well as a special kind of expressive verbal fluency.

In reply to a number of similar reactions, Kirk and Kirk (1978) have responded that the major dissatisfactions expressed have been the result of the misuse of the ITPA rather than uses intended for the test. For example, they stress that the major intent of the instrument was to determine differential abilities and disabilities (intraindividual differences) rather than an overall level of functioning.

> Using the overall score to evaluate a child to compare his with other children rather than to compare his own subtest scores with each other are common misconceptions of the use of the test. (p. 61)

and further (p. 70):

> . . . its main function is to help assess discrepancies in cognitive and perceptual functioning, and in some aspects of language and memory performance.

We have paid considerable attention to the ITPA in terms of detailed description. It has been a frequently used—and frequently abused and misused instrument in the evaluation of language remediation programs. Therefore it seems appropriate to repeat that the ITPA was designed primarily as an educational psychometric tool for assessment of intraindividual variations. The ITPA score does maintain a high correlation with intelligence test results, but language skills, at least in the normal range of intelligence, are usually not in high agreement with intelligence.

Illinois Children's Language Assessment Test (ICLAT)

The *Illinois Children's Language Assessment Test* (Arlt 1977) is another instrument which includes a broad range of skills in its assessment. It is described as a children's version of the Schuell (1957) *Short Examination for Aphasia* and was designed "to evaluate the language performance of children who exhibit auditory dysfunctions, visual disturbances and speech and language dysfunctions" (Arlt 1977, p. 1.). The test sections cover the matching of colors and forms; auditory retention; auditory comprehension; recognition and naming; matching of objects to test pictures; evaluation of oral musculature; evaluation of articulatory and stimulability skills; free association; mean length of response; body concept; and copying of geometric forms. With 18 "variables" the test result presents a profile in six response areas: expressive, receptive, visual, auditory, symbolic, and motor function. Some of the test sections mentioned need further definition. For example, the free association subtest asks the child to place doll house furniture in a doll house. The scoring is presumably by the appropriateness of the association of the furniture. Body concept is assessed by an adaptation of the Goodenough-Harris "Draw-A-Man" test (Harris 1963), and articulation is assessed with a single-phoneme imitative test. The Draw-A-Man score and the articulation test score are recorded separately from the rest of the ICLAT.

Test score norms were developed from a population of 240 normal children: 20 boys and 20 girls at 3-0, 3-6, 4-0, 4-6, 5-0, and 5-6 age levels. The children were all selected from the Champaign-Urbana, Illinois area. The manual includes individual subtest norms and total test score norms for boys and girls separately for the six-month age separations from 3-0 to 6-0. Girls consistently showed higher scores than boys at all age levels. Differences were small between sexes and generally small between age separations. No statistics were included to determine significance of differences, or for determination of the contribution made by the array of subtests.

Little statistical detail was included in the manual to illustrate reliability and validity. Concerning reliability, Arlt retested 56 of the 240 children and reported (p. 3): "The test reliability coefficient ranged from zero to 1.00. Correlation coefficients of 1.00 were yielded by 33 percent of the total population, with 67 percent of this population yielding correlation coefficients ranging from 0.50 to 1.00." Validity is less well documented. The manual reports a "positive correlation" between the ICLAT and PPVT scores, and a "comparison" made with teacher evaluations for 80 subjects of the ICLAT preschool sample, but no data were reported to show the value of the comparisons.

Our concern with statistical evaluation of this test was prompted by the model from which it was drawn, and therefore, the types of items included. There are virtually no test items which would yield a linguistic-form analysis and relatively few which relate to language function. The bulk of the items seem to relate more closely to intellectual functioning and neurological integrity than to language skill. Insofar as that is true, the ICLAT may separate more accurately between normal and abnormal children than between language-skill groups of intellectually normal children. There are no data available on which to make or to refute this speculation.

Sequenced Inventory of Communication Development (SICD)

The SICD (Hedrick, Prather, and Tobin 1975) is a revision of the *Sequenced Inventory of Language Development* (Hedrick and Prather 1970). It was designed to assess children's growth in communication skills from 4 to 48 months of age. Items for the SICD were adapted from the REP Scale (D'asaro and John 1961), the *Denver Development Scale* (Frankenberg and Dodds 1967), the ITPA (Kirk, McCarthy, and Kirk 1968), plus some additional items and procedures generated by the authors. It is a receptive and an expressive instrument and contains subtest areas not frequently included in language tests. Figure 5-5 illustrates the test model.

The receptive scale subtests include: awareness, discrimination, and understanding. Levels within these subsets are concerned with both sounds (localization) and words (discrimination and understanding). Some items are scored

Receptive Scale						
Awareness		Discrimination		Understanding		
Sound	Speech	Sound	Speech	Words+	Words	
						4 months Age levels 48 months

Expressive Scale											
Expressive Behaviors									Expressive Measurements		
Imitating			Initiating			Responding			Verbal Output		Articulation
Motor	Vocal	Verbal	Motor	Vocal	Verbal	Motor	Vocal	Verbal	Quant.	Descrip.	

Figure 5-5 Test model of the Sequenced Inventory of Communication Development

(From Hedrick, Prather, and Tobin, 1975)

by a behavioral response; others are scored from parental report. The test items are sequenced according to the chronological age at which 75 percent of the standardization sample exhibited these behaviors.

Expressive-scale subtests include both expressive behaviors and expressive measurements. Expressive behaviors are categorized as imitating, initiating, and responding. These three are further subdivided as motor response, vocal response, and verbal response. Motor in this sense refers to pointing, gesturing, or manipulating responses; vocal indicates a sound not classifiable linguistically; and verbal refers to words or linguistically classifiable sounds. Initiating behaviors are scored primarily from parental report, since test situations usually generate responding behaviors. The expressive measurements included are verbal output and articulation. The quantitative portion of verbal output is obtained from MLR and SCS scores for 50 responses; the descriptive portion includes information on emergence of parts of speech, such as prepositional phrases, adverbs, third person pronouns, and so on, and is also obtained from the MLR protocol. Articulation is assessed for children two years and older with items selected from the *Photo Articulation Test* (Pendergast and others 1969). Fifty consonant productions in initial and final word positions and 18 vowels are included.

The standardization test sample included 252 children, 21 at each of 12 discrete age levels at four-month intervals from four to 48 months. All children were from the greater Seattle, Washington area; Caucasian; equally divided at each age level into high, middle, and low socioeconomic groups; approximately equally divided between boys and girls; and judged to be normally developing. Testing time was reported to take from 30 minutes for infants to 75 minutes for children 24 months and older.

Scoring of SICD. Two primary age scores are computed: Receptive Communication Age (RCA), and Expressive Communication Age (ECA). Item numbers are listed in chronological order on the score sheet under the appropriate areas. The examiner circles the item numbers crediting receptive and expressive behaviors to a child and computes the percentage of items credited at each age level. Generally, the child is assigned an RCA or an ECA at the older of two consecutive levels on which he has successfully completed more than 75 percent of the items. More detailed descriptions for scoring and interpretation can be found in the manual (1975).

Reliability and Validity. Reliability was reported primarily in terms of stability (test-retest) and is appropriately high. Validity, or the degree to which a test actually samples behaviors it purports to measure, is always a function of the comparator instrument or judgment. The verbal output portion of the SICD was computed with MLR and SCS data. None of these measures purport to test exactly the same attributes, but the correlations ranged from 0.75 to

0.80. The highest correlation was between RCA and ECA (r = 0.95), which would indicate an overall consistency of the test. A possibly more important supporting estimate of validity was high agreement between RCA, ECA, and chronological age in the test subjects. We have already discussed the difficulty in interpreting MLR and SCS data, but those measures would appear to be more corroborative than essential to the SICD profile.

Utah Test of Language Development (UTLD)

The UTLD (Mecham, Jex, and Jones 1967, 1978) is a "direct-test" version of the *Verbal Language Development Scale* (Mecham 1958, 1971) which we discussed in Chapter II. In addition to items abstracted from the test, items for the UTLD were taken from or modeled after items from the *Vineland Social Maturity Scale* (Doll 1946), the *Peabody Picture Vocabulary Test* (Dunn 1965), and geometric designs and digit repetition tasks from an intelligence test (Terman and Merrill 1937). With such a diverse base of test items, it is readily apparent why the UTLD has been described as a general test of language development.

Like the earlier *Verbal Language Development Scale,* items on the UTLD are arranged by age levels. The age span of the test is from 1 to 15 years. The entire test contains 51 items with an unequal number of items per age; the first two age levels (I-II, and II-III) contain 15 test items; the last five years (X-XV) are accomplished with 8 items. Test instructions give one point credit for each item passed. The basal level of performance is eight consecutive correct responses; the ceiling is eight consecutive incorrect or no-credit responses. The basal score plus additional points scored yields a total score. A table in the *Manual of Directions* converts the total raw score to a Language-Age-Equivalent. Language Age divided by chronological age yields a Language Quotient. Reliability and validity data are primarily from comparisons of the UTLD with the *Verbal Language Development Scale* and both statistics are high for these comparisons.

As with the ITPA and the ICLAT, however, some of the types of items included in the UTLD appear to test general developmental skills rather than skills which are language specific. For example, there is little doubt that fine visual-motor coordination is related to neurological maturation and neurological integrity, but if visual or visual-motor skill per se were prerequisite to language, blind people would not talk. Similarly, the applicability of auditory-memory tasks depends on the stimuli used. Digit repetition tasks are frequently included in intelligence testing (for example, the Wechsler intelligence tests for children and adults, or the Stanford-Binet batteries). Miller (1956) stated that approximately seven items can be remembered as separate units; and more than seven discrete pieces presented one at a time would have to be coded in order to be retained. Underwood (1966) described the difference between pure item-retention tasks and coded-retention tasks as first and second-order learning habits. In a first-order learning habit, there are no restrictions placed on the positions that can be occupied by the discrete units; this would be analogous to repetition of a series of digits or unrelated words. A second-order habit (1966, p. 106) "... determines the category or class of response at any moment but doesn't determine the specific instance of the class or category." The later definition is analogous to a language code. If you were asked to go to the store to get: "a pound of butter, a dozen eggs, and a loaf of bread," you would not have to store 12 words (13 morphemes) but only *butter, eggs,* and *bread* in your short-term memory storage. Because you know the linguistic code, or the order of the language elements, you would "fill-in" *pound of, dozen,* and *loaf of* in the appropriate spots. Fillenbaum (1973) has persuasively argued that syntax is not merely a memory skill.

Sylvester (1969) utilized the UTLD in a comparison of language skills in two groups of first-grade children; one group with good articulation (above the *Templin-Darley Screening Test of Articulation* cut-off score) and the other with poor articulation (below the cut-off score for their age). The two groups of 6½-year-old children, matched for age, sex, intelligence, and socioeconomic status did differ in their UTLD scores. The only modification in the administration of the UTLD was that testing was begun at the four-year level (item 20) for all children and continued through the limit of the test (item 51 is placed at the 16-year level). The good-articulation children's mean score was at approximately the 9-5 age level (according to the UTLD conversion chart) and the poor articulators' mean was 7-3. Those conversion-chart age scales represent a mean difference of approximately six correct items. This difference was significant at the 0.05 level of confidence.

More important for the purposes of this comparison, the test items were not equally efficient at discriminating between the two groups. The items were operationally defined as consisting of six types of tasks: perceptual-motor, receptive vocabulary, academics, retention span, coded retention span, and coded language.

Perceptual-motor tasks, operationally defined as copying geometric figures and drawing pictures (four items on the test), were those tasks which required coordination of the child's visual perceptions and her motor skill. The two groups did equally well with these items.

Receptive vocabulary (five items) were vocabulary-recognition tasks where the child was asked to point to common pictures named by the examiner. On three of the five items in this group, the good-articulation children did slightly better than the poor-articulation children—an average of two more words correctly identified.

Academic tasks were operationally defined as those nine items which required the child to name colors, to count, and to read and write numbers and simple words. The two groups were very similar on these tasks, with an average difference of less than one point in favor of the good-articulation children.

Retention span included four items which required digit and unrelated word-series repetition. On the two longer items there was a separation between the two groups in favor of the good-articulation children.

Coded retention span (7 items) was the operational rubric given to what was previously described as those tasks which required second-order habit learning. These primarily included repetition of sentences. The separation for the two groups was slightly greater and more consistent than for simple retention-span (first-order habit) tasks, and was again in favor of the good-articulation children.

Coded language. For want of a better term, two items which required the child to tell a familiar story (for example, The Three Bears, Goldilocks) and to rhyme words were designated as "coded language." It is assumed that these two tasks required more language abstraction. The two groups separated by a difference of four points and three points respectively.

Although Sylvester did not statistically treat these subgroup data, the trend of separation indicates that the most consistent differences are on those items which require language abstraction as opposed to academic, perceptual-motor, and vocabulary skills.

Houston Test for Language Development

The *Houston* test has two parts. Part I (Crabtree 1958) was designed as a direct test of children from 6 to 36 months of age. Part II (Crabtree 1963) extended the scale from three years through six years of age. Part I test items are further divided by age categories and might be described at the youngest age levels as "awareness" or "readiness" demonstrations such as "returns a smile" and "attends to voice." Higher level functions may be termed interactive, such as "gives four lines from memory," or "gives full name." An articulation (single-phoneme, word-repetition) test and a vocabulary test (the child is asked to name 20 pictures of common objects) are also included in Part I.

Scoring on the *Houston* is limited to the responses that are observed by the examiner. Test items are arranged at age levels: 6, 12, 18, 24, 30, and 36 months. Each item in an age group is given the same weight. Three of the six age levels each have nine items; therefore, each item is weighted as 0.66 in terms of language months. If all nine items were credited (9 × 0.66), the child would be given six points (six-month credit). The other three age levels have six items each; therefore, each item is given one-month credit. The total score represents all points credited at all age levels and is equivalent to a "Language Age" score.

Test-retest reliability (with a "portion of the sample") in terms of inter-examiner reliability was reported (Crabtree 1958, p. 1) as a Pearson r = 0.84. Validity was apparently assumed by a growth in the percentage of children passing the total number of items with increasing age, from an average of 19 percent of the six-month-old children passing all items to 89 percent at the thirty-six-month level.

Part II of the *Houston* is more varied in the types of items included. *Vocabulary* items requiring a naming or descriptive performance; *body parts* and *gesture* items; *communicative behavior* which allows a description of language function as well as structural complexity (based on a suggested total of 10 responses); *counting* or number concept; *geometric drawing* or copying of geometric designs; and repetition of *melody patterns* are all included.

Each part of the test may be used separately. If the two parts are used together, either part may be used at the three-year level. There are no reliability or external validity measurements reported. Validity was again assumed by an increase in percentage of the initial sample of children passing the test items at progressive chronological ages. The trial studies for the *Houston, Part II* utilized 211 white children from the greater metropolitan area of Houston, Texas.

The four age ranges sampled with Part II (3, 4, 5, 6 years) have a range of 13 to 17 total possible points per age. The score for each age range is obtained by counting the failures in each age column and subtracting from the possible score for that age. The basal age is the lowest age at which all items were passed; the upper age is the highest age at which any items were passed. The Language Age is obtained from the sum of the scores. The test pattern of responses should be completed by listing items under age of highest success in order to show areas of weakness and strength. It is also expected that the clinician will describe any unusual or significant behaviors under a "Comments" section. The age levels resulting from this test profile are expected to be broad rather than specific. Deviations of one year from chronological age are considered within normal range; deviations of two years from chronological age are considered significant (Crabtree 1963, p. 12).

Preschool Language Scale (PLS)

The *Preschool Language Scale* (Zimmerman and others 1979) is based on maturational and developmental aspects of language competence. The PLS was designed to evaluate ". . . maturational lags, strengths, and deficiencies as they pertain to developmental progress." Changes from 1969 to the 1979 version include a simplified scoring system and some repositioning of items to reflect children's developmental progression. The PLS samples behaviors from age 1½ to seven years at half-year levels to age five and one-year separations beyond that point (1½, 2, 2½, 3, 3½, 4, 4½, 5, 6, 7). The 1979 manual includes data on reliability, validity, and item analysis.

The PLS includes two discrete scales: Auditory Comprehension and Verbal Ability. There are four items for each age level on each scale. As with most age-scale measurement devices, it is suggested that the examiner begin approximately one year below where the child is expected to perform. If the child misses an item at that age level, the administration has begun at too high a level. The examiner must go back in the scale until the child has passed all four items at one age level. That will be the child's basal age. Continue testing forward from that point. Each of the scales is discontinued at the point where the child misses all four items on an age level. To score the PLS, the basal age for each section is entered on the score sheet followed by the number of items passed at each succeeding level. The four items on each level from 1½ through five years are to be multiplied by a credit of 1½ months; the four items at age levels six and seven are multiplied by 3-month credit. The resulting sum is added to the basal age for each section. These age totals for both the Auditory Comprehension (AC) and the Verbal Ability (VA) scales represent the equivalent language ages for each. A quotient can be derived from either age score by dividing AC or VA by chronological age. The average of AC plus VA yields an overall language age score; this result divided by chronological age is a language age quotient.

Auditory Comprehension subtests cover a wide range of tasks which utilize (primarily) auditory input to measure understanding of words. For example, pictured objects must be identified by use ("Show me what we use to comb our hair"; "What do we use to sweep the floor?"), pictures for recognition of time ("Which one tells you it is nighttime?"); grouping of colors, shapes, and sizes; tapping a rhythm in imitation; and counting and simple arithmetic skills (defined as concepts of quantity and operational correspondence). In other words, the emphasis is on comprehension of concepts and appropriate performance.

The *Verbal Ability* scale also has a broad definition. Examples of items include digit and sentence repetition; use of plurals, prepositions, tenses; understanding of opposites (called relational thinking: "Brother is a boy, sister is a ____"; "The sun shines during the day, the moon at ____"); knowledge of the names of coins; and an articulation subtest with imitation of single-phoneme consonants in simple words, and correct repetition of short sentences.

The examples mentioned are not inclusive but are meant to be illustrative of the breadth of items included in the PLS definitions of comprehension and verbal ability. As with most measurement scales, more information of a diagnostic nature will be gathered from a description of the behavior than from a simple reporting of age level of performance.

McCarthy Scales of Children's Abilities (MSCA)

The MSCA (McCarthy 1972) is also more generally developmental than specific to language in children. It is included here, in spite of some redundancy with tests already discussed, because it has some uniqueness and precision in description. The MSCA contains six scales: Verbal, Perceptual-Performance, Quantitative, General Cognitive, Memory, and Motor. The tests involve language, numerical concepts, motor coordination, and other skills to reflect cognitive and motor ability. The six scales are composed of 18 separate tests but with considerable overlap on some subtests for the areas to which they contribute. The five verbal tests, seven perceptual-performance, and three quantitative scales do not overlap in abilities tested, and these three areas make up the General Cognitive Tests. Memory (four tests) and motor (five tests) are overlapping with other scales. All of the memory tests are included on the General Cognitive scale. Three of the five motor tests are independent of General Cognitive (do not overlap with other tests) and two overlap with perceptual-performance items.

Test scores are assigned weighted values. Weighted raw scores are derived by multiplying the child's raw score by the tests assigned weight. A composite raw score for a scale equals the sum of the child's weighted raw scres on all of the tests comprising that scale. Scaled scores are provided according to chronological age of the child tested, as well as percentile ranking for General Cognitive Index and the MSCA indices. These scaled scores therefore provide a profile of the child's abilities on the six scales included. Comparisons would then be possible with other children of the same age, as well as within the child for relative ability within the areas tested.

The test was designed for children ranging from 2½ to 8½ years of age. There are standardized instructions for administering the scale and test-retest reliability data reported are high. Validity was not reported in the manual. In terms of comparison with other general developmental scales, the MSCA would at least appear to have high face validity.

COGNITIVE/SEMANTIC OR CONCEPT TESTS

Language Assessment Tasks (LAT)

Earlier in this chapter we commented that there were no available standard measures of semantics. To the degree that semantics is represented by language-function and language-content judgments, the Language Assessment Tasks (Kellman, Flood, and Yoder 1977) is an exception to that statement, although the LAT is not standardized. The LAT is unique in one other respect—it was designed primarily to provide a description of language function for the child from nine to fourteen years of age. The bulk of the language descriptions available are for younger children. We know of no other measure which provides a similar breadth of language description for this age range.

The LAT is divided into sections to provide measures of comprehension, production, language content, and a judgment of communicative function. Subtest results are plotted as a function of age scores to develop a profile of abilities for comparison with Piaget's cognitive levels.* According to Kellman, Flood, and Yoder (1977, p. xi):

*The Piaget divisions or stages of cognitive development used by the LAT include: Sensorimotor period, birth to 2 yrs.; Preoperational period, 2-7 yrs.; Early Preoperational period, 2-4 yrs.; Late Preoperational period, 4-7 yrs.; Concrete Operations period, 7 to 11 or 12 yrs.; Formal Operations, 12 yrs.-adulthood.

> If the level of language development is approximately equal to the cognitive level, it suggests that there is not a language delay, even though the language development level may be below chronological age. If the language development level is below the cognitive level, it suggests there is a delay in language development. The degree of language delay is determined by the gap between the cognitive level and the language development level.

Subtests include functional tests of syntax and semantics for both comprehension and production areas. For example, in the comprehension of syntax section the child is asked to demonstrate, by her actions, an understanding of *before* and *after* ("Clap your hands after you sit down"). Comprehension of semantics includes the child's expressed understanding of the meaning of idioms ("What does 'feeling blue' mean?") and her explanation of riddles. Also included in the comprehension section is a subtest entitled "Para-linguistics" (identified as intonation, stress, and junction) in which, for example, the child must distinguish between *green house* and *greenhouse.*

In the production section, syntax judgments are made from elicited oral (and written) language samples. Semantics includes vocabulary, word definitions, and the use of *wh* questions in eliciting information. Language content items incorporate both labels and concepts expressed in subtest areas identified as *temporal* (for example, order and duration), spatial (for example, right-left), classification (for example, "A radish, lemon, beets, carrots. Which one doesn't belong? Why?" and "What do they have in common"), and causality ("What causes day and night?"). The communicative function area is a judgment of how well the child uses language to gain or give information, to express beliefs or feelings, to entertain, to interact—in short, how well can she use language to solve problems?

Year and month norms are provided for some of the subtest areas; other subtest results are interpreted by the Piaget cognitive divisions with an age spread of two to three years. In the LAT authors' introductory statement they agree that "... The LAT is not a polished tool. It is still rough, and may continue to be so for a long time. . . ." They have, however, collected a number of language tasks from available literature and created a few more for the purpose of the test profile—some of these have been normed, and some have not. The validity of the composite has not been determined, but there does appear to be considerable language-function description available from this protocol for the age range at which it is directed—and we know of no other test like it.

Basic Concept Inventory (BCI)

The *Basic Concept Inventory* (Engelmann 1967) is identified as a criterion-referenced measure rather than a norm-referenced achievement test. It was designed for children who are preparing for beginning academic tasks. A norm-referenced measure is used to make comparisons among a group of children or to make predictions about a population. A criterion-referenced measure (Glaser

1963), on the other hand, should indicate *why* a child failed a particular task which is expected of him and is required in order to move to the next academic level.

A quote from the *Teacher's Manual* (1967, p. 6) may serve to illustrate this point:

> The Basic Concept Inventory, like any other criterion-referenced measure, is based on the assumption that a child has received certain instruction, and that the instruction may or may not have been adequate in teaching the skills that are prerequisite to certain types of academic performance. The culturally disadvantaged child has received instruction in the use of language and in perceiving conceptual dimensions of his world, just as the middle-class youngster has. However, the instruction given the disadvantaged child may have failed to teach him some of the specific skills that were taught to the middle-class child. Similarly, the instruction of the middle-class child may also have failed on the basis of certain criteria. The Inventory is designed to identify the effectiveness of children's previous instruction in certain skill areas. After the children have received direct instruction in the basic skill areas, the Inventory can be administered again to evaluate certain components of the direct instruction.[2]

To at least some degree, the *Basic Concept Inventory* is therefore a test of language function. What is being assessed is whether the child can understand and profit from classroom instruction; specifically, whether he can undersand the type of verbal instructions commonly given in early elementary classrooms.

There are three parts to the BCI:

1. Basic instructions that test the child's ability to handle different types of selection criteria. Included are uncomplicated criteria such as naming (find the boy); plurals; *not* criteria (find the balls that are *not* white); compound criteria (find the one that does not talk and does not bark); and selectional criteria that do not provide enough information to identify a particular object (for example, an illustration showing three boxes, for which the child is told "There is a ball in one of these boxes. The ball is not in this box. Do you *know* where the ball is? Don't guess.").

2. Items which evaluate the ability of the child to repeat statements and to answer questions that are *implied* by these statements. For example, "A boy is not walking when he is running." "What is a boy not doing when he is running?"

3. Pattern awareness tests that assess the child's ability to perceive a pattern or rule and asks him to expand, or complete a sequence. For example, the child is asked to repeat a simple digit series–7, 4. Then he is asked to repeat the series, 7 - 7, 4 - 4, and on through 7 - 7 - 7, 4 - 4 - 4, and so on. The series is not random. The child should be able to repeat the series if he has perceived a pattern; if he has not perceived the pattern, he probably could not repeat the series.

[2] S. Engelmann, *Basic Concept Inventory.* Copyright © 1967 by Follett Educational Corporation. Used by permission of the author.

Scoring procedures and interpretations of items are included in the manual. The purpose of the scoring, as stated previously, is not for comparison with other test populations but purely for the purpose of determining concepts which the child can handle in a classroom situation. That is, the testing is not to determine "capacity" or personal adequacy but to determine level of instruction for the classroom. That being the case, there are no age norms or achievement norms for comparison. Administration of the *Basic Concept Inventory,* however, should result in identification of the types of linguistic tasks which may interfere with the child's educational achievement.

SUMMARY

When Sir Henry Head published his text on *Aphasia and Kindred Disorders of Speech* in 1926 he entitled the chapter on aphasia language testing "Chaos." The same might be said a half-century later of testing of language acquisition. The chaos that Head referred to, and the chaos of language-development testing that is apparent from the parade of language scales we have discussed (see Table 5-3) is due to an awkward blending of divergent theories and empiricist biases. Some of the tests we have reviewed have been based on specific theoretical viewpoints; some have been constructed to reflect what their authors thought was important for their therapy regimes. Relatively few have been developed from theoretical biases which are compatible with current linguistic theories. Only one of the measures we have reviewed (the ITPA) claims to be based on a specific psycholinguistic model, and very few linguists or psychologists find that model to be an adequate explanation of language development.

Language-related children are an extremely heterogeneous group, and no one test, or small group of tests, is most descriptive for all the population with a diversity of etiologies and linguistic behaviors. The tests of verbal output, included at the beginning of this chapter, may hold the greatest potential for description of a child's language. It is also appropriate to reiterate that the circumstances of the child-adult interview may not indicate all that the child knows about language. Controlled-circumstance test situations, which comprise the bulk of this chapter, are an attempt to determine *what* the child knows, or what she *does* in the specified circumstances but the circumstances are restricted. The prerequisite for obtaining information about a child's language skills is the requirement that the clinician knows what he is looking for. There is no substitute for that prerequisite. Without that knowledge, the examiner can determine only a score; with that knowledge the clinician can gain a sufficient understanding to plan an appropriate therapeutic regime.

At the beginning of this chapter we very briefly mentioned the concept of language function—the communicative intent or the purpose that one has in talking. We mentioned the term pragmatics, and defined it as communicative

Table 5-3 Summary of language tests

Name	*Ages*	*Type of Norms*	*Skills Tested (Scoring)*
Mean Length of Response (MLR)	1½-4½ yrs. (McCarthy) 3-8 yrs. (Templin)	Means and standard deviations	Expression–words per response.
Mean Length of Utterance (MLU)	–	–	Expression–morphemes per response.
Structural Complexity Score (SCS)	3-8 yrs.	Means and standard deviations	Expression–weighted score for complexity of utterance in simple to compound, etc. terms.
Developmental Sentence Scoring (DSS)	2-7 yrs.	Percentile rankings	Expression–values for words and types of words.
Developmental Sentence Types (DST)	–	–	Expression–relative description but no scores.
Length-Complexity Index (LCI)	–	–	Expression–values for linguistic complexity of phrases.
Peabody Picture Vocabulary Test (PPVT)	2-18+ yrs.	Intelligence quotient, mental age, and percentile rankings	Receptive vocabulary.
Vocabulary Comprehension Scale (VCS)	2-6 yrs.	Mean ages for individual words sampled	Vocabulary comprehension–receptive.
Morphology (Berko or Berry-Talbot)	–	–	Expressive–regular morphologic past tense, plural, possessive, progressive, and comparative endings.
Northwestern Syntax Screening Test (NSST)	3-8 yrs.	Percentile rankings	Expressive and Receptive.

Table 5-3 Summary of language tests (continued)

Name	*Ages*	*Type of Norms*	*Skills Tested (Scoring)*
Carrow Elicited Language Inventory (CELI)	3-8 yrs.	Means, percentile ranks Standard scores for total and subgroup scores	Expressive.
Assessment of Children's Language Comprehension (ACLC)	3-6½ yrs.	Mean percentage for subparts of test	Receptive (vocabulary only for items used in other three sections).
Michigan Picture Language Inventory (MPLI)	4-6 yrs. (Wolski) 3-9 yrs. (Lerea)	Means and standard deviations	Vocabulary, Expressive, Receptive.
Bankson Language Screening Test (BLST)	4-8 yrs.	Means and standard deviations plus percentile ranks	Expressive.
Test for Auditory Comprehension of Language (TACL)	3-7 yrs.	Means, standard deviations, and percentiles	Receptive—for total and subgroups.
Illinois Test of Psycholinguistic Abilities (ITPA)	2-10 yrs.	Language age by category subtest and total	Receptive and Expressive subtests.
Illinois Children's Language Assessment Test (ICLAT)	3-5½ yrs.	Mean scores	Receptive and Expressive subtests.

Table 5-3 Summary of language tests (continued)

Name	*Ages*	*Type of Norms*	*Skills Tested (Scoring)*
Sequenced Inventory of Communication Development (SICD)	4-48 mo.	Age scores	Receptive and Expressive.
Utah Test of Language Development (UTLD)	1-15 yrs.	Age scores	General–not separated by modality or type.
Houston Test for Language Development	Part I- 6-36 mo. Part II- 3-6 yrs.	Age scores	General development–not separated by modality or type.
Preschool Language Scale (PLS)	1½-7 yrs.	Age scores	Receptive and Expressive.
McCarthy Scale for Communication Assessment (MSCA)	2½-8½ yrs.	Standard score (weighted scale & scores)	General developmental with separate sub-test area profile.
Language Assessment Tasks (LAT)	9-14 yrs. (grades 4-8)	Age scores	Profile of Receptive and Expressive plus Content and Communicative function.
Basic Concept Inventory (BCI)	1st. gr.	Criterion referenced	General–school development based on *Reception* of linguistic concepts.

interaction. Insofar as interaction may be measured in degrees of effectiveness, pragmatics, or communicative interaction, may be measurable on a continuum from "good" to "poor." Communicative interaction and language content are obviously important concerns in our definition (diagnosis) of language abilities and disabilities, but we have not yet, as a profession, agreed on critical aspects of pragmatic language or on definition of the points along the presumed continuum.

The tests we have discussed, as examples of the kinds of information that can be obtained from available controlled-circumstance situations, primarily are tests of language form rather than language function. The language tests discussed were listed, in order of discussion, in Table 5-3. Age ranges for which the tests were designed, types of normative comparisons available (mean scores for ages, age scores, and percentile ranks), and types of skills tested (expressive, receptive) are tabulated. This type of listing does not make a qualitative judgment for a clinician in search of "the best" test. It is not intended to.

The tests reviewed were included as examples, rather than as an exhaustive listing. The descriptions given of the tests were meant to provide some basis for the clinician's judgment in choosing among them. No one test will provide all of the necessary information for a remediation regimen if a problem has been determined to exist. The age, the area of concern, and the capability of the child in question, are all important factors in your test selection. Some of the tests described are linguistically specific. Some are general. Some are better than others in terms of economy of effort, of time, of effectiveness in identifying particular problems. The primary misuse of the diagnostician's responsibility, however, would be in the assumption that any one test is "all good" and another is "all bad."

The presentation of language tests has assumed that a judgment of "language disorder" must be based on an understanding, in both form and function, of what is to be expected with chronological age. The description available, from an appropriate combination of test results, should give an indication of the child's abilities and disabilities within his language system.

REFERENCES

Arlt, P. B., *Illinois Children's Language Assessment Test, Instruction Booklet.* Danville, Ill.: The Interstate Printers and Publishers, Inc., (1977).

Arndt, W. B., A psychometric evaluation of the Northwestern Syntax Screening Test. *J. Speech Hearing Dis.*, 42, 316-319 (1977).

Bankson, N. W., *Bankson Language Screening Test.* Baltimore: University Park Press, (1977).

Bangs, T. E., *Vocabulary Comprehension Scale.* Lamar, TX: Learning Concepts, (1975).

Bates, E., *Language and Context: The Acquistion of Pragmatics.* New York: Academic Press, (1976).

Berko, J., The child's learning of English morphology. *Word,* 14, 150-177 (1958).

Berry, M. F., and R. Talbot, *Exploratory Test for Grammar.* Rockford, Ill.: Berry and Talbot, 4322 Pine Crest Road, (1966).

Bliss, L. S., and D. V. Allen, A story completion approach as a measure of language development in children. *J. Speech Hearing Res.,* 20, 358-372 (1977).

Bloom, L., Talking, understanding, and thinking, Chap. 11, in *Language Perspectives–Acquisition, Retardation, and Intervention,* eds. R. L. Schiefelbusch and L. L. Lloyd. Baltimore: University Park Press, (1974).

Boehm, A. E., *Boehm Test of Basic Concepts* (Manual). New York: The Psychological Corporation, (1971).

Brown, R., *A First Language: The Early Stages.* Cambridge, Mass.: Harvard University Press, (1973).

Brown, R., and C. Fraser, The acquisition of syntax, in *Verbal Behavior and Learning,* eds. C. N. Cofer and B. S. Musgrave. New York: McGraw-Hill, (1963).

Carroll, J. B., Review of Illinois Test of Psycholinguistic Abilities: Revised Edition, in *The Seventh Mental Measurements Yearbook,* ed. O. K. Buros. Highland Park, N.J.: The Gryphon Press, (1972).

Carrow, E., *Test for Auditory Comprehension of Language.* Lamar, TX: Learning Concepts, (1973).

Carrow, E., *Carrow Elicited Language Inventory Manual.* Lamar, TX: Learning Concepts, (1974).

Carrow, E., and J. Lynch, Comparison of semantic versus syntactic comprehension in three groups of linguistically deviant children. Unpublished manuscript cited in E. Carrow. *Test for Auditory Comprehension of Language.* Lamar, TX: Learning Concepts, (1973).

Carrow, M. A., The development of auditory comprehension of language structure in children. *J. Speech Hearing Dis.,* 33, 99-111 (1968).

Chomsky, N., *Aspects of the Theory of Syntax.* Cambridge, Mass.: MIT Press, (1965).

Crabtree, M., *The Houston Test for Language Development, Manual of Directions.* Part I (1958) and Part II (1963). Copyright by Margaret Crabtree, Houston, TX.

Darley, F. L., and K. L. Moll, Reliability of language measures and size of language sample. *J. Speech Hearing Res.,* 3, 166-173 (1960).

D'asaro, M. J., and V. John, A rating for evaluation of Receptive, Expressive and Phonetic language development of the young child. *Cerebral Palsy Review,* 22, no. 5 (1961).

Dean, E. A., Language comprehension as a predictor of articulation skills in kindergarten-age children. Unpublished Master's thesis, University of Tennessee, Knoxville, (1975).

Dever, R. B., A comparison of the results of a revised version of Berko's test of morphology with the free speech of mentally retarded children. *J. Speech Hearing Res.,* 15, 169-178 (1972).

Doll, E. A., *The Vineland Social Maturity Scale.* Minneapolis: American Guidance Service, Inc., (1946).

Dunn, L. M., *Expanded Manual for The Peabody Picture Vocabulary Test.* Circle Pines, Minn.: American Guidance Service, Inc., (1965).

Engelmann, S., *The Basic Concept Inventory, Teacher's Manual.* Chicago: Follett Educational Corporation, (1967).

Fillenbaum, S., *Syntactic Factors in Memory.* The Hague: Mouton, (1973).

Fillmore, C. J., The case for case, in *Universals in Linguistic Theory,* eds. E. Bach and R. T. Harms. New York: Holt, Rinehart and Winston, (1968).

Foster, R., J. J. Giddan, and J. Stark, *Assessment of Children's Language Comprehension, Manual.* Palo Alto, Calif.: Consulting Psychologists Press, Inc., (1973).

Frankenberg, W. K., and J. B. Dobbs, Denver Developmental Screening Test. *J. Pediatrics,* 71, 181-191 (1967).

Fraser, C., U. Bellugi, and R. Brown, Control of grammar in imitation, comprehension, and production. *J. Verb. Learn. Verb. Behav.,* 2, 121-135 (1963).

Glaser, R., Instructional technology and the measurement of learning outcomes: Some questions. *Amer. Psychol.,* 18, 519-521 (1963).

Hahn, E., Analyses of the content and form of the speech of first grade children. *Quart. J. Speech,* 34, 361-366 (1948).

Halstead, W. C., and J. M. Wepman, The Halstead-Wepman aphasia screening test. *J. Speech Hearing Dis.,* 14, 9-15 (1949).

Harris, D. B., The Goodenough-Harris Drawing Test, *Children's Drawings as Measures of Intellectual Maturity.* New York: Harcourt Brace Jovanovich, (1963).

Head, H., *Aphasia and Kindred Disorders of Speech, Vol. I.* London: Cambridge University Press, (1926).

Hedrick, D. L., and E. M. Prather, *Sequenced Inventory of Language Development (SILD), Experimental Edition.* Child Development and Mental Retardation Center, University of Washington, Seattle, (1970).

Hedrick, D. L., E. M. Prather, and A. R. Tobin, *Sequenced Inventory of Communication Development Examiner's Manual.* Seattle: University of Washington Press, (1975).

Kellman, M., C. Flood, and D. Yoder, *Language Assessment Tasks.* Copyright Kellman, Flood, Yoder, (1977).

Kirk, S. A., and W. D. Kirk, Uses and abuses of the ITPA. *J. Speech Hearing Dis.,* 43, 58-75 (1978).

Kirk, S. A., J. J. McCarthy, and W. D. Kirk, *Illinois Test of Psycholinguistic Abilities (Examiner's Manual).* Urbana, Ill.: The University of Illinois Press, (1968).

Lee, L. L., Developmental sentence types: A method for comparing normal and deviant syntactic development. *J. Speech Hearing Dis.,* 31, 311-330 (1966).

Lee, L. L., *Northwestern Syntax Screening Test.* Evanston, Ill.: Northwestern University Press, (1969, 1971).

Lee, L. L., *Developmental Sentence Analysis.* Evanston, Ill: Northwestern University Press, (1974).

Lee, L. L. Reply to Arndt and Byrne. *J. Speech Hearing Dis.*, 42, 323-327 (1977).

Lee, L. L., and S. M. Canter, Developmental sentence scoring. *J. Speech Hearing Dis.*, 36, 315-340 (1971).

Leonard, L. B. and others, Understanding indirect requests: An investigation of children's comprehension of pragmatic meanings. *J. Speech Hearing Res.*, 21, 528-537 (1978).

Leonard, L. B., J. G. Bolders, and J. A. Miller, An examination of the semantic relations reflected in the language usage of normal and language-disordered children. *J. Speech Hearing Res.*, 19, 371-392 (1976).

Lerea, L., Assessing language development. *J. Speech Hearing Res.*, 1, 75-85 (1958).

Marquardt, T. P., and J. H. Saxman, Language comprehension and auditory discrimination in articulation deficient kindergarten children. *J. Speech Hearing Res.*, 15, 382-389 (1972).

McCarthy, D., *McCarthy Scales of Children's Abilities.* New York: The Psychological Corporation, (1972).

McCarthy, D., The language development of the preschool child. *University of Minnesota Institute of Child Welfare Monograph,* No. 4, Minneapolis: University of Minnesota Press, (1930).

McCarthy, D., Language development in children, in *Manual of Child Psychology,* ed. L. Carmichael. New York: John Wiley, (1954).

McCarthy, J. J., and S. A. Kirk, *The Illinois Test of Psycholinguistic Abilities, Examiner's Manual.* Urbana: University of Illinois Press, (1961).

Mecham, M. J., *Verbal Language Development Scale.* Minneapolis: American Guidance Service, Inc., (1958, 1971).

Mecham, M. J., J. L. Jex, and J. D. Jones, *Utah Test of Language Development: Manual of Directions.* Salt Lake City: Communication Research Associates, (1967, 1978).

Messer, S., Implicit phonology in children. *J. Verb. Learn. Verb. Behav.*, 6, 609-613 (1967).

Miller, G. A., The magical number seven, plus or minus two: Some limits on our capacity for processing information. *Psych. Res.*, 63, 81-97 (1956).

Miller, L., Pragmatics and early childhood disorders: Communicative interactions in a half-hour sample. *J. Speech Hearing Dis.*, 43, 419-436 (1978).

Miner, L., Scoring precedures for the Length-Complexity Index: A preliminary report. *J. Commun. Dis.*, 2, 224-240 (1969).

Minifie, F., F. L. Darley, and D. Sherman, Temporal reliability of seven language measures. *J. Speech Hearing Res.*, 6, 149-156 (1963).

Newfield, M. U., and B. B. Schlanger, The acquisition of English morphology by normal and educable mentally retarded children. *J. Speech Hearing Res.*, 11, 693-706 (1968).

Nice, M. N., Length of sentences as a criterion of a child's progress in speech. *J. Ed. Psych.*, 16, 370-379 (1925).

Nicolosi, L., and J. D. Krescheck, Variability in test scores, Form A and Form B on the Peabody Picture Vocabulary Test. *J. Lang., Speech, Hearing Serv. Schools,* 3, 44-47 (1972).

Olswang, L. B., and A. L. Carpenter, Elicitor effects on the language obtained from young language-impaired children. *J. Speech Hearing Dis.* 43, 76-88, (1978).

Osgood, C. E., A behavioral analysis of perception and language as cognitive phenomena, in *Contemporary Approaches to Cognition,* ed. J. S. Bruner. Cambridge, Mass.: Harvard University Press, (1957).

Paraskevopoulos, J. N., and S. A. Kirk, *The Development and Psychometric Characteristics of the Revised Illinois Test of Psycholinguistic Abilities.* Urbana: University of Illinois Press, (1969).

Pendergast, K. and others, *Photo Articulation Test.* Danville, Ill.: The Interstate Printers and Publishers, Inc., (1969).

Prutting, C. A., T. M. Gallagher, and A. Mulac, The expressive portion of the NSST compared to a spontaneous language sample. *J. Speech Hearing Dis.,* 40, 40-48 (1975).

Ramer, A. L. H., and N. S. Rees, Selected aspects of the development of English morphology in Black American children of low socioeconomic background. *J. Speech Hearing Res.,* 16, 569-577 (1973).

Ratusnick, D. L., and R. A. Koenigsknect, Internal consistency of the Northwestern Syntax Screening Test. *J. Speech Hearing Dis.,* 40, 59-69 (1975).

Schlesinger, L. M., Production of utterances and language acquisition, in *Ontogenesis of Grammar,* ed. D. L. Slobin. New York: Academic Press, (1971).

Schuell, H., A short examination for aphasia. *Neurology,* 7, 625-634 (1957).

Scott, C. M., and A. E. Taylor, A comparison of home and clinic gathered language samples. *J. Speech Hearing Dis.,* 43, 482-495 (1978).

Shriner, T. H., A review of mean length of response as a measure of expressive language development in children. *J. Speech Hearing Dis.,* 34, 61-68 (1969).

Shriner, T. H., and D. Sherman, An equation for assessing language development. *J. Speech Hearing Res.,* 10, 41-48 (1967).

Siegel, G. M., and P. A. Broen, Language assessment, in *Communication Assessment and Intervention Strategies,* ed. L. L. Lloyd. Baltimore: University Park Press, (1976).

Slobin, D. I., Imitation and grammatical development in children, in *Contemporary Issues in Developmental Psychology,* eds. N. S. Endler, L. R. Boulter, and H. Osser. New York: Holt, Rinehart and Winston, (1968).

Slobin, D. I., and C. A. Welsh, Elicited imitation as a research tool in developmental psycholinguistics, in *Studies of Child Language Development,* eds. C. A. Ferguson and D. I. Slobin. New York: Holt, Rinehart and Winston (1973).

Smith, C., An experimental approach to children's linguistic competence, in *Studies of Child Language Development,* eds. C. A. Ferguson and D. I. Slobin. New York: Holt, Rinehart and Winston, (1973).

Sylvester, N. C., A comparison between defective and normal articulation groups on morphological skill and general language development. Unpublished Master's thesis, University of Tennessee, Knoxville, (1969).

Templin, M. C., *Certain Language Skills in Children,* University of Minnesota Institute of Child Welfare Monograph, No. 26. Minneapolis: The University of Minnesota Press, (1957).

Templin, M. C., The study of articulation and language development during the early school years, in *The Genesis of Language,* eds. F. Smith and G. A. Miller. Cambridge, Mass.: The MIT Press, (1966).

Terman, L. M., and M. A. Merrill, *Measuring Intelligence.* Boston: Houghton Mifflin, (1937).

Underwood, B. J., The language repertoire and some problems in verbal learning, in *Directions in Psycholinguistics,* ed. S. Rosenberg. New York: Macmillan, (1966).

Wall, L. L., A study concerning linguistic skills and three levels of articulation proficiency. Unpublished Master's thesis, University of Tennessee, Knoxville, (1970).

Wechsler, D., *The Measurement and Appraisal of Adult Intelligence.* Baltimore: Williams and Wilkins, (1958).

Weiner, P. S., The perceptual level functioning of dysphasic children: A follow-up study. *J. Speech Hearing Res.,* 15, 423-438 (1972).

Weiner, P. S., and W. C. Hoock, The standardization of tests: Criteria and criticisms. *J. Speech Hearing Res.,* 16, 616-626 (1973).

Wepman, J. M., and L. V. Jones, *The Language Modalities Test for Aphasia.* Chicago: University of Chicago Education-Industry Service, (1961).

Whitacre, J. D., H. L. Luper, and H. R. Pollio, General language deficits in children with articulation problems. *Lang. Speech,* 13, 231-239 (1970).

Whorf, B. L., *Language, Thought and Reality: Selected Writings.* Cambridge, Mass.: Technology Press, (1956).

Williams, H. M., An analytical study of language achievement in preschool children, Part 1, (and) An analytical scale of language achievement, in *Development of Language and Vocabulary in Young Children. University of Iowa Studies in Child Welfare.,* 13, 9-18, and 49-77 (1937).

Winitz, H., Language skills of male and female kindergarten children. *J. Speech Hearing Res.,* 2, 377-386 (1959).

Wolski, W., Language development of normal children four, five, and six years of age as measured by the Michigan Picture Language Inventory. Unpublished Doctoral dissertation, University of Michigan, Ann Arbor, (1962).

Zimmerman, I. L., V. G. Steiner, and R. L. Evatt, *Preschool Language Manual.* Columbus, Ohio: Chas. E. Merrill, (1969, 1979).

Evaluation of Developmental Skills

VI

Normally, growth and maturation proceed at characteristic rates for each developmental aspect.

Eric H. Lenneberg
The Natural History of Language

In many ways language maturation parallels motor and physical maturation. For more than half a century (Abt, Adler, and Bartelme 1929), it has been recognized that early language development was a predictive yardstick for general development. At the same time, motor development has sometimes been used as a predictor* of the child's general and intellectual potential (Gesell and Amatruda 1941). This is not to say that a causal relationship exists between motor and speech development, but in the absence of specific etiologies which may affect skills differentially, there is a pattern of consistency in normal behavioral evolution (Lenneberg 1966; McGraw 1963; Gesell and Amatruda 1947). Our consideration of developmental skills in this chapter is an outgrowth of the recognition that motor and perceptual functioning as well as language skills provide information on neurological integrity and maturation.

We will review only a small number of developmental, motor, and visual perceptual assessment instruments and will assume some consistency among the tests in terms of the items and areas evaluated. It is pertinent to note that many of these tests rest more firmly in the province of the occupational therapist and/

*For a more complete review of perceptual-motor programs and test instruments, what predictions can be made, and what predictions cannot be made, see Cratty (1970).

or psychometrist and will not consistently be used as appraisal instruments by the speech-language clinician. Observations of particular interest to the speech-language clinician in developing a more comprehensive picture of infants and very young children (for example, Bayley 1935) include skills such as maintaining balance in sitting, standing unsupported, and hopping on one foot. They give way to an interest in fine motor skills in the use of the hands and eye-hand coordination in older children.

DEVELOPMENTAL SCALES

Gesell and his associates (1939, 1940, 1941, 1947, 1948) were concerned with four fields of developmental behavior: motor, adaptive, language, and personal-social. The *Gesell Scales* are an empirically based product of their twenty-year study of normal children aimed at the development of a system of developmental diagnosis for infants and children. The scales assume that motor, adaptive, language, and social behaviors are all a function of mental growth and require progressively more coordinated patterning of behavior based upon neurological integrity and maturation. In other words "We cannot or need not separate or distinguish physical patterns and behavior patterns. The child is a unitary organism, and from the very beginning is growing as a single unit" (Gesell and Ilg 1947, p. 16).

Since we have previously discussed language and personal social behaviors, the primary focus insofar as the Gesell Scales are concerned, will be on motor and adaptive behaviors. The *Gesell Motor and Adaptive Scales* are not measures of intelligence, and the age-scale items of the instrument are not to be taken as specific rules of thumb. Rather, the scales are designed to yield a very general picture of the child's growth in adaptive behaviors primarily during the first five years of life. Both the motor and adaptive scales span the ages from 18 to 72 months at six month divisions, but Gesell considered five to be the "nodal" age (Gesell and Ilg 1947, p. 251). Items on the scale are listed as age norms but were designed to be used for general orientation and interpretation, rather than as standards of behavior that the child must meet.

The *Motor Scale* consists largely of walking and balance activities; for example, the child runs without falling at 24 months, alternates feet going up stairs at 36 months; walks downstairs with the last few treads one foot to a tread at 48 months. The *Adaptive Scale* has a number of eye-hand coordination tasks, especially at the earlier age divisions. For example, a tower of six or seven blocks is to be built at 24 months, eight blocks at 30 months, and a tower of nine blocks at 36 months. Many drawing and counting tasks are also included, such as copying geometric figures, draw-a-man, and counting objects. These are age-related tests which means that the total number of correct responses credits the child with a year-month age score for Motor Age Level or Adaptive Age Level.

There is also a *Preliminary Behavior Inventory* (Gesell and Amatruda 1947) which is a screening test of observations for motor, adaptive, language, and personal-social behaviors. This abbreviated scale with one or two items per age designation at intervals from four weeks to six years is not to be used as a diagnostic inventory. Suggested use of the instrument is for the examiner to check the most advanced behaviors in each field. Gross deviations or disparities indicate the need for a diagnostic behavior examination.

The *Denver Developmental Screening Test* (Frankenburg and Dodds 1967) is essentially a display of the Gesell test items is a different form. A few of the test items, however, are placed at slightly different age levels than on the Gesell Scales. For example, building a tower of eight cubes is shown on the Gesell Adaptive Scale at the 30-month level. According to the Denver chart, 25 percent of children 21 months of age can build a tower of eight cubes, 75 percent can perform the task at between 24 and 30 months, and 90 percent have accomplished this feat at approximately 39 months.

Behaviors to be evaluated on the test are segmented into four categories: gross motor, language, fine-motor adaptive, and personal-social. Items are arranged on an age scale with one month separations from one to 24 months and by half-year divisions from 2-5 to 6 years. For convenience in deriving an approximate developmental age for each of the four categories, the Denver response sheet is marked with ages along the horizontal axis. Developmental item skills are shown horizontally on bar graphs beginning in line with the age-scale markers where 25 percent of the standardization population of 1,036 children had mastered the skill. The bar graph becomes shaded at the point where 75 percent of the tested children performed the test item and terminates where 90 percent of the children satisfied the criterion item. Many of the items are directly tested, but some items, especially at the earlier age levels, are keyed to allow credit by parental report. Items passed are marked with "P," refused items by "R," failed items by "F," and no opportunity by "N.O." Failure or delay is defined as failure to successfully perform an item at an age level at which 90 percent of comparably aged children passed. Normal children are expected to show a scattering of successes and failures on items within an area and between categories. The manner in which the items are displayed on the response sheet allows the examiner to more easily make informed judgments of the overall developmental picture presented by the child. Test-retest and inter-examiner reliability have been established at 0.95 and 0.90, respectively.

TESTS OF MOTOR SKILL

The *Oseretsky Test of Motor Proficiency* was originally published in Russian in 1923. It was adapted into Portuguese and later translated into English (Doll 1946). It was designed for children from four to sixteen years of age and was described as "... a year-scale of tests of motor maturation for measuring genetic levels of motor proficiency (and) ... affords a standard means for the clinical evaluation of behavioral development." The test was designed to evaluate manual abilities, motor skills, and motor equilibrium; that is, to show the value of children's motor reactions and their causes so that they could be trained to control and coordinate movements. The test is composed of 85 items divided into six groups for each age level: (1) tests for general static coordination (balance), (2) tests for dynamic coordination of the hands, (3) tests for general dynamic coordination, (4) tests for motor speech, (5) tests for simultaneous voluntary movement, and (6) tests for synkinesia (associated involuntary movements). The original Oseretsky test suffered from significant procedural shortcomings. For example, Doll (1946, p. 2) noted that:

> It is not clear from most of the test directions to what extent the examiner may assist the child by supplementing the verbal directions with demonstration. Since many of the test directions presumably would not be clearly understood without demonstration, the lack of which increases the intellectual requirements of the tests, it may be assumed that demonstrating the tasks is not only permissable but desirable or even imperative ... the tests are not free from a rather marked intellectual loading since the problem of comprehending the task and to some degree responding to it is inherent in the testing.

These procedural shortcomings have lead to two notable adaptations of the test.

Sloan (1955) modified and adapted the Oseretsky Scale and his experimental results were published as the *Lincoln-Oseretsky Motor Development Scale.* A total of 380 boys and 369 girls between the ages of six and fourteen were tested on the 85 original Oseretsky items. The number of subjects at the various age levels ranged from 39 to 46. All subjects were obtained from the public schools in small towns in central Illinois and were from moderate to "low-moderate" socioeconomic-level families. They were selected on the basis of age and grade placement alone. None were reported to have a marked intellectual deficiency, but individual intelligence tests were not administered.

On the basis of statistical analyses of the performance of the children on the Oseretsky scale, test items were eliminated which did not contribute to the total score, and the format of the test was changed. The six types of items used by Oseretsky were maintained, but the 36 items retained are structured as a single order of difficulty rather than represented at each age level. As with the original Oseretsky scale, varying amounts of credit are given for speed of performance, dominant and nondominant hand performances are weighted differently, and boys and girls are scored separately. An example of an item from the test is the act of throwing a ball. Equipment necessary includes a ball and a ten-inch square target placed eight feet in front of the child at chest height. With both right hand and left hand separately, the subject is asked to bring his hand to the shoulder (as in a shot put) and throw the ball at the target. Scoring is based on the number of times the target is hit. An improper throw (overhand, or underhand, for example) is not counted. If the child hits the target four times (out of five), he is given three points; three hits or two hits, two points; one hit, one point; and no hits, no points. Consequently, scoring is determined by how many points are credited to the child on the item and not whether he passed or did not pass.

The directions for the Lincoln-Oseretsky Scale are concise, the amount of credit per item is explicitly stated, and the total number of points for the child's age and sex can be interpreted according to means, standard deviations, and percentile scores provided for children 6 to 14 years of age. As a validity statement, Sloan reported that the test correlated well with chronological age and was capable of discriminating between children of different ages. Split-half reliability ranged from a low of 0.59 (for 14-year-old girls) to a high of 0.94. For the nine age groups on which data were collected, reliability coefficients were 0.80 and above, except for the 13- and 14-year-old boys (0.72 and 0.78, respectively) and the 14-year-old girls.

The *Bruininks-Oseretsky Test of Motor Proficiency* (Bruininks 1978) is an expansion as well as an adaptation of the Oseretsky scale. The test is designed to assess the motor skills of children from 4-5 to 14-5 years of age. The battery includes eight subtests comprised of 46 items to provide an index of motor proficiency for both gross and fine motor skills. The short form contains 14 items and serves as a survey of general motor proficiency.

Four subtests of the battery (running speed and agility, balance, bilateral coordination, and strength) assess gross motor skills; three subtests (upper limb coordination, response speed and visual motor control) measure fine-motor skills, and one subtest (speed and upper-limb dexterity) tests both gross and fine motor skills. Approximately 40 percent of the items are revised tasks from the *Oseretsky Tests of Motor Proficiency,* and the test includes three subtests not included in the original Oseretsky version.

Performance on each item is scored according to the time required to complete the task, the number of units completed per unit time, the number of errors observed during performance of the task, or as pass or fail based upon established criteria. The raw scores are converted to scale values which can then be totaled. The test was standardized on 765 subjects between 4-6 and 14-6 years of age. The sample included approximately an equal number of boys and girls, and racial and community size representation were considered in the subject selection.

The raw scores are converted to point scores, and point scores are converted to derived scores based on chronological age. Norms are expressed as four types of derived scores: subtest standard scores at 6 month intervals from 4-6 years to 14-5 years, percentile ranks, stanines, and age equivalents. By comparing the derived scores with the scores of subjects from the standardization, the subjects performance can be compared to the reference group. The complete battery yields three estimates of motor proficiency: a gross motor composite score, a fine motor composite score, and a battery composite score. The performance on each composite is expressed as a standard score with a mean of 50 and a standard deviation of 10 for each age level. The test appears to have adequate construct validity. Test-retest reliability based upon results from 63 second graders and 63 sixth graders was found to be 0.77 for the gross motor composite, 0.88 for the fine motor composite, and 0.89 for the battery composite.

The *Motor Problems Inventory* (Riley 1972) is primarily an empirically based test. It consists of 15 items which are described as included in "traditional examination procedures used by speech and language pathologists, traditional psychological observations, and the traditional neurological examination." The items are categorized as small muscle coordination, laterality, gross motor coordination, and general observations. No special equipment is required except for a stop watch and a room sufficiently large to allow gross muscle activities, such as hopping, skipping, and running.

Small-muscle coordination includes items such as finger snapping and diadochokinetic movements of the tongue and lips. Laterality items include lateral alternating movements of the tongue, slapping the thighs with the hands bilaterally, and hand-eye-foot preferences. Gross-motor coordination is observed in hopping, balancing, and walking and running activities. General observations are concerned with hyperactivity, perseveration, distractability, and legibility of handwriting.

Each of the fifteen items is scored as "no problem", "some problem," or "much problem" according to criteria shown with each of the items. These three terms are given weights of 0, 1, and 2 respectively. The range of scores for the 15 items is therefore 0 to 30. Normative comparisons are based upon the range of scores for children of preschool, kindergarten, and first through fifth grade. The standardization population consisted of 209 children with from 30 to 60 children at each of the grade levels except that there were no children included at the second and fourth grade levels. The normal-range, significant-problem, and severe-problem designations for these two ages were by interpolations of the curves.

Validity and reliability data are based upon comparison of the instrument to "soft" neurological signs and test-retest consistency. The test is reported to be of value for screening special education classes, selecting children to be referred for neurological examination, and as a measurement of the motor component in speech, language, and education disorders. However, no statistics are cited for the agreement of the test scores with speech and language disorders.

The motor development-proficiency scales we have discussed have one assumption in common. That is, that coordination skills and patterns of behavior reflect the integrity of the neurological system. Children on the low end of the coordination continuum will tend to be classified differently according to the theoretical biases favored in the academic or clinical environment in which the clinician finds herself. These children have been variously categorized with terms ranging from aphasoid to clumsy. To explore the rationale for the variety of terms used would require more a defense of theoretical biases than a listing of diagnostic criteria. Our purpose is not to argue whether one term is better than another for describing a syndrome, but rather to provide a rationale for appraisal instruments that aid in establishing a more complete description of the patient and problem referred. For the same reason, we will include several examples of scales which provide measurements of visual perception.

TESTS OF VISUAL PERCEPTION

Tests of visual-perceptual skills are expected to have diagnostic relevance to children with learning disabilities, especially those problems related to reading and assigning meaning to visual symbols. The *Developmental Test of Visual Perception* (Maslow and others 1964; Frostig and others 1966) has five major components: eye-hand coordination; figure-ground perception; form constancy; position in space; and spatial relationship.

Tests of eye-hand coordination require the child to draw straight and curved lines between narrow boundaries or to draw straight lines to a target. Figure-ground tasks require the child to discriminate between intersecting shapes and to find hidden figures. Form constancy requires a discrimination of circles and squares in different sizes, positions and shading among other figures on the page. Position in space is a test of directionality. The differentiation required is to separate figures in a like position from those which are reversed or rotated. In the spatial relationship subtest, the task is to copy patterns by linking dots.

The 1963 standardization (Maslow and others 1964) is based on the performance of over 2,100 unselected nursery school and public school children from three to nine years of age. The five subtest areas are considered relatively distinct. Each can be converted to a perceptual age equivalent, and a total perceptual age and quotient can be derived. Maslow and others (1964) reported that the perceptual quotient was more informative than the perceptual age. Means, standard deviations, and upper and lower quartile rankings are provided at half-year levels between five and eight years of age.

Validity has been expressed in terms of agreement with Goodenough (1955) intelligence test results and with beginning reading scores in early elementary classrooms. The correlations ranged from 0.31 to 0.50. Measures of reliability were generally higher.

The *Developmental Test of Visual Motor Integration* (Beery 1967) was devised as a measure of visual perceptual and motor behavior integration in young children. It is geared toward academic assessment, rather than clinical diagnosis, and its primary users are elementary school teachers. The test is composed of 24 geometric forms to be copies with pencil and paper. The forms are arranged in the order of increasing difficulty and can be administered to children from 2 to 15 years of age, individually or by group administration. The recommended procedure is to evaluate the child's reproduction of a form accordng to a series of criteria provided using illustrations to aid in doubtful cases. At the corner of each scoring-criteria page are notations of age norms for a particular form. For example, male 5-6 means that 50 percent or more of the boys from the standardization population succeeded on the form at approximately five years and six months of age. Testing is discontinued after the child has failed on three consecutive forms although he may be allowed to attempt more difficult items. Age equivalents from raw scores are provided for boys and for girls from 2-10 to 15-9 years.

A validity estimate was derived from correlations between the test scores and age. The correlation between chronological age and test scores was 0.89 and was higher for mental age. Correlations were found to be higher in first-grade children than in older children. Test-retest reliability from a sample of 171 subjects was 0.83 and 0.87 for boys and girls, respectively.

The *Motor-Free Visual Perception Test* (Colarusso and Hammill 1972) purports to test visual perception without confounding by motor activity. The test is composed of 37 items selected to assess spatial relationships, visual discrimination, figure-ground, visual closure, and visual memory. The items are individually administered and are multiple choice. The only response required from the child is that she point to the one of four alternatives that she thinks is the correct response. The child is not allowed to trace any figures and generally is given 15 seconds to make a selection although it is not a time test.

The test was standardized on an unselected sample of 881 normal children age 4 to 8 years and who resided in 22 states. Included were children from all races, economic levels, and residential areas. Perceptual age estimates for each possible raw score are provided and include upper and lower ages based on the standard error of measurement for the entire test. Therefore, if a child's raw score is 22, it is likely that his true raw score is between 20 and 24, his perceptual age is between 5-8 and 6-5 and the best estimate is 6-0. A perceptual quotient is derived in a similar manner. Perceptual quotients are provided for children at a one-year interval between 4-0 and 4-11 and at 6-month intervals from 5-0 to 8-11. The perceptual age and the perceptual quotient, then, should not be interpreted without considering the standard error of measurement for the raw scores.

Test-retest reliability was found to range from 0.77 to 0.82, split-half from 0.81 to 0.84 and Kuder-Richardson from 0.71 to 0.82. Construct validity was evaluated by means of age differentiation, correlations with similar tests, and internal consistency. The test correlated higher with other measures of visual perception (0.49) than it did with tests of intelligence (0.31) or school performance (0.38). The authors indicated that these findings support the validity of the measure because it would be expected to correlate higher with visual perception devices than with measures of intelligence and school performance.

Our discussion of developmental tests would not be complete unless we considered the *Bender Visual Motor Gestalt Test* (Bender 1938). The test is composed of nine designs selected by Bender from figures used by Wertheimer (1923) to study visual perception. The patient's task is to reproduce the nine figures which are then scored for imperfections. A separate set of instructions for the test was published along with the figures by Bender in 1946. Since its inception, the test has received intensive study and has proven useful for investigating adults (for example, Pascal and Suttell 1951) and children (for example, Clawson 1962) with disorders ranging from psychiatric disturbances to mental retardation and brain damage. Koppitz (1963; 1975) has devoted two volumes to reviews of the accumulated work with the test.

Since our concern is with visual-motor integration as a developmental skill, we will not consider the use of the test as an indicator of brain damage or emotional disturbance. Similarly we will not review the several scoring systems for the test or the relationship of test results to intelligence, school achievement, mental age, or learning ability. Our focus will be on the scoring system developed by Koppitz (1963; 1975) and the results of the test as estimators of visual motor maturity.

The Developmental Bender Test Scoring System (Koppitz 1963; 1975) contains 30 items which are used to quantify the imperfections in the reproductions of the nine gestalt designs.The total score is based on the distortion of shape, rotation, failure to integrate design parts, and perseveration in the copying of the figures. Theoretically the score can range from 0 to 30 although scores of more than 20 are unusual. It is important to point out that the score is indicative of negative aspects of the copied designs; that is, with improved copying accuracy, the score will decrease rather than increase.

Koppitz (1975) has noted that by the age of nine, the average child will make few if any errors and that below the age of five, the designs are difficult to score. Consequently, the age range of the test is approximately 5 to 9 years although it may be of use for children above nine if they are markedly immature or have significant visual-motor integration problems.

The 1974 standardization of the test on 975 children yielded means and standard deviations at half-year intervals from five to twelve years; age equivalents from less than 4 to 12 years; and percentiles as a function of chronological age levels. For example, if a seven-year-old child received a score of 12, he would be functioning at the tenth percentile for children of his age which is equivalent to the visual-motor integration of a child five years and two months of age. The score of 12 falls more than one standard deviation below the mean for his age, and he would be considered to have "extremely poor" visual-motor integration.

The Bender Gestalt Test appears to have adequate although not high test-retest reliability. Koppitz (1975) reviewed nine studies which found reliability coefficients fom 0.53 to 0.87 although additional instability would be expected in brain-damaged and emotionally disturbed children. Correlations between the Bender and the *Frostig Developmental Test of Visual Perception* are not high (0.39 to 0.52) although the test results do correlate more positively (0.82) with the *Beery Developmental Test of Visual-Motor Integration* (Krauft and Krauft 1972).

SUMMARY

There is considerable commonality in the test observations and theoretical bases of developmental tests. Motor and perceptual measures have been reviewed because motor coordination, perception, and early language development are all assumed to be a function of neurological integrity. Therefore, measures of these skills provide a more complete description of the child's behavioral development. A summary of the tests discussed follows (Table 6-1) along with the age ranges for which each was designed.

Table 6-1 Summary of Developmental Tests

Tests	*Ages*
Developmental Scales	
Gesell Scales	1-72 months
Denver Developmental Screening Test	1-72 months
Motor Skills Tests	
Oseretsky Test of Motor Proficiency	4-16 years
Lincoln-Oseretsky Motor Development Scale	6-14 years
Bruininks-Oseretsky Test of Motor Proficiency	4.5-14.5 years
Motor Problems Inventory	Preschool-Fifth grade
Visual-Motor Perception Tests	
Developmental Test of Visual Perception	3-9 years
Developmental Test of Visual Motor Integration	2-15 years
Motor-Free Perception Test	4-8 years
Bender Visual-Motor Gestalt Test	5-9 years

REFERENCES

Abt, I. A., H. M. Adler, and P. Bartelme, The relationship between the onset of speech and intelligence. *J. Amer. Med. Assoc.,* 93, 1351 (1929).

Bayley, N. A., The development of motor ability during the first three years. *Monogr. Soc. Res. Child Develop.,* 1, 1-26 (1935).

Beery, K. E., *Developmental Test of Visual Motor Integration: Administration and Scoring Manual.* Chicago: Follett Publishing Co., (1967).

Bender, L., A visual motor Gestalt test and its clinical use. *The Amer. Orthopsychiat. Assoc. Res. Monogr.,* no. 3 (1938).

Bender, L., *Bender Motor Gestalt Test: Cards and Manual of Instructions.* New York: The American Orthopsychiatry Association, (1946).

Bruininks, R. H., *Bruininks-Oseretsky Test of Motor Proficiency: Examiner's Manual.* Circle Pines, Minn.: American Guidance Service, Inc., (1978).

Clawson, A., *The Bender Visual Motor Gestalt for Children: A Manual.* Beverly Hills, Calif.: Western Psychological Services, (1962).

Colarusso, R., and D. Hammill, *Motor-Free Visual Perception Test.* San Rafael, Calif.: Academic Therapy Publications, (1972).

Cratty, B. J., *Perceptual and Motor Development in Infants and Children.* New York: Macmillan, (1970).

Doll, E. A., *The Oseretsky Tests of Motor Proficiency: A Translation from the Portuguese Adaptation.* Minneapolis: Educational Test Bureau, (1946).

Frankenburg, W. K., and J. B. Dodds, *The Denver Developmental Screening Test.* Denver, Colo.: University of Colorado Medical Center, (1967).

Frostig, M., W. Lefever, and J. Whittlesey, *Developmental Test of Visual Perception: Administration and Scoring Manual.* Palo Alto, Calif.: Consulting Psychologists Press, (1966).

Gesell, A., *The First Five Years of Life.* New York: Harper & Row, (1940).

Gesell, A., *Studies in Child Development.* New York: Harper & Row, (1948).

Gesell, A., H. Thompson, and C. Amatruda, *Infant Behavior: Its Genesis and Growth.* New York: McGraw-Hill, (1934).

Gesell, A., and C. S. Amatruda, *Developmental Diagnosis.* New York: Hoeber, Inc., (1941).

Gesell, A., and C. S. Amatruda, Developmental diagnosis: Normal and abnormal child development, in *Clinical Methods and Pediatric Applications* (2nd ed). New York: Hoeber, (1947).

Gesell, A., and F. L. Ilg, *Infant and Child in the Culture of Today.* New York: Harper & Row, (1947).

Goodenough, F. L., *Measurement of Intelligence by Drawings.* New York: Harcourt Brace Jovanovich, (1955).

Koppitz, E., *The Bender Gestalt Test for Young Children.* New York: Grune and Stratton, (1963).

Koppitz, E., *The Bender Gestalt Test for Young Children. Vol. II: Research and Application, 1963-1973.* New York: Grune and Stratton, (1975).

Krauft, V., and C. Krauft, Structured vs. unstructured visual-motor tests for educable retarded children. *Percept. Motor Skills,* 34, 691-694 (1972).

Lenneberg, E. H., The natural history of language, in *The Genesis of Language*, eds. F. Smith and G. A. Miller. Cambridge Mass.: M.I.T. Press, (1966).

Maslow, P. and others, The Marianne Frostig Developmental Test of Visual Perception, 1963 Standardization. *Percep. Motor Skills*, 19, 463-499 (1964).

McGraw, M. D., *The Neuromuscular Maturation of the Human Infant*. New York: Hafner, (1963).

Pascal, G., and B. Suttell, *The Bender-Gestalt Test: Quantification and Validity for Adults*. New York: Grune and Stratton, (1951).

Riley, G. D., *Motor Problems Inventory: Manual*. Los Angeles: Western Psychological Services, (1972).

Sloan, W., The Lincoln-Oseretsky Motor Development Scale. *Genetic Psych. Monogr.*, 51, 183-252 (1955).

Wertheimer, W., Studies in the theory of Gestalt Psychology. *Psychol. Forsch*, Vol. 4 (1923).

PART III

Examination of the Speech-Production Mechanism

VII

Physiology without anatomy is unfounded, anatomy without physiology is useless.

Franz Joseph Gall

The examination of the speech-production mechanism is very much a descriptive task. There are observations to be made and behaviors to be quantified, but there are no psychometrically based tests to aid in these tasks. Similarly, the data obtained typically does not allow a determination of adequacy from computation of a derived score that can be compared to normative data because the reference for adequacy lies within the experience of the examiner and not within the numbers tables. It is of paramount importance, then, that the examiner make his observations systematically and with an understanding of why the patient is asked to perform each task.

Two evaluations are made as part of the examination. The first entails a determination of structural integrity. This involves a careful description of the size, shape, and relationship of the speech-production structures. Functional integrity, the second consideration, involves determining the adequacy of the system for producing speech-related movements. Structure and function are not separable, but we have divided the evaluation into these two parts because some of the observations are made of skeletal, dental, and muscular structures at rest while others are made while the structures are executing speech-related movements.

Few aspects of the appraisal of speech disorders are treated in such a cursory and perfunctory manner as the speech mechanism examination. This relatively superficial treatment of an integral part of the appraisal has resulted because clinicians frequently do not have a clear understanding of what they are looking for and the inferences they are to draw from what they find. The examination does not take long to complete, is not unusually difficult, and is as important and should be as routine as the audiological evaluation.

The idea that the oral-peripheral examination of the patient is as integral a part of patient assessment as auditory testing brings up an important point. Audiological procedures are geared toward determining the anatomic and functional integrity of the hearing mechanism. An otoscopic examination and tympanometry are carried out to determine the status of the tympanic membrane-ossicular chain system, and test batteries are used to assess the integrity of the auditory nerve and higher neural functions of audition. The audiologic examination, then, is essentially an evaluation of a set of structures and the neural mechanisms that subserve them. Likewise, an examination of the speech-production mechanism is an evaluation of structures and the neural mechanisms responsible for their innervation.

Perusal of any standard neurology text (DeJong 1958; Brain and Walton 1969; Alpers and Mancall 1971) quickly reveals the close similarity between procedures used by the speech pathologist during the course of the oral-peripheral examination and the cranial nerve examination of the neurologist. The two examinations have similarities, but they are by no means identical. The cranial nerve examination involves testing the sensory and/or motor functions of each of the highly specialized cranial nerves for evidence of peripheral or central nervous system damage. The oral-peripheral examination entails the evaluation of only some of the nerves. It is abbreviated to the extent that some motor functions, such as eye movements, and some sensory processes, such as olfaction and taste, are omitted or only screened while highly integrated execution of speech movements are evaluated in detail. It is an extension of the cranial nerve examination as well because respiratory muscles, whose innervation is by means of the spinal nerves, also are examined. A listing of the cranial nerves and an abbreviated description of their functions are provided in Table 7-1.

Before considering the procedures of the oral examination, several aspects of speech production need to be examined. First, speech is an overlaid function since the primary role of the respiratory, laryngeal, and articulatory systems are the maintenance of life-support systems by means of vegetative breathing and feeding. Consequently, it is readily apparent that the speech mechanism is capable of producing muscular forces and structural displacements, velocities and accelerations considerably greater than are normally necessary for speech production. Two examples may suffice to demonstrate this point. We have all seen the circus performer who hangs by her teeth from the high trapeze. She is capable of developing enough force between her teeth to support her weight. Speech

Table 7-1 The cranial nerves and their functions (abbreviated)

Cranial Nerve	Function
I. Olfactory	Sense of smell
II. Optic	Vision
III. Oculomotor	Eye movement
IV. Trochlear	
VI. Abducens	
V. Trigeminal	Jaw movements Sensation for face
VII. Facial	Facial movements Taste for anterior two-thirds of tongue
VIII. Auditory	Hearing Maintenance of equilibrium
IX. Glossopharyngeal	Pharyngeal movements Sensation to soft palate and pharynx Taste to posterior third of tongue
X. Vagus	Sensation for pharynx, larynx Thoracic and abdominal viscera Pharyngeal and laryngeal movements
XI. Spinal Accessory	Shoulder girdle movements
XII. Hypoglossal	Tongue movements

activities, in comparison, never approximate these maximal abilities of the masticatory musculature. Similarly, if we examined the average subglottal pressure needed for speech production, we would find it to be approximately 5 to 10 cm H_2O while the respiratory unit is capable of producing pressures in excess of 50 cm H_2O, such as during heavy lifting. We must be aware then that the tasks we ask the patient to perform are well within the physiological capabilities of a normal adult or child.

In light of the significant differences between typical and maximal performance, it is not surprising that the speech-production apparatus is capable of substantial compensations for structural or functional inadequacies. Examples are readily available for both speech-impaired and normal speakers. Children with repaired cleft lip who have reduced lip tissue and scarring continue to produce bilabial plosives. In fact, bilabial plosives are one of the least frequent types of errors for repaired-cleft speakers. Similarly, speakers with partial or complete glossectomy (partial or complete resection of the tongue) may produce speech that is only minimally reduced in intelligibility.

The functional compensatory abilities of normal speakers also have been demonstrated. Lindblom and Sundberg (1971) and Lindblom, Lubker, and Gay

(1978) have shown that normal speakers can produce formant frequencies with bite blocks between their teeth, at the first glottal pulse of a vowel, that approximate those of an unimpeded condition. This suggests that the speech-production mechanism is capable of substantial and immediate reorganizational abilities. Moreover, Hixon, Mead, and Goldman (1976) observed that subjects maintained a relatively constant subglottal pressure during speech, using widely varying patterns of muscular forces while standing and sitting, positions in which the force of gravity would have considerably different effects. More informal examples are the ability to produce speech while eating or with a pipe between the teeth without a significant reduction in intelligibility. The point to be made is that the speech-production mechanism is capable of significant compensation for typical or novel constraints imposed on its activity.

When maximal compensation has been reached, it appears that any additional psychological or physiological loading has the effect of deteriorating performance. Indirect evidence is readily available for aphasic patients who demonstrate reduced performance when fatigued or under emotional stress and for stutterers who typically have a greater number of disfluencies when in situations of great communicative demand. Knowledge of the patient's condition at the time of testing is therefore important to making inferences regarding the integrity of the speech-production apparatus and may offer information on probable prognosis as well.

Articulatory structures are variable even in a "normal" group of speakers. If dental configurations were used as an example, it would be found that less than half the population has what could be described as "normal" dentition. Likewise there are variations in tongue size, palatal vault height, and size of the mandible. More than for almost any other group of judgments to be made, the variations on normal will have to be considered in determining the anatomic integrity of the patient being examined, as well as the significance of the deviations in relation to the speech presented.

Finally, the entire examination should be completed even if only a part of the speech-production apparatus is involved. If you have a medical examination, the physician will evaluate a number of systems: neurological, cardiovascular, genito-urinary, and so on, whether you have an ulcer or head trauma, which points out the fact that no system of an organism is functionally independent. The examination should be completed in its entirety, whether the source of the problem is limited, such as in acquired quadriplegia due to an upper spinal cord lesion, or involves the entire speech-production system, such as in Parkinson's disease.

We will present some procedures for evaluating the speech-production mechanism including the voice evaluation and oral-peripheral examination. The descriptions should not be considered exhaustive, but rather, representative. Other descriptions of these examinations are provided by Darley, Aronson, and Brown (1975), Dworkin (1978), Mason (1969), and Mason and Simon (1977).

EVALUATION OF RESPIRATORY AND LARYNGEAL SYSTEMS

The respiratory system is relatively resistant to disease processes and traumatic lesions that would affect the development of air pressures and air flows necessary for speech production. This is perhaps related to the crucial role of respiration for the maintenance of an oxygen supply to the cells of the body. Witness to this is the patient with a traumatic lesion to the spinal cord at the fifth cervical vertebrae. Although the affects of this type of lesion are to produce a quadriplegia with paralysis of some of the respiratory muscles, the patient continues to be able to produce speech with only a minimal impairment since intelligible speech does not require more than tidal volume. Respiratory deficits that effect phonation and articulation relate more to the inability to coordinate respiratory activities with laryngeal and upper airway functions. Consider the patient with congenital cerebral palsy of an athetoid type who begins expiration and then suddenly stops due to involuntary movement resulting from contraction of the inspiratory musculature. This patient has sufficient respiratory activity to maintain life and to generate pressures and flows but cannot adequately control the input and output of the respiratory unit for speech production. Since the respiratory and laryngeal processes are so closely related, they are typically examined together as part of the evaluation of the speech-production mechanism.

THE VOICE EVALUATION

Evaluation of voice disorders can be divided into two broad categories: history of the problem and examination of the respiratory-phonatory system. It is assumed that a general history will have been obtained by interview so that this portion of the history will relate specifically to the voice disorder itself. It is also assumed that patients with voice disorders will be evaluated for other than respiratory and laryngeal dysfunction. An example of a voice evaluation form is included in Figure 7-1.

History of the Problem. The case history information we discussed in Chapter II was general in purpose. Voice and a number of other problems require further specific background. A voice history will entail a self-description of the problem by the patient and a general history of the problem as deduced from the patient's history and collateral information, such as results of medical examinations, vocational and family history, and so on.

The self-description of the voice problem should include questions regarding the nature of the problem–what does the voice problem sound like and feel like; the severity of the problem–how significantly does it effect the communication process; the effect of the problem–how "bad" is the problem, and how

VOICE EVALUATION

A. HISTORY OF SPEECH DISORDER

1. Patient's description of the problem
   Severity____
   Effect on communication______________________________
   Etiology ____
2. Development of the Problem
   Onset____
   Progression ____
   Consistency ____
   Duration ____
3. Previous Voice Evaluations or Therapy
   ____
4. Vocal Habits
   Occupation____
   Vocal Abuse ____
5. Additional Significant History
   Familial____
   Medical ____
   Social____
   Emotional (concern for problem)_____________________
   ____

B. RESPIRATORY AND LARYNGEAL EXAMINATION

1. Respiratory Efficiency

   Observations of breathing: Clavicular ______________
   Abdominal ____________________Thoracic______________
   Shortness of breath_________________________________
   Audible breathing___________________________________

   Breath Control:
   Counts on one breath________________________________
   Sustain a, i, or u: Trials _____ _____ _____
   Prolong voiceless fricative /s/_____ _____ _____
   Prolong voiced fricative /z/ _____ _____ _____

   Muscular tension of the chest and neck which appear to be related to breath supply and control?_____________________________
   ____

2. Laryngeal Observations

   Tension____
   Muscular contractions exhibited during phonation which are similar to those exhibited during swallowing___________________
   ____
   Indirect Laryngoscopy _______________________________
   ____

Figure 7-1 Example Voice Evaluation Form

C. PHONATION

1. Pitch
   Subjective appropriateness ______________________
   Habitual Pitch ______________________
   Pitch Range (# of notes) ______________________
   Optimum Pitch ______________________

   Pitch Control
   Discrimination ______________________
   Imitation of high, medium, and low pitches ______________________
   ____
   Production of a tone ______________________
   Imitation of upward and downward inflectional patterns ______________________
   ____
   Ability to maintain steady pitch ______________________
   ____

2. Loudness
   Subjective appropriateness for situations

   Ability to alter loudness:
   Imitate soft, medium, and loud sounds ______________________
   ____
   Glide from loud to soft during production of vowels ______________________
   ____
   Discrimination of loudness ______________________

3. Quality
   Type of Disorder

Breathy	________	Harsh	________	Hoarse	________
Denasal	________	Nasal	________	Aphonia	________

   Severity ______________________

Changes in Quality during:	Reading	Prolonging Vowels
Vary Pitch	________	________
Vary Loudness	________	________
Vary Rate	________	________
During Physical Exertion	________	________
During Exaggeration of Articulatory Movements	________	________

4. Related Observations
   Pitch Breaks ________ Phonation Breaks ________
   Hard Glottal Attack ________ Glottal Fry ________
   Spastic Dysphonia ________ Other ________
   ____

D. Oral Peripheral Examination

E. Hearing Screening

Figure 7-1 Example Voice Evaluation Form (continued)

"different" does the voice sound; and the etiology of the problem according to the patient. The purpose of this portion of the history taking is to evaluate the patient's view of the nature, severity, etiology, and effect of the voice problem. Murphy (1964) has developed a series of twenty questions (see list that follows) to explore the vocal psychodynamics of the patient.

Questions to Elicit Patient's Self-Description and Self-Perception of His Problem*

1. What do you think about your voice?
2. What do others think about your voice?
3. Do you pay attention to the voices of others? What do you notice?
4. Do you think you can learn about others through their voices?
5. How do you judge other people's voices?
6. Do you compare your voice with the voices of others?
7. What kind of voices do you like? Dislike? Why?
8. What would you like others to think about your voice?
9. What impression does your voice really make?
10. Is your voice different with people who are older? Younger? Males? Females? How? Why?
11. Should a man's voice be masculine?
12. Should a woman's voice be feminine?
13. What do you think about the strength of your voice?
14. What do you think about the health of your voice box (throat, larynx, vocal folds)?
15. What should a good voice be?
16. What kind of voice do you want?
17. Do you think you can improve your voice?
18. How important is it to you to improve your voice?
19. What do you think caused or is causing your voice difficulty?
20. Anything else about your voice we haven't mentioned?

The general history of the voice problem will explore other aspects of the development of the voice problem. When did it begin? Was there a sudden or gradual onset? Has the problem become progresssively worse, or has the course of the problem been characterized by plateaus and intermittent remissions? Has the problem been previously evaluated and treated? If so, by whom? Is the problem consistent or does it appear to be affected by voice usage, time of day, and so forth? The patient's voice usage habits should be explored in detail if there appears to be hyperfunction. The results of medical examinations, previous therapy, general medical history, and social familial history should be explored with care. The important thing for you to remember in obtaining information is that you want to gain all the information possible about the patient and her disorder before, during and following its onset. The importance of this exploration of the problem cannot be underestimated because of the host of metabolic, traumatic, neurologic, and emotional factors that produce voice disorders.

*From Albert T. Murphy, *Functional Voice Disorders,* p. 92. Copyright 1964 by Prentice-Hall, Inc., Englewood Cliffs, New Jersey. Reprinted by permission.

The interview process also allows the examiner to note important aspects of the voice disorder that will require further exploration. For example, is habitual pitch appropriate to the patient's age and sex? Is loudness suitable to the situation? Is the patient breathy, hoarse, harsh? What are voice usage patterns?

Physical Examination. The examiner should carefully observe respiratory and laryngeal characteristics. The type of vegetative and speech respiratory patterns should be noted. Normally, the only respiratory pattern of particular concern is the use of clavicular breathing. Clavicular breathing involves upward movement of the clavicles to increase the size of the respiratory unit. It is of concern because it is less efficient than thoracic-abdominal breathing patterns and because it may bring about tension in extrinsic laryngeal muslces. Any shortness of breath and struggle to breath should be noted. The tension in the accessory (extrinsic) muscles of the larynx should be observed because vocal hyperfunction is frequently evidenced by an increase in extrinsic laryngeal muscle tension. The tension can be noted by palpation of the neck musculature during phonation of vowels, counting, and conversational speech.

Considerable controversy exists regarding the role of the speech pathologist in the indirect examination of the larynx. Needless to say, every individual with a voice problem that you are asked to examine should be evaluated by a laryngologist before proceeding with therapy since it is the physician's task to differentially diagnose the disorder and to provide surgical and drug therapy if deemed necessary. In some cases medical treatment must proceed any direct voice therapy that may be considered. This point is made by Boone (1977):

> No voice therapy should begin in any setting, with any aged patient until a laryngologist has examined the patient's vocal apparatus and recommended such therapy.

What then is the speech pathologist's role in indirect observation of laryngeal structure and function? We agree with the statement of Moore (1957):

> The (indirect laryngoscopy) examination technique can and should be learned by the voice pathologist, since it is a help to be able to observe laryngeal conditions and to follow the changes which occur in the course of therapy. It should be emphasized, however, that the diagnosing of laryngeal diseases and disorders is the province and responsibility of the laryngologist.

The physical examination, therefore, should involve a careful observation of respiratory patterns, laryngeal extrinsic musculature tension, and indirect laryngoscopy. Indirect laryngoscopy is utilized to note the status of the larynx and to follow the course of laryngeal changes resulting from therapy, but is never utilized to make differential diagnoses which are clearly the province of the physician. Indirect laryngoscopy requires a minimum of time, a limited number of inexpensive instruments, and an average degree of dexterity. The patient is seated with knees together, head tilted slightly forward and chin up. The examiner is seated on a stool approximately level with the patient's knees and directly in front. A light is positioned behind and slightly to the right of the patient's head. A head mirror is worn by the examiner and is used to focus a beam of light on to a laryngeal mirror introduced into the oral cavity. With the tongue firmly held with a piece of gauze by the examiner and with the back of the mirror lifting the soft palate, a slight rotation of the mirror will allow visualization of the laryngeal structures. Structures should be examined in a serial order. A detailed discussion of these procedures is provided by Netter (1964). The student should practice these procedures with careful attention to detail and under the direct supervision of a physician or speech pathologist trained in these techniques before attempting to utilize it in the course of therapy or diagnosis.

Determining Respiratory Efficiency. Several tasks may be utilized to provide information about the efficiency with which the patient utilizes the respiratory system for phonation. One method is to ask the patient to count as far as possible on one breath after being provided with a rate-of-count model of approximately three digits per second (Boone 1977). The length of time she is able to count and the number of digits produced is recorded. Additionally, information regarding total performance is noted such as how does the patient maximally inspire and how well does she sustain exhalation. A similar task is to ask the patient to prolong a vowel such as /a/, /i/ or /u/ as long as possible at a comfortable pitch and loudness level. The average of three productions then can be compared to norms available regarding maximal performance (Ptacek and Sander 1963; Yanagihara and Koike 1967; Yanagihara and others 1966). For example, Ptacek and Sander found maximum phonation time for vowels averaged 25 seconds for men and 17 seconds for women. The presence of voice tremor, intermittent arrests of the voice, and intermittent waxing and waning of loudness are noted. Another method of determining the ability to sustain expiration is to ask the patient to read as many words as possible from a selected passage without renewing his air supply. A related task is to ask the patient to prolong the voiceless fricative /s/ as long as possible. This provides information on how well the patient can maintain expiration without phonation. The patient is then asked to produce the voiced cognate /z/ as long as possible. Typically the patient without vocal pathology will be able to maintain each of the fricatives the same length of time while the patient with vocal-fold pathology will be unable to maintain the voiced fricative as long as the voiceless due to reduced phonatory efficiency, assuming that velopharyngeal functioning is within normal limits. Boone (1977) suggested this as a rapid method of determining how much of the phonation problem is related to poor respiratory control.

Several types of information can be obtained from these procedures. First, the ability of the patient to sustain a controlled exhalation with and without phonation can be discussed. Second, the relative efficiency of phonation can be determined by comparing the duration of sustained productions of voiced and voiceless fricatives. Third, reductions in maximal performance can be noted for sustained vowels. Although this information may be of some value, remember that normal speech production typically does not require a maximal effort on the part of the patient.

Evaluation of Aspects of Phonation. Several important aspects of the phonatory process typically are examined as part of the voice evaluation. These include pitch, loudness, and quality. Each of these parameters of voice production will be considered individually although the reader should be aware that these processes are intricately related.

Pitch. Earlier in our discussion we noted that you should make some judgment during the initial interview as to whether the voice pitch of the patient is "too high" or "too low" in relation to the patient's age and sex. Additionally, you will want to obtain information regarding the patient's habitual pitch, optimal pitch, and pitch range.

Habitual pitch is the central tendency of pitches used by an individual (Fairbanks 1960). As such, it represents a range that may be influenced by situational variables and the emotional status of the patient. Several methods may be utilized to determine habitual pitch. One suggested by Boone (1977) as the easiest and most valid involves the recording of conversational speech and oral reading from the patient during the first visit to the clinic. The speech sample is then analyzed by stopping the tape recorder at selected points and attempting to match the patient's habitual pitch by means of a pitch pipe. This is accomplished by starting at approximately the mean fundamental frequency of male or female speakers (128 Hz or C_3 for males, 213 Hz or A_3 for adult females, 256 Hz or C_4 for prepubertal child) and then moving by gradations (sharps and flats) until the habitual pitch is approximated (the distribution of fundamental frequency for males and females is presented in Figure 7-2). This procedure should be repeated seven or eight times or more during the course of analyzing the speech sample. The modal pitch (most frequently occurring) is determined and designated as the patient's habitual pitch. Boone suggests that utilizing modal rather than mean pitch offers a more valid estimate of habitual pitch.

Another method of determining habitual pitch has been suggested by Fairbanks (1960). A reading sample of approximately 180 words is selected. The selection is divided into three 60 word segments. During the reading of the first 60 words, normal inflectional patterns are utilized by the patient. During the reading of the second 60 words, the patient is asked to compress the range

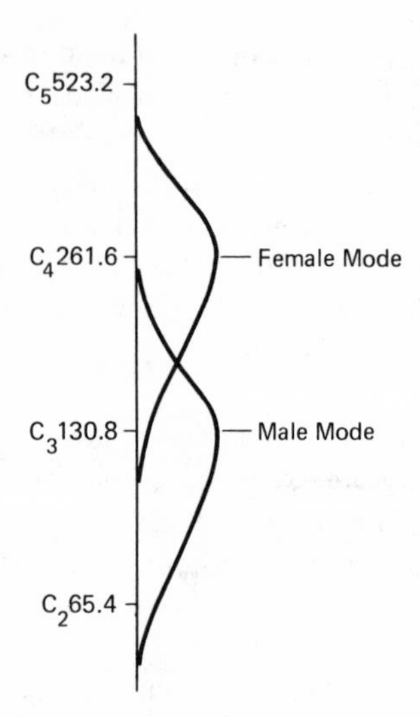

Figure 7-2 Distribution of Fundamental Frequency for Males and Females. (From W. Zemlin, ***Speech and Hearing Science.*** Englewood Cliffs, N.J., Prentice-Hall, Inc., 1968. By permission.)

until by the end of this section he is chanting in a monotone. He should then complete the reading utilizing this monotone and finish with a humming or singing of notes equal to his habitual pitch. A pitch pipe or piano then can be utilized to identify the habitual pitch. The whole procedure may be repeated to determine the accuracy of the estimate. Other procedures utilized to determine habitual pitch include asking the patient to sing a tone without a model and then attempting to match the produced tone on a pitch pipe or piano. Similarly, the patient can be asked to count to ten and then to prolong a vowel, the pitch of the vowel being determined with a pitch pipe. Repetition of these procedures will allow a determination of modal habitual pitch.

The total pitch range can be determined by asking the patient to sing up and down the scale. Boone (1977) suggested that this be accomplished by providing the patient with three-second models of the tones to be produced (recorded by a male, female, or child). The patient is asked to match each tone and to take a breath between each production. The patient is first asked to match notes to the lowest tone, then to go up the scale to the highest notes she can produce including the falsetto, matching tones back down to the lowest note and then back up to the highest note again. This procedure provides an estimate of the total pitch range of the patient. The total number of tones is recorded. The examiner should be aware, however, that patients will not be equally skilled in matching tones.

Optimum pitch is the perceptual correlate of the maximal efficiency of vibration of the vocal folds. This suggests that the vocal folds have an optimal rate of vibration determined by their length, mass, and natural elasticity. A number of methods have been suggested for estimating the optimal frequency of vibration.

1. Determine the total pitch range including falsetto. Optimum pitch is located one-fourth of the way from the bottom of the pitch range. For adult females, it may be one to two notes below the one-fourth level (Fairbanks 1960).
2. Determine the total pitch range excluding falsetto. One-third of the distance from the bottom of the pitch range will be the optimum pitch.
3. Ask patient to take a deep breath and intone "ah" on expiration (Murphy 1964).
4. Ask patient to grunt "ah" or "oh," gradually prolonging the utterances until a passage is chanted at the original grunt pitch level (Murphy 1964).
5. Ask patient to stop up his ears and sing "ah" or hum "m" up and down the scale until the pitch level at which the tone swells or is louder is identified (Murphy 1964).
6. Cough sonorously on an /i/ sound (Murphy 1964).
7. Yawn and sigh should produce optimum pitch (Boone 1977).
8. Say "un'huh" and note pitch (Boone 1977).

After an optimal pitch level has been determined the patient may be asked to produce several vowels and words to help substantiate the determined pitch. These procedures will reveal approximately the same optimal pitch level. Fisher (1966) suggests that the optimal pitch in normal speakers fulfills several requirements: (1) it is within the pitch range where maximal vocal fold efficiency of vibration is located; (2) there are at least four notes below the modal optimum pitch for downward intonations; and (3) there is at least an octave above modal optimum pitch for upward intonations. She suggested further that the habitual (modal) pitch should be changed if it is less than four notes above the lowest note that can be phonated clearly or if the modal pitch is as much as two notes from optimum pitch. Finally, she suggested that ten notes is the minimal range of intonation required for production of "factual" speech. This range will include three notes below the modal pitch and six notes above the optimal modal pitch. Moreover, she suggests that an increase in the upper range interval (from modal optimal pitch to the highest pitch) will increase the effectiveness of speech more surely than any other one device. Wilson (1978) has provided composite tables of mean fundamental frequency and acceptable fundamental frequency limits for males and females between one and 18 years of age that the examiner may find of value in determining the appropriateness of habitual pitch levels (see Table 7-2).

Pitch-control skills also are evaluated if the habitual pitch of the patient is to be changed to optimal pitch. Van Riper (1978) recommended that the following pitch skills be examined: (1) ability to discriminate between two pitches which differ in a single note (these can be sung or played on a piano or

Table 7-2 Fundamental frequency and acceptable ranges of fundamental frequency for males and females from one to eighteen years of age (Wilson 1978). Values at eighteen years would be expected to approximate fundamental frequency for adults.

	Age	*Fundamental Frequency*	*Acceptable Limits of Fundamental Frequency*	*Nearest Musical Note to Fundamental Frequency*	*Acceptable Limits of Fundamental Frequency in Musical Notes*
		Hz	*Hz*		
	1 & 2	445	370-525	A_4	$F\#_4$-C_6
	3	400	340-460	G_4	F_4-$A\#_4$
	4	375	320-425	$F\#_4$	$D\#_4$-$G\#_4$
	5	350	300-390	F_4	D_4-G_4
	6	325	280-365	E_4	$C\#_4$-$F\#_4$
	7	295	260-330	D_4	C_4-E_4
	8	295	260-330	D_4	C_4-E_4
Male	9	260	220-300	C_4	A_3-D_4
	10	235	195-275	$A\#_3$	G_3-$C\#_4$
	11	225	185-260	A_3	$F\#_3$-C_4
	12	210	170-245	$G\#_3$	F_3-B_3
	13	195	155-230	G_3	$D\#_3$-$A\#_3$
	14	190	155-220	$F\#_3$	$D\#_3$-A_3
	15	165	130-195	E_3	C_3-G_3
	16	150	120-180	D_3	$A\#_2$-$F\#_3$
	17	135	110-170	$C\#_3$	A_2-F_3
	18	125	100-155	B_2	G_2-$D\#_3$

pitch pipe); (2) ability to hum at high, medium, and low pitches after they are presented by the examiner; (3) ability to produce a tune alone or in conjunction with the examiner; and (4) ability to follow upward and downward inflectional patterns. Finally, the ability to maintain a steady pitch for a specified period of time should be examined.

Loudness. Loudness can be defined as the perceptual correlate of acoustic energy produced by the speech mechanism. Two aspects of the loudness parameter are considered in the voice evaluation: (1) its suitability to the conversational setting, and (2) the ability of the patient to volitionally alter it. Appropriateness of the loudness level used by the patient can be assessed by requesting that he produce levels consistent with situations. For example, the examiner should gradually move away from the patient and ask him to produce speech consistent with the distance from the examiner. Ability to control loudness can be assessed by asking the patient to sustain tones at soft, medium,

Table 7-2 Fundamental frequency and acceptable ranges of fundamental frequency for males and females from one to eighteen years of age (Wilson 1978). Values at eighteen years would be expected to approximate fundamental frequency for adults. (continued)

	Age	*Fundamental Frequency*	*Acceptable Limits of Fundamental Frequency*	*Nearest Musical Note to Fundamental Frequency*	*Acceptable Limits of Fundamental Frequency in Musical Notes*
		Hz	*Hz*		
Female	1 & 2	445	370-525	A_4	$F\#_4$-C_6
	3	380	335-475	$F\#_4$	E_4-$A\#_4$
	4	355	310-450	F_4	$D\#_4$-A_4
	5	335	290-425	E_4	D_4-$G\#_4$
	6	315	270-395	$D\#_4$	$C\#_4$-G_4
	7	280	245-310	$C\#_4$	B_3-$D\#_4$ (F_4)[a]
	8	290	245-350	D_4	B_3-F_4
	9	275	235-335	$C\#_4$	$A\#_3$-E_4
	10	265	225-320	C_4	A_3-$D\#_4$
	11	265	220-310	C_4	A_3-$D\#_4$
	12	260	220-310	C_4	$G\#_3$-D_4
	13I[b]	260	235-295	C_4	$A\#_3$-D_4
	13II[b]	245	210-295	B_3	$G\#_3$-D_4
	14	235	195-270	$A\#_3$	G_3-$C\#_4$
	15	220	185-260	A_3	$F\#_3$-C_4
	16	215	185-260	A_3	$F\#_3$-C_4
	17	210	175-245	$G\#_3$	F_3-C_4
	18	205	175-245	$G\#_3$	F_3-B_3

[a] Preferred upper limit.
[b] 13I = premenarche; 13II = postmenarche.

From D. Kenneth Wilson, Voice Problems of Children *2nd ed. Baltimore: Williams and Wilkins, (1978). By permission.*

and high intensity levels, to imitate loudness of sustained sounds and words presented by the examiner, and to glide from loud to soft during production of vowels. Finally, the ability to discriminate different loudness levels can be determined by presenting two tones of differing loudness and asking the patient to judge which of the two was louder. This procedure is facilitated by having pairs of words or vowels tape-recorded and ready for use. Reduced variation in loudness during conversational speech also is noted. Typically, loudness problems are indicative of psychological or organic problems. The examiner also should remember that there is no optimal loudness level for an individual—loudness depends upon the situation in which the patient finds herself.

Quality. A wide variety of terms have been utilized to describe voice quality problems. We will utilize only four: breathiness, harshness, hoarseness, and nasality. Breathiness is voice quality characterized by an audible escape of air. Harshness is typified by aperiodicity of vocal-fold vibration and is usually accompanied by hard glottal attacks and low pitch. Hoarseness is defined as a combination of breathiness and harshness with both audible escape of air and aperiodicity of vocal-fold vibration.

Two types of abnormal nasal resonance typically are identified as part of the voice evaluation. Hypernasality is a voice-quality disorder due to abnormal coupling of the oral and nasal cavities and is characterized acoustically by anti-resonances and reduced formant frequencies. Denasality is produced by abnormal reduction in the amount of coupling typically utilized for production of nasalized consonants such as /m/ and /n/. Insofar as voice-quality disorders are due to problems at the level of the larynx, hyper- and hyponasality are not voice problems but articulation problems. That is, the phonemes are inappropriately articulated–either as nasal resonance where oral resonance is expected, or as a lack of nasality on intended nasal phonemes. Fairbanks' (1960) definition, for example, was:

> The test of the existence of a voice quality disorder is whether or not the quality that is heard is independent of phonemes, or, in other words, whether or not the phenomenon heard can be superimposed upon a good example of a voiced sound.

By that definition, hyper- and hyponasality are *not* voice-quality disorders. From a remediation standpoint, the therapeutic regime for abnormalities of nasal resonance will usually have some features common to articulation therapy, and some procedures similar to voice therapy.

Several procedures should be utilized to estimate voice-quality disturbances. By this time in the evaluation you will have collected and taped a number of speech samples from the patient and should be able to describe and estimate the severity of the disorder from these samples. If these samples are insufficient, you may wish to obtain a sample of connected speech, oral reading, and isolated production of vowels and voiced continuants. From careful listening an estimate of the disorder can be obtained and recorded on a rating scale which considers breathiness, hoarseness, and harshness.

Secondly, the effects of varying pitch, loudness, and rate on voice quality should be evaluated. Ask the patient to read a speech sample and prolong vowels at lower and higher than habitual pitch levels, at higher and lower than habitual loudness levels and at faster and slower than habitual rates. Examine the effects of physical exertion and relaxation on voice quality by requesting that the patient produce words or an extended vowel during pushing or pulling activities and during relaxation. Finally, note whether voice quality is improved when articulatory movement is exaggerated during the reading of a passage. Pay careful attention to the presence of laryngeal extrinsic musculature tension during these activities. Also carefully note the presence and frequency of hard glottal attacks during production of conversational speech and reading. Wilson (1978) provides rating scales for estimating the amount of vocal abuse produced by a patient. The scales include vocal abuse categories of shouting, screaming, cheering, excessive talking, strained vocalizations, reverse phonation, explosive release of vocalizations, abrupt glottal attack, throat clearing, coughing, talking in noise, and other factors. Each category is rated in amount (0 = none; 1 = little; 2 = frequent; 3 = excessive) and degree (1 = mild; 2 = moderate; 3 = severe). Although these ratings can be completed as part of the voice evaluation, other persons acquainted with the patient such as teachers, friends, and relatives may also need to be interviewed.

Summary of Voice Evaluation. These procedures should yield a large body of information regarding the patient's voice problem including presenting complaint, history of the disorder, habitual pitch, pitch range, optimal pitch, habitual loudness level and ability to alter loudness, type of voice-quality disturbance, and the effects of rate, loudness, and pitch on overall quality, respiratory and laryngeal efficiency, and the types of abusive vocal behavior utilized by the patient. From the information gained a prognosis should be made and appropriate therapy instituted, if warranted.

Prognosis in Voice Disorders. Prognosis will depend on many factors including the etiology of the disorder, the duration of the problem, the severity of the disorder, and the motivation of the patient. Obviously all medical, social, vocational, and speech and language evaluation results must be considered carefully in order to determine prognosis. A sample behavioral prognostic checklist for "functional" voice disorders has been developed by Murphy (1964). The checklist include eleven vocal (for example, severity and complexity of the voice disorders, loudness level, respiration, articulation), five auditory (hearing acuity, sound discrimination, ability to imitate vocal sounds, ability to carry a melody, auditory memory span), fourteen psychosocial (for example, general level of emotional adjustment, absence of associated symptoms, self-defensive behavior, general nonverbal spontaneity), and three miscellaneous criteria (intelligence, general physical condition, other) which are rated as inferior, below average, average, above average, or superior. The checklist also includes a rating of overall prognosis for improvement. Murphy indicated that the rating scale is for "discussion" purposes only. However, if it is coupled with other information about the patient and his problem, it may prove to be a valuable tool. An accurate prognosis can only be made by someone with "all the facts" and the clinical experience to evaluate them.

EXAMINATION OF THE ORAL-FACIAL SPEECH MECHANISM

The purpose of the examination of the speech mechanism is to describe the status and function of the articulatory and resonatory systems. As such, it is an important part of *any and all* speech and language evaluations and should be carried out in a systematic and efficient fashion. This section will describe the procedures involved in conducting this portion of the examination. An example of an oral-peripheral examination form is included in Figure 7-3.

Positioning of the Client. Mason (1969) has described how the patient should be positioned. He should be in a posture that most clearly approximates that which he uses during speaking. Typically, this involves positioning the client in an erect position in a chair, with eyes focused directly forward. Except when we are making structural evaluations of the palate, the client should not tilt his head backward for the intraoral examination. Studies (McWilliams, Musgrave, and Crozier 1968) have shown that modifications of a "natural" head posture can distort normal muscle relationships in the head and neck and produce physiologic differences which do not reflect normal function during speech production. Therefore, the patient should sit with the head in a natural upright position with his mouth aligned on a horizontal plane with the eye level of the examiner.

Facial Musculature. The head and neck should be examined carefully. Any scars on the side of the head and neck should be noted. The symmetry of the face should be examined at rest. Drooping of the corner of the lip, or ptosis (partial or complete closure of the eyelid) may indicate weakness. If upper-lip scarring is observed, the amount of upper-lip tissue, shape of the scar, and tightness of the upper lip should be recorded. Drooling, lack of forehead wrinkling on one side, and incomplete labial closure also are indicative of muscle weakness.

Voluntary nonspeech movements should be tested. Ask the patient to smile, and note if the corners of the lips move equally on each side. Request she pucker her lips, and note if this activity is symmetrical. Reduced movement is suggestive of weakness. Ask her to blow out her cheeks and seal air in her mouth. Press gently on each cheek to determine if the labial seal is broken and air escapes. Reduced ability to maintain intraoral pressure is suggestive of weakness on that side of the face.

Mandibular Musculature. At rest, the mandible is examined to determine if it droops on one side compared to the other. If the jaw deviates to one side or the other when it is maximally opened, it suggests weakness on the side toward which it deviates. The examiner should also test the strength of jaw depressors and elevators by requesting that the patient overcome the resistance

Name:______________________________Sex:____________Birthdate:_________Case No:_______

Referral reason:__________________________________By:_______________________________

Examiner:____Date:_____________________________

STRUCTURE (JUDGEMENT)

L	T	Te	A	P	
					Normal Structure
					Slight deviation--probably no adverse effect on speech
					Moderate deviation--possible adverse effect on speech; remedial services may be required, particularly if other structures of speech are also deviant
					Extreme deviation--sufficient to prevent normal production of speech; modification of structure required, either with or without clinical speech services

(L-Lips; T-Tongue; Te-Teeth; A-Dental Arch; P-Palate)

FUNCTION--Diadochokinesis

Average of three trials of 5 second duration each.

Single syllables: puh, tuh, kuh
Lip Approximation:
(puh) ____, ____, ____, average per second ____

Tongue-tip-alveolar:
(tuh) ____, ____, ____, average per second ____

Back-tongue-palate:
(kuh) ____, ____, ____, average per second ____
Combined syllables: (puh-tuh-kuh) ____, ____, ____ average per second ____
Gag reflex ___________ (present or absent)

****

If no significant deviations in structure or function, the form can be discontinued at this point. Continue with following page for more description, especially when deviations are noted.

Figure 7-3 Sample Oral Examination Form

From W. Johnson, F. L. Darley, and D. C. Spriestersbach, ***Diagnostic Methods in Speech Pathology.*** New York: Harper & Row, 1963. By permission.

(Indicate severity of deviation with description)
NOSE - structural deviations____
Function______________________________(structure, etc.)______________

LIPS - structural deviations ____________________(repaired) ____________
cleft: Right___Left ____Bilat. ______Includes premaxilla______________
corners retract: bilaterally ___________symmetrically___________________
Unilaterally: Right ___________Left ____________________

MANDIBLE AND DENTAL STRUCTURES:
Mandible: Normal ________Prognathic ___Retruded______
Occlusion: Normal ______Neutrocclusion ___Distocclusion ______
Mesiocclusion ______(relative to first molars)
Lateral relationship: Normal _____Crossbite R____L______
Overbite: Normal ____Open ____Closed______
Condition of teeth:____

PALATE:
Hard palate: shape ______ arch_______width _______
cleft ______
Soft palate: short _____tight_______blue ________cleft_________
movement _________(gag______"ha" ________)
Uvula: bifid________ absent _______normal ________

TONSILS: absent ______normal ______ enlarged _____ inflamed ______infected _______

ORO-PHARYNX: size _____; movement: mesial _____lateral ______none evident _____

TONGUE: Size _______; tremor: (rest) ________(protruded) _______
Function; curl _______, point ________
move voluntarily; up _________down________right _______left ________
sweep lips smoothly ________move independently of mandible __________
tongue-thrust swallow _______

COMMENTS:

Figure 7-3 Sample Oral Examination Form (continued)

offered by the examiner to jaw opening when it is elevated (occluded) or to jaw closing when it is depressed. Weakness is estimated by the difficulty the patient has in overcoming the resistance presented by the examiner. It should be remembered, however, that the jaw-closing muscles are capable of producing considerably more force than the jaw-opening muscles because of their role in mastication.

The Dentition and Alveolar Ridge. To evaluate dental occlusal relationships, the clinician instructs the patient to bite down on his back teeth and spread his lips. This procedure usually results in a normalized pattern of jaw closure rather than a thrusting forward of the mandible with contact of maxillary and mandibular incisors which frequently occurs if the patient is simply asked to "bite down." With the teeth in contact, the examiner can observe the posterior and anterior occlusal relationships and the bony framework of the dental arch. The occlusal relationship should be described as well as the condition of the teeth, presence of misaligned and extraneous teeth, and edentulous space. A number of terms have been developed to aid in this descriptive process. These terms are based on variations from the normal occlusional pattern.

In normal adults, the maxillary arch has a slightly larger diameter than the mandibular arch. Therefore, the upper arch overlaps the lower arch such that the maxillary anterior teeth are labial (anterior) to the mandibular teeth. The teeth of the lower and upper arches are arranged so that each tooth is opposed by two teeth of the opposite arch except for the upper third molars and the lower central incisors (Zemlin 1968). The point of reference for describing malocclusions is the oppositional relationship of the first upper and first lower molars; that is, the first lower molar is one cusp anterior to the upper oppositional molar. *Neutrocclusion* is used to describe a malalignment of individual teeth when the anteroposterior (front-back) and lateral (side-side) relationship of the upper and lower dental arches are normal. *Distocclusion* is an abnormal retrusion of the mandible so that the lower dental arch is too far posterior in relation to the upper arch. *Mesiocclusion* refers to an excessive protrusion of the mandible in relation to the maxilla so that the lower arch overlaps the upper arch.

Several other terms may be of value in describing dental abnormalities. *Openbite* refers to the lack of contact between the upper and lower anterior teeth when the posterior teeth are in occlusion. Conversely, *closebite* refers to an excessive overlap of the lower teeth by the upper anterior teeth. *Crossbite* is used to describe a lateral overlap of the upper and lower arches, rather than the normal parallel alignment. In addition to describing the relative positions of the upper and lower arches, it is also useful to describe the relative position of individual teeth. *Labioversion* is a tilting of a tooth toward the lip; *buccoversion* is the deflection of the tooth toward the cheek; *linguaversion* is the tilting of the tooth toward the tongue. *Mesioversion* means that the tooth is medial to its normal position, and *distoversion* indicates that it is distal from normal position. *Edentulous* spaces refer to missing teeth, and *supernumerary* refers to extra or additional teeth. For a rather extensive discussion of dental malocclusions, the interested reader is referred to Bloomer (1971).

The Hard Palate. When a patient is requested to open his mouth, he usually depresses the mandible maximally to allow the examiner a clear view of the oral cavity. This is only appropriate for a view of palatal or dental structure. It is not the recommended posture for a functional examination since when the mouth is opened as wide as possible, the musculature of the pharynx is immobilized due to the communication between oral and pharyngeal rings of musculature at the pterygomandibular joint (Mason 1969). The recommended mouth opening during the intraoral examination, according to Mason, is three-fourths of the maximal distance.

The hard palate is inspected with the patient's head tilted backward so that the entire hard palate is exposed at one time. This posture can be assumed for inspection of the hard palate because it is a rigid structure not distorted by head position. The primary features of the hard palate to be assessed as reviewed by Mason (1969) include midline coloration, location of its posterior border, and size and shape of the palatal vault. Normal midline colors are pink and white. A bluish coloration should raise suspicion about the adequacy of the bony framework of the palate, such as the possible presence of a submucous cleft. The posterior border of the hard palate can be located by drawing an imaginary line across the palate to join the posterior borders of the maxillae. This is approximately the posterior border of the palantine bone and is useful for evaluating the length of the hard palate and the point at which palpation for the posterior nasal spine should be performed in cases of suspected submucous clefts. The size and shape of the palatal vault should be carefully noted and recorded if it deviates significantly from "normal."

The Palatopharyngeal Musculature. When examining this area, the examiner will want to assess the coloration of palatal and pharyngeal structures, the anatomic integrity of these structures, and the function of the palatopharyngeal musculature during voluntary and reflex activity. The normal coloration of the velum is similar to that of the hard palate. Any inflammation or marked redness of the velopharyngeal area should be referred to a physician for further examination. The size of the faucial tonsils also should be noted. Tonsillitis is evidenced by redness and engorgement of blood vessels of the tonsillar tissues.

The uvula at the posterior end of the soft palate usually is observable during the intraoral examination. It should be examined carefully since a bifid uvual may appear intact until it is separated with a tongue blade.

The soft palate should be carefully observed at rest. Unilateral weakness will be evidenced by one side of the palate resting at a lower level. Bilateral weakness usually is evidenced by both sides of the soft palate resting at a lower than normal level (near the dorsum of the tongue). Any signs of scars should be carefully recorded.

Only limited information can be obtained about the effectiveness of palatopharyngeal structures in gaining velopharyngeal closure because of the limited access of the examiner to a view of their size, shape, and function. The overall size and length of the soft palate are of importance, but these dimensions are difficult to ascertain because they depend upon the depth of the nasopharynx. A large nasopharynx can make a normal-sized soft palate appear small.

The effective length of the soft palate is a critical feature to be noted since that is the portion of the elevated velar tissue used to obturate the nasopharyngeal opening. Another way to define effective velar length is the amount of tissue filling the distance between the posterior border of the soft palate and the posterior pharyngeal wall on the horizontal plane of the soft palate (Mason 1969). Effective length is judged by asking the patient to say "ha" while the tongue is gently depressed. A judgment should be made by the examiner regarding the adequacy of velar movement for gaining obturation of the nasopharynx after she has observed the size of the nasopharynx and the effective length of the soft palate. The contribution of the faucial pillars to velopharyngeal closure also should be noted as the patient phonates. We will have more to say about evaluating velopharyngeal closure in Chapter VIII which deals with instrumental approaches to diagnosis of speech disorders. Finally, a word of caution. The adequacy of the velopharyngeal mechanism should not be evaluated with the tongue protruded since the anatomic connection of the tongue and palate by means of the palatoglossus muscles will restrict soft-palate elevation during phonation. The symmetry of the soft-palate movement should be noted during phonation. If there is unilateral weakness, the uvula will tend to move toward the intact side. If there is bilateral weakness, production of a syllable such as "ha" results in a minimum of palatal movement.

The pharyngeal gag reflex also is elicited routinely as part of the examination. The reflex typically is elicited by gently placing pressure on the back of the tongue or by stroking the soft palate or pharyngeal wall with a tongue depressor. A normal response is a symmetrical posterior-superior movement of the soft palate and mesial movement of the faucial pillars. Asymmetrical movement or reduced movement of the palate or faucial pillars are suggestive of weakness. An inability to elicit a gag reflex is to be noted, but the examiner should be aware that a small percentage of normal subjects do not have a gag reflex. Significant differences in movement between the habitual movement associated with phonation of a vowel or syllable and movement noted during the gag reflex provide an esimate of potential for responding to speech therapy in cases of velopharyngeal insufficiency.

Tongue Musculature. The tongue is examined at rest and during voluntary activities. First, examine the tongue as it lies in the mouth. Note its size and whether it is shrunken or furrowed on one side. Also look for the presence of involuntary contractions or twitchings of muscle fibers around the edges of the tongue, and inspect it for signs of involuntary movement. Muscle atrophy and fasciculations are suggestive of peripheral nervous system damage to the hypoglossal nerve. Next, ask the patient to protrude the tongue as far as possible. If there is unilateral weakness, the tongue will deviate toward the side of dysfunction; in bilateral weakness, the patient will be able to protrude the tongue little if at all. Lingual strength can be tested by asking the patient to resist the examiner's attempts to force the tongue to the left, right, or inward with a tongue depressor. Tongue strength (lateral) also can be tested by asking the patient to place his tongue against the inside of the cheek and then to resist attempts of the examiner to move it medially. Weakness is evidenced by greater ease in forcing the tongue medially on the side opposite the weakness. In cases of facial weakness, the lips should be manually retracted on the weakened side, and the examiner should evaluate lingual deviation by comparing the midline of the tongue with the middle of the jaw. Lingual range of motion is tested by asking the patient to touch the upper lip and alveolar ridge, corners of the mouth, and a point at the midline of the lower lip with the tip of his tongue. Finally, the patient is asked to move his tongue from side to side as quickly as possible. The rate and regularity to these movements are carefully observed and noted. The examiner may also be interested in the status of the lingual frenulum. The frenulum is considered adequate for speech production if the patient can touch the alevolar ridge with her tongue tip when the mouth is held half open. However, the anterior attachment of the frenulum to the under surface of the tongue and a "heart-shaped" appearance of the tongue upon protrusion also may reveal evidence of a restrictive frenulum.

Diadochokinesis. Diadochokinesis is the ability to make rapid alternating movements. Establishing the ability of the patient to produce rapid speech and nonspeech movements frequently is performed as part of the intraoral examination. For example, the examiner may ask the patient to move her tongue back and forth as quickly as possible or to repeat syllables at maximum rates. The important thing to remember is that reduced diadochokinetic rates in themselves are not important since we rarely produce syllables at the maximum rates physiologically allowable. Rather, the importance of diadochokinetic testing is to evaluate the ability of the patient to make consistent articulatory contacts without articulatory breakdowns and significant variations in rate. Typically, diadochokinetic rates are determined by asking the patient to produce the syllables /pa/, /ta/, and /ka/ and the syllable series /pataka/ as quickly as possible over three trials. The average of the three trials is then compared to established norms. The norms for boys and girls nine, ten, and eleven years old are presented in Table 7-3 (Bloomquist 1950). If a nine-year-old boy produced less than 3.8 repetitions per second (two standard deviations below the mean of 4.8), we might conservatively judge his performance to be "inadequate." Additional

Table 7-3 Mean number of sounds repeated per second in three trials, and standard deviation, subjects grouped according to age and sex

	Age 9				*Age 10*				*Age 11*			
	Girls		Boys		Girls		Boys		Girls		Boys	
Sound	M	SD	M	SD	M	SD	M	SD	M	SD	M	SD
p	4.4	.47	4.8	.49	4.7	.76	4.9	.64	5.2	.52	5.5	.64
t	4.5	.65	4.6	.50	4.9	.82	5.0	.98	4.9	.47	5.5	.99
k	4.1	.53	4.2	.51	4.4	.53	4.6	.92	4.6	.55	4.9	.44
ptk	4.8	.72	4.3	.68	5.0	.47	5.0	.80	5.3	.58	5.0	.54

From Bloomquist 1950.

norms are available for children three to five (McKelvey 1976), nine to eleven (Lundeen 1950), and six to fifteen (Irwin and Beckland 1953).

Swallowing. Swallowing also is evaluated as part of the oral-peripheral examination. In a later chapter we will discuss dysphagia evaluation. In this section we will briefly review procedures for determining the presence of a reversed tongue-thrust swallow (tongue-thrusting). Fletcher, Casteel, and Bradley (1961) suggest that this disorder be evaluated in the following manner. Tell the patient you want to observe how he swallows. Place fingers of both hands on the anterior portions of the masseter and over the hyoid bone so that muscle movement can be noted. At the same time, depress the lower lip with the thumbs to break the labial seal and to expose the tongue if it is protruded during swallowing. Ask the child to swallow several times. Criteria for the tongue-thrusting pattern include absence of masseter action during swallowing, difficulty swallowing when the labial seal is broken, and tongue protrusion beyond the edges of the incisors. Although tongue thrusting may be examined, Mason and Proffit (1974) suggest that swallowing therapy is not indicated before puberty.

SUMMARY

This chapter has briefly reviewed procedures for evaluating the anatomic and structural integrity of the speech apparatus. These procedures are not to be used only in cases of obvious structural and functional dysfunction, but rather to be used as an integral part of the evaluation of patients regardless of the suspected speech and language problem. As mentioned earlier, the voice evaluation and oral examination forms included in this chapter are examples or guides for your evaluation.

REFERENCES

Alpers, B., and E. Mancall, *Essentials of the Neurological Examination.* Philadelphia: F. A. Davis Co., (1971).

Bloomer, H., Speech defects associated with dental malocclusions and related abnormalities, in *Handbook of Speech Pathology,* ed. L. Travis. Englewood Cliffs, N.J.: Prentice-Hall, Inc., (1971).

Bloomquist, B., Diadochokinetic movements of nine-, ten-, and eleven-year-old children. *J. Speech Hearing Dis.,* 15, 159-164 (1950).

Boone, D., *The Voice and Voice Therapy,* 2nd ed. Englewood Cliffs, N.J.: Prentice-Hall, Inc., (1977).

Brain, L., and J. Walton, *Brain's Diseases of the Nervous System.* London: Oxford University Press, (1969).

Darley, F., A. Aronson, and J. Brown, *Motor Speech Disorders.* Philadelphia: W. B. Saunders, (1975).

DeJong, R., *The Neurologic Examination.* New York: Hoeber-Harper, (1958).

Dworkin, J., II. Differential diagnosis of motor speech disorders: The clinical examination of the speech mechanism. *J. National Student Speech Hear. Assoc.,* 6, 37-59 (1978).

Fairbanks, G., *Voice and Articulation Drillbook.* New York: Harper & Row, (1960).

Fisher, H., *Improving Voice and Articulation.* Boston: Houghton Mifflin, (1966).

Fletcher, S., R. Casteel, and D. Bradley, Tongue-thrust swallow, speech articulation, and age. *J. Speech Hearing Dis.,* 26, 201-208 (1961).

Hixon, T., J. Mead, and M. Goldman, Dynamics of the chest wall during speech production: Function of the thorax, rib cage, diaphragm, and abdomen. *J. Speech Hearing Res.,* 19, 297-356 (1976).

Irwin, J., and O. Becklund, Norms for maximum repetitive rates for certain sounds established with the Sylrater. *J. Speech Hearing Dis.,* 18, 149-160 (1953).

Lindblom, B., and J. Sundberg, Neurophysiological representation of speech sounds. Paper presented at the XVth World Congress of Logopedics and Phoniatrics. Buenos Aires, Argentina, (1971).

Lindblom, B., J. Lubker, and T. Gay, Formant frequencies of some fixed-mandible vowels and a model of speech motor programming by predictive simulation. *J. Phon.,* 7, 147-161 (1979).

Lundeen, D., The relationship of diadochokinesis to various speech sounds. *J. Speech Hearing Dis.,* 15, 54-59 (1950).

Mason, R., Improving the efficiency of the intraoral examination. *J. Tenn. Speech Hearing Assoc.,* 14, 4-10 (1969).

Mason, R., and W. Proffit, The tongue thrust controversy: Background and recommendations. *J. Speech Hearing Dis.,* 39, 115-132 (1974).

Mason, R., and C. Simon, An orofacial examination checklist. *J. Lang. Speech, Hear. Serv. Schools,* 8, 155-164 (1977).

McKelvey, J., Performance of normal three and four year old children on ten selected oral motor tasks. Unpublished Masters thesis, University of Texas, Austin, (1976).

McWilliams, B., R. Musgrave, and P. Crozier, The influence of head position upon velopharyngeal closure. *Cleft Pal. J.*, 5, 117-124 (1968).

Moore, G., Voice disorders associated with organic abnormalities, in *Handbook of Speech Pathology*, ed. L. Travis. Englewood Cliffs, N.J.: Prentice-Hall, Inc., (1957).

Murphy, A. *Functional Voice Disorders.* Englewood Cliffs, N.J.: Prentice-Hall, Inc., (1964).

Netter, F., The larynx. *Clinical Symposia.* Summit, N.J.: CIBA Pharmaceutical Company, (1964).

Ptacek, P., and E. Sander, Maximum duration of phonation. *J. Speech Hearing Res.*, 3, 227-244 (1963).

Van Riper, C., *Speech Correction: Principles and Methods,* 6th ed. Englewood Cliffs, N.J.: Prentice-Hall, Inc., (1978).

Wilson, D., *Voice Problems of Children,* 2nd ed. Baltimore: Williams and Wilkins, (1978).

Yanagihara, N., and Y. Koike, The regulation of sustained phonation. *Folia Phon.*, 19, 1-18 (1967).

Yanagihara, N., Y. Koike, and H. von Leden, Phonation and respiration: function study in normal subjects. *Folia Phon.*, 18, 323-340 (1966).

Zemlin, W., *Speech and Hearing Science.* Englewood Cliffs, N.J.: Prentice-Hall, Inc., (1968).

Instrumental Approaches to Assessment of Speech Disorders

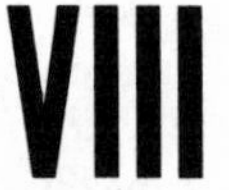

In the laboratory, or by means of laboratory techniques, clinical diagnoses of speech disorders are made.

M. D. Steer and T. D. Hanley, "Instruments of Diagnosis, Therapy, and Research," *Handbook of Speech Pathology (1957)*

Instrumentation extends the senses of the observer and objectifies his observations. Its utilization for the disgnosis of speech disorders is in its infancy; its potential appears limited only by the creativity of the engineer and the interpretive powers of the diagnostician. Its usefulness lies in the ability of the diagnostician to gather detailed information directly from the abnormal speech apparatus rather than relying on perceptual information. This deductive shortcut might be likened to a mechanic's efforts to diagnose the problem of a malfunctioning car motor. If he knows nothing about engines, it does not matter whether he listens to it, acoustically analyzes the noise of the troubled engine, or takes the motor apart, he will not be able to diagnose the problem even though evidence of its malfunctioning is available at each stage of his examination. If he knows how engines operate when in good repair, he may be able to diagnose the problem through listening or acoustical analysis, but he can make his best estimate of its dysfunction by taking it apart, examining each of the components, and inferring why the engine is not working properly.

Two features of this analogy from Netsell (1975) are important to instrumental approaches to the diagnosis of speech disorders. First, we must have some knowledge of normal processes in order to judge *if* the speech-production apparatus is disordered. This is an important point we made in our discussion of standardization of tests on "normal" subjects in order to make decisions whether a communicative problem exists. The comparative process of determining normalcy is rendered considerably more difficult in instrumental analysis, however, by the lack of a large physiological data base to aid in making our decisions. The process is complicated further by the variability demonstrated by normal speakers when electromyographic, structural movement, aerodynamic, and acoustical data are examined. The large variations in normal performance, coupled with the lack of a significant normative data base, make diagnostic interpretations and decisions difficult based on instrumental data alone. Physiological data from disordered speech processes are an aid to diagnosis and appraisal; they are not the only information available and cannot be relied upon exclusively for making our decisions.

Secondly, collection of physiological data has the advantage of investigating the source of the disorder by allowing us to examine the problem more directly. If we wish to determine the physiological origin of a particular type of dysarthria from perceptual analysis, for example, we must make inferences across the levels of the speech-production process. We listen to the acoustic output from the patient which is based on the resonant characteristics and sound generation sources of the vocal tract; the sound sources are developed by changes in air pressure and flows within the vocal tract produced by alterations in structural movement. The movements, in turn, are produced by changes in muscular activity controlled by the nervous system. Given that the disorder has a neuromuscular origin, we are required to make inferences across several stages of the speech-production process. The inferential leap from perceptual information to the underlying neuromuscular pathology is no mean task for even the well-trained clinician; it is even more formidable because the movements of the articulatory structures cannot be separated from the constrictions that serve as sound sources or the movements that control vocal tract resonance (Abbs and Watkin 1976). Even though the experienced diagnostician can make inferences from perceptual judgments of the acoustic waveform to the underlying neuromuscular pathology, she must, as we mentioned earlier, have a knowledge of normal functioning to determine the extent to which the patient's speech production differs from normal. The advantage of instrumental approaches is that we can get closer to the source of the problem and can quantify our observations in a highly detailed fashion; comparisons with normal performance then become more reliable and valid.

The ability to gather objective data closer to the source of the problem is not purchased without cost. As we seek to examine earlier stages of speech production, less and less of the process is available for measurement at one point in time. For example, spectrographic analysis allows us to display most of the acoustic information available in the speech waveform at one time. A complete aerodynamic description requires that we monitor approximately seven relevant variables. Structural-movement data may be collected from ten or more articulators, and muscle function, if we attempt to describe the entire speech activity, requires examining approximately a hundred muscles. Since there are a finite number of parameters that can be recorded and interpreted at one time, as we move toward the origins of the speech-production process, we are able to monitor less and less of the total activity. This situation is comparable to a wedge-shaped piece of pie that gets tastier as we eat toward the point. We get a lot of pie at the periphery, but it does not taste very good. As we eat toward the point it gets better and better, but we have less and less of it. The only wise course for the hungry man is to eat the entire piece, of course. Likewise, the diagnostician will want to use information from each stage of the speech-production process even if only a limited number of variables are available for study at each level.

The purpose of this chapter is to describe instrumentation useful for collecting information about disordered speech processes. It is understood that much of this instrumentation may not be readily available to the diagnostician; knowledge of its operation, however, may provide important insights for the student of differential diagnosis.

INSTRUMENTAL APPROACHES

The stages of the speech-production process along with some instrumental approaches to the study of each stage are presented in Figure 8-1. It should be obvious that the schematic diagram is a highly simplified graphic display of a very complex process and does not include feedback systems or interactive effects between the stages. Moreover, we have not attempted to list all possible investigative techniques, but only a representative sample of those most commonly employed in speech research. Reviews of physiology instrumentation and their advantages and disadvantages are provided by Strong (1970), Abbs and Watkin (1976), Warren (1976), Hardy (1965), and Hixon (1972), and of speech acoustics instrumentation by Wakita (1976).

MUSCLE ACTION POTENTIALS

We shall begin our discussion with electromyography because it allows examination of one of the earliest stages of the speech-production process. This is not to say that attempts have not been made to directly measure central or peripheral nervous system activity during speech production. Electromyography, however, is the first instrumental approach that can provide readily interpretable information.

Electromyography (EMG) is a method of displaying the time varying electrical activity associated with muscle contraction (Harris 1970). The source of the electrical activity is the resting potential of living mammalian cells; that is, the potential difference between the inside and outside of an active cell.

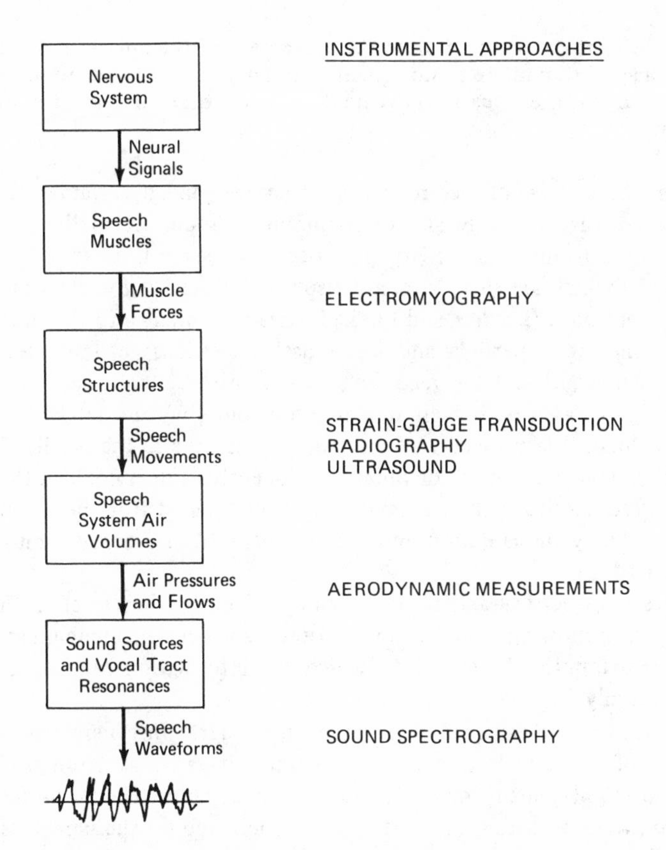

Figure 8-1 Stages of the speech production process and instrumental approaches to the study of each stage.

(Adapted from J. Abbs and K. Watkin, Instrumentation for the study of speech physiology, in ***Contemporary Issues in Experimental Phonetics,*** ed. N. Lass. New York: Academic Press, 1976. By permission.)

Muscle fibers are functionally arranged such that a large number of fibers lie in parallel, enclosed within a sheath. Groups of fibers within the muscle are connected to a single neuron and thereby comprise a motor unit. Each muscle is made up of a number of these motor units. When a suprathreshold stimulus is delivered to a motor unit, a wave of depolarization sweeps down the muscle fibers. The momentary changes in electrical activity can be recorded by use of electrodes or "probes" placed next to each other within or overlying the muscle.

Surface, needle, and hooked-wire electrodes are utilized for monitoring speech muscle activity. No matter which are chosen, they must meet several requirements according to Abbs and Watkin (1976):

> . . . it is obvious that electrodes for measurement of speech muscle activity must (1) allow for placement in confined spaces (such as the oral cavity),

(2) be light enough to follow the movement of the muscle and yet remain in place (to minimize movement artifacts), and (3) be unobtrusive in relation to the speech movement activity that one is attempting to observe.

In general, each type of electrode has advantages and disadvantages. Surface electrodes are easy to apply and offer minimal discomfort to the patient but cannot be used to monitor activity from deep muscles or those muscles (such as the mentalis) which are small in comparison to the size of the electrode. Intramuscular electrodes (needles and hooked-wires implanted into the muscle) can be used to monitor superficial and deep muscles as well as small muscles because they are lightweight and the recording area is small. There tends to be some discomfort associated with their implantation, but they are relatively painless once embedded. The hooked-wire electrode is superior to the needle electrode because it is smaller and more flexible. Consequently, it does not load the muscle as much while retaining the advantages normally gained from needle-electrode use; that is, easy implantation and measurement from a specific muscle area (Basmajian 1967).

Since the electrical activity recorded by the electrode is small, it first must be amplified. Following amplification, various types of signal manipulation may be used to maximize the ease with which the information can be interpreted when graphically displayed.

So what is the value of electromyographic data? In general, the absolute magnitude of the signal is of little value since it varies as a function of the electrode used, placement location, and tissue impedance. The magnitude of the signals from two muscles cannot be directly compared for the same reason. The value of electromyography lies in two areas. First, it is useful in examining the time relationship between muscle activity and associated speech gestures, and second, it provides information on the status of the neuromuscular system, such as the presence of hypertonicity or abnormal variations in the activation and inhibition of muscle activity.

STRUCTURAL MOVEMENT

Several techniques have been employed for the measurement of structural movement. Typically, the use of these procedures is mutually exclusively and employment of more than one method at a time is a rarity. As with electromyography, there are advantages and disadvantages associated with the use of each technique.

Three primary instrumental approaches as reviewed by Moll (1965) and Bzoch (1970) are considered under the rubric of *radiography* including "still" X-ray, laminography, and cinefluorography. Their common feature is that they each use X-rays, a form of electromagnetic radiation with defined wavelengths.

The X-rays are directed toward the subject's body and penetrate all structures to varying degrees. The resulting image can be made visible on film or visualized on a fluoroscopic screen and then videotaped or photographed.

Still X-rays most often have been used to visualize speech structures from the lateral view. They appear to be of limited utility in speech research since they yield a static rather than a dynamic portrayal of the speech structures. Laminography is similar to still X-ray but offers the advantage of visualizing only the structures within a given plane.

Cinefluorography involves the photographing of the intensified image so that dynamic speech processes, rather than a single position, is monitored. Radiation effects are reduced by synchronizing the X-ray generator and the camera shutter. To analyze movement of the articulatory structures, sequences of individual cinefluorographic frames are traced, and measurements are made from the tracings utilizing radiopaque beads, skeletal structures, and/or articulators covered with a radiopaque substance as referents.

There are a number of problems associated with the use of radiographic techniques which have been reviewed by Bzoch (1970). Danger from radiation exposure requires strict limitations on the speech sample, and the actual acquisition of the data must be under the supervision of a radiologist. The requirement that the body be stabilized limits observations of articulators to a single body position while the same function may differ in other postures due to changes in antigravity muscles.

There also are data-reduction problems. Variations in radiopacity from individual to individual results in reduced reliability of the data measurements. Straight-line emission characteristics of X-rays cause relative enlargement of the periphery which necessitates the use of correction factors in measurement. Subject instability errors may arise from small movements of the subject's head which alter the positional relationships between reference skeletal structures and articulators. Errors also may occur in the measuring of frames because anatomical structures which have no functional relationship to speech production are used as reference points. Finally, there is the problem of which measurements to make.

In spite of these limitations, cinefluorography offers a view of dynamic activity from a number of articulators at the same time, an important advantage. It is the procedure of choice for investigating structures such as the velopharyngeal mechanism and tongue which are relatively inaccessible by other techniques.

Ultrasound is useful for observing the dynamic activity of structures without interfering with their activity or exposing the patient to irradiation. Ultrasound is produced by exciting a crystal with an electrical field which changes the crystal's dimensions and produces waves. The ultrasonic waves have the property of being reflected back at the interface (boundary) between two mediums such as the lateral pharyngeal wall and the pharyngeal airspace. The reflected wave is converted into a time-amplitude display since the time between the initiation of the ultrasonic pulses and their return is proportional to the distance from the transmitter to the boundary. This technique has been used to monitor pharyngeal wall (Kelsey, Minifie, and Hixon 1969), tongue (Watkin and Zagzebski 1973), and vocal fold movement (Minifie, Kelsey, and Hixon 1968). The problems with the technique are that the experimenter is not exactly sure of the point on the structure that she is measuring from and the transmitter-receiver must be at a ninety degree angle with the interface. Moreover, in disorders characterized by structural anomalies (cleft palate, partial glossectomee), it may be particularly difficult to identify the point on the structure being monitored.

Strain-gauge transduction theoretically can be used to monitor displacement of any speech structure. In actuality, transducers of this type have been utilized primarily to investigate movements of the jaw (Sussman and Smith 1970a; Abbs and Gilbert 1973; Abbs 1973), velum (Christiansen and Moller 1971), and lips (Sussman and Smith 1970b; Abbs and Gilbert 1973). Strain gauges (Abbs and Watkin 1976) operate on the principle that as a wire is stretched, it is reduced in diameter and increased in length, thus offering greater resistance to the flow of current. Conversely, when these conductors are compressed, there is decreased resistance to current flow. Strain-gauge elements are bonded to a thin metal beam (cantilever) and attached to the structure of interest. Resistance changes proportional to the deformation of the strip occur when the structure is displaced. The resistance changes modulate the current across an amplifier thereby varying the voltage. The time varying voltage resulting from the structural displacement is graphically displayed.

The advantages of this technique are the ease with which the cantilever beams can be attached to the structures and the absence of subject discomfort. The primary disadvantage is that cantilevers cannot be attached to structures such as the tongue without impeding normal articulatory activity.

We have briefly reviewed only three methods for monitoring structural movement. Descriptions of other techniques, such as high-speed photography, electromagnetic induction, and photoelectric techniques, are available in Abbs and Watkin (1976), Hanley and Peters (1971), Hixon (1972), and Harris (1970).

AIR PRESSURE–AIR FLOW

Structural movements induce volume changes and produce variations in air pressure and air flow in the speech system. The pressures and flows of interest are displayed in Figure 8-2. The pressures include intraoral, intranasal, subglottic, and atmospheric. The flows are those across the glottis, the nasal cavity, and oral cavity. Integration of volume velocity of air flow provides an estimate of volume.

One means of determining lung volume is the *spirometer*. A wet spirometer consists of a bell inverted in a tank of water. Movement of the bell is recorded by a stylus on a slowly revolving drum of paper. The movement of the

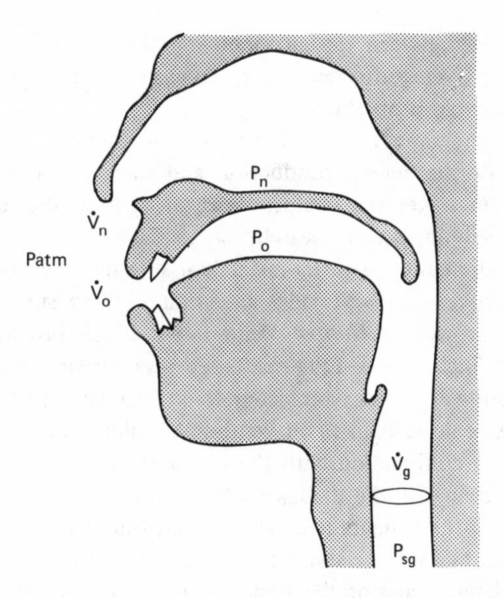

Figure 8-2 Speech air pressures and airflows. Air pressures include oral (Po), nasal (Pn), subglottic (Psg), and atmospheric (Patm). Airflows include glottal ($\dot{V}$g), oral ($\dot{V}$o), and nasal ($\dot{V}$n).

(Adapted from R. Netsell, Speech Physiology. In F. Minifie, T. Hixon, and F. Williams, eds., ***Normal Aspects of Speech, Hearing and Language.*** Englewood Cliffs, N.J.: Prentice-Hall, Inc., 1973. By permission.)

bell is caused by the subject's breathing through a tube which forces air into the bell. A spirometer can be used to measure lung volumes and capacities. One major drawback of the device is that the magnitude of some measures, such as inspiratory capacity, are highly dependent on the amount of effort expended by the subject. Therefore, multiple trials are usually performed, and the maximum value obtained is considered to be the most valid indicant of performance. A second limitation is that the variables cannot be measured during speech production unless the instrumentation is adapted.

A second means of determining lung volumes is through the use of a *body plethysmograph* (Hixon 1972). It measures air volume as a function of the pressure differential between a chamber in which the subject is placed and the outside atmosphere. The subject is seated in a booth completely enclosed except for the head and neck which are allowed to project through the top of the chamber. The neck collar provides an airtight seal for the air enclosed in the chamber. During breathing activities, the pressure in the chamber increases and decreases with net inspiratory and expiratory volume changes. With each volume change, gas is displaced through a fine metal screen located in the front wall of the chamber. The flow through the screen is directly proportional to the pressure differential between the chamber and the atmosphere. By integrating the flow sensed by a pressure transducer, a measure of the volume displaced in and out of the chamber is obtained.

The plethysmograph has the advantage of allowing a determination of volume changes during speech production and therefore appears to be much more valuable than a wet spirometer. However, it is cumbersome and has not been used extensively in speech research.

Static measurements of intraoral air pressure may be obtained with a *U-tube water manometer* which provides an estimate of pressure in centimeters of water displaced, or with a *Hunter Manometer,* which provides a reading in ounces per square inch. The U-tube manometer is constructed of a flexible tube into which the subject blows, connected to a U-shaped glass tube filled with colored water. A scale is marked in centimeters along the side of the tube. A leak-tube is used in conjunction with the manometer both to simulate air flow and to prevent valving of the tube with the tongue. Netsell and Hixon (1978) have described a U-tube manometer with a leak tube which simulates pressure and flow values normally associated with phonation. It thereby serves to approximate the glottal resistance of the upper airway. The subject is instructed to blow into a tube for a specified duration while maintaining a prescribed pressure level. Assuming velopharyngeal closure and a tight lip seal around the tube, the method offers an estimate of subglottal pressure. It may be used to differentiate respiratory from laryngeal involvement by estimating the ability of the patient to develop and maintain subglottic pressure under a simulated phonation condition.

The Hunter Manometer works on the same principle as the U-tube. Readings appear on three calibrated dials, and there is a manually operated bleed (leak) valve. Indications of velopharyngeal adequacy are obtained by dividing the reading obtained during a trial with the nares open compared to that obtained with the nares occluded. Theoretically, the ratio should be 1.0. If there is a leak through the velopharyngeal opening with the nares unoccluded, lower ratios are obtained and are an indication of inadequacy. A ratio of 0.89 or less is considered inadequate velopharyngeal closure (Spriestersbach and others 1961).

Dynamic air pressures are monitored by means of a pressure transducer which converts pressure into voltage. This is accomplished by a diaphragm within a transducer. When pressure is exerted on the diaphragm, it is displaced with a resultant change in voltage. The voltage is amplified and displayed on an oscillograph. The intraoral pressure is coupled to the pressure transducer by means of a tube inserted into the oral cavity. The tube is positioned so that its opening is oriented perpendicular to flow to reduce flow artifacts. To obtain bilabial plosive pressure, the tube is entered into the corner of the mouth. To obtain pressues for a large number of consonants, the tube with an oropharyngeal balloon attached to the end is passed through one of the nares to a point below the velopharyngeal space. Another alternative is to place the tube in the dental-gingival sinus so that it enters the oral cavity from behind the last upper molar. Nasal pressure is obtained by sealing the tube to a nasal olive inserted into one of the nares. Subglottic pressure can be obtained by puncturing the trachea between the second and third rings with a hypodermic needle and attaching it to a pressure transducer. These techniques have the advantage of monitoring dynamic pressures during speech production.

Two systems described by Lubker (1970) are generally used to measure air-flow rates occurring during speech. The difference between the systems is in the choice of the sensing device. The sensing element most commonly used to measure airflow is the *pneumotachograph.* This device is based on the principle that as air flows across a resistance; the air-pressure drop is proportional to the rate of flow. The pressure drop, or differential, is sensed by a transducer, converted to an electrical signal, amplified, and graphically displayed. This technique for monitoring airflow has the advantage of easy calibration, stability, and it can be used to detect and differentiate between ingressive and egressive flow. The primary disadvantage is that a face mask must be used to trap the flow of air through the device which places certain restrictions on articulatory movements. Lubker and Moll (1965) have suggested that these restrictions are limited primarily to lip and jaw movements and are highly phoneme-dependent.

The second airflow measuring technique reviewed by Lubker, the *warm wire anemometer,* uses a heated wire as the air-flow sensing element. He noted that "the basic principle involves the cooling effect of a flow of air on a heated wire through which an electric current is flowing. As the wire is cooled, its resistance to current flow is altered in a systematic manner. The variations in the electrical signal passing through the heated wire, when amplified, recorded, and calibrated, provide a record flow rate." The primary advantage of this system is that no face mask is needed to channel the flow of air. Although applications have been made of a single heated wire placed in a tube similar to a pneumotachograph and attached to a mask (Van Hattum and Worth 1967), more recent use has involved the suspension of a series of wires in front of and close to the oral and nasal ports without a mask (Subtelny, Worth, and Sakuda 1966; Subtelny and others 1969). The warm wire or wires must be arranged rather close to the subject's mouth, and their distance must be constant throughout the experiment. Consequently, the subject's head movements need to be restricted, or the apparatus must be attached to the face, or both. The warm wire system has a number of disadvantages including inability to differentiate between ingressive and egressive flow, poor linearity and frequency response, and difficulties in calibration (Lubker 1970).

These methods allow some means of determining the volume velocity of air flow through the oral cavity and nasal passages. Transglottal air flow can be determined through the use of a plethysmograph (Hixon 1972).

ACOUSTIC ANALYSIS

The *sound spectograph* is an instrument which visually presents information about the frequency, intensity, and duration of the speech waveform. The speech sample is introduced into the spectrograph via microphone or tape recorder. As the signal is analyzed, a hot-wire stylus records a "picture" of the sound wave on a rotating drum. The spectrogram produced provides a display of frequency on the vertical axis, duration on the horizontal axis, and intensity by the darkness of the trace. Two filter bandwidths may be used for the analysis. A broad band filter provides the best pictoral representation of the waveform for determining formant frequencies, glottal pulse, and segment duration. The narrow band filter is used for determining fundamental frequency, harmonics, and intonational contours. The spectrograph also can be used to obtain line spectra for selected portions of a signal and amplitude and intensity displays. The sound spectrograph has been used extensively in research examining acoustic aspects of both speech production and speech perception. It is an important tool in correlating elements of the acoustic signal with perceived qualities and with acoustic correlates of articulatory gestures. Spectrograms are potentially useful in the diagnosis of voice disorders, where they can be used to supplement other sources of information. Spectrographic data affords physical evidence of perceived vocal abnormalities, such as perturbations of the glottal pulse.

Another device for evaluating the acoustic waveform is the *fundamental frequency indicator* (Hanley and Peters 1971). This instrument is specifically designed to extract the fundamental frequency from the speech waveform. The device may be of value in correlating the maturational development of the larynx and in assessment of voice disorders related to pitch.

A *Probe Tube Microphone Assembly* permits the simultaneous recording of oral and nasal acoustic energy in decibels. A probe tube is inserted into the nasal meatus, while the oral signal is recorded by means of a condenser microphone a short distance from the lips. The greater the nasal air flow, the less the difference between the nasal and oral sound pressure levels. This relationship may indicate the degree to which the nasal and oral tracts are coupled during speech and thereby provides an estimate of the adequacy of velopharyngeal closure. A review of this technique is provided by Counihan (1979).

SOME CONSIDERATIONS IN THE SELECTION OF INSTRUMENTATION

We have reviewed only a few of the many instrumental devices available for diagnosis and appraisal of speech disorders. Others run the gamut from the tongue depressor and flashlight to computer analysis of the acoustic signal. A number of factors must be considered before selecting the instrumentation to be used.

1. *The device should be minimally invasive of the patient.* Any instrument that causes the patient discomfort or invades the body should be used with great caution. For example, the implantation of needle or hooked-wire electrodes and the positioning of a nasopharyngeal balloon may be painful, and in most cases should be done under the supervision of a physician. This point is doubly important when instruments of this type are used with patients who have chronic debilitating conditions, such as Parkinson's disease.
2. *The procedures should minimally endanger the patient.* This is a postulate of the first point. Some procedures such as cinefluorography produce potentially hazardous radiation and should be used only with qualified personnel available. A basic consideration for all such procedures is that the benefit to be gained must outweigh the risks involved.
3. *The instrumentation should not impede normal speech production.* Some devices may effectively load the structure or structures under study and bring about compensatory articulatory activity. The instrumentation chosen should not alter "typical" or "normal" speech production.
4. *The instrumentation should allow an adequate sampling of connected speech.* Devices such as the oral manometer and wet spirometer cannot be used during connected speech and therefore can only be used in a secondary capacity.
5. *If possible, information should be provided about several stages of the speech-production process.* Abbs and Watkin (1976) noted:

> Electromyographic and aerodynamic monitoring represent micro and macro poles in the specification of speech production activity. . . It would appear worthwhile to observe the mediating variable (viz., structural movement) simultaneously with EMG or air pressures and air flows to facilitate interpretation of these aerodynamic or electromyographic indices of speech system activity.

   Moll (1965) made a similar observation when he emphasized that photographic and radiographic procedures provide information only on structural positions and should be utilized in conjunction with other physiologic research techniques and acoustic and perceptual analyses. The point to be made is that considerable ambiguity may result from attempts to make inferences from only a single stage of the speech-production process.
6. *The speech sample and variables to be measured should be selected with care.* It would seem of little value to measure lower lip electromyographic activity in a patient with velopharyngeal inadequacy. Likewise, measurement of nasal air flow during production of a bilabial nasal consonant would offer little information about this patient's hypernasality.

AN EXAMPLE OF INSTRUMENTATION USED FOR CLINICAL DIAGNOSIS

A review of studies utilizing instrumental approaches to the diagnosis of speech disorders quickly reveals that research, rather than clinical assssment, has been the primary goal of the investigations. In some cases the two objectives (research and diagnosis) overlap, but the intent usually is to discover characteristics of speech production in a particular disordered group of patients. Our purpose here is to provide an example of data collected for research purposes but which contains valuable clinical information and demonstrates the potential of instrumentation.

The example is from Netsell (1969) who recorded intraoral air pressures (using a pressure transducer), rate of nasal airflow (via a pneumotachograph), and the speech signal to determine velopharyngeal competence in cerebral-palsied children. The speech sample included the consonants /t/, /d/, and /n/ to represent voiceless, voiced, and nasal contrasts. The sample was produced under several rate and context conditions.

Speech audio, nasal airflow rate, and intraoral air pressure for a neurologically normal and a dysarthric subject are presented in Figure 8-3. Examination of the figure reveals that except for a slight burst on the initial utterance, no nasal air flow is seen in the production of /ʌtʌdʌ/ by the dysarthric subject. However, during each repetition of /ʌtʌnʌ/, there are two bursts of nasal flow—one for /t/ and one for /n/. It is evident that this patient opened the velopharynx early in anticipation of the /n/ with resultant inappropriate nasal airflow during the /t/. Velopharyngeal closure was achieved during production of /t/ as evidenced by the peaks of intraoral pressure. Since the subject appeared to be able to develop intraoral pressure during production of plosives, the problem is one of timing and not of inability to decrease the area of the velopharyngeal opening during speech production. This finding is important to clinical assessment since remedial procedures vary as a function of the diagnosis. If timing is the problem, as in this example, then a palatal lift may be the optimal form of treatment. If the problem had been due to an inability to adequately close the velopharyngeal port due to a congenitally short palate, then obturation or surgical intervention would be the rehabilitation procedure of choice.

Many other examples of instrumental assessment are available for dysarthria, stuttering, cleft palate, laryngectomy, and voice disorders.

SUMMARY

Instrumental approaches to the diagnosis of speech disorders extend the senses of the clinician and objectify her observations. Many types of instrumentation are available including devices to monitor and record electromyographic, structural movement, aerodynamic, and acoustic variables. Each instrumental

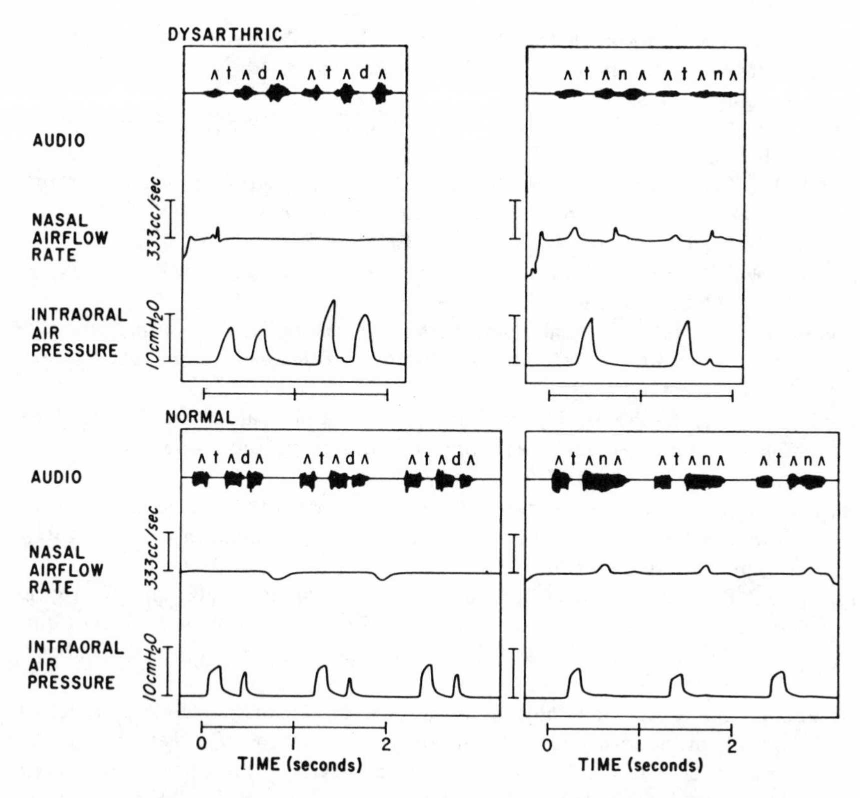

Figure 8-3 Oscillographic recordings of the speech signal (audio), nasal air flow rate, and intraoral air pressure from a dysarthric female and a normal female repeating the utterances /ʌtʌdʌ/ and /ʌtʌnʌ/ (left and right side of the figure, respectively) to illustrate an inappropriate opening of the velopharynx.

(From R. Netsell, Evaluation of velopharyngeal function in dysarthria. *J. Speech Hearing Res.,* 34, 113-122, 1969. By permission.)

device has advantages and disadvantages. The instrumentation you choose will be based on your purposes in testing and what you want to know. The information obtained must be integrated with data from other appraisal procedures, however, because instrumentally obtained information is only a component, and not the entire data base, for diagnosis.

REFERENCES

Abbs, J., Some mechanical properties of lower lip movement during speech production. *Phonetica,* 28, 65-75 (1973).

Abbs, J., and B. Gilbert, Strain gauge transducer system for lip and jaw motion in two dimensions. *J. Speech Hearing Res.,* 16, 248-256 (1973).

Abbs, J., and K. Watkin, Instrumentation for the study of speech physiology, in *Contemporary Issues in Experimental Phonetics,* ed. N. Lass. New York: Academic Press, (1976).

Basmajian, J., *Muscles Alive–Their Functions Revealed by Electromyography.* Baltimore: Williams and Wilkins, (1967).

Bzoch, K., Assessment: Radiographic techniques. *Proceedings of the Workshop: Speech and the Dentofacial Complex; The State of the Art.* Washington, D.C.: ASHA Reports Number 5 (1970).

Christiansen, R., and K. Moller, Instrumentation for recording velar movement. *Amer. J. Orthod.,* 59, 448-455 (1971).

Counihan, D., Oral and nasal sound pressure measures, in *Communicative Disorders Related to Cleft Lip and Palate* (2nd ed.), ed. K. Bzoch. Boston: Little, Brown, (1979).

Hanley, T., and R. Peters, The speech and hearing laboratory, in *Handbook of Speech Pathology and Audiology,* ed. E. Travis, Englewood Cliffs, N.J.: Prentice-Hall, Inc., (1971).

Hardy, J., Air flow and air pressure studies. *Proceedings of the Conference: Communicative Problems in Cleft Palate.* Washington, D.C.: ASHA Reports Number 1 (1965).

Harris, K., Physiological measures of speech movements: EMG and fiberoptic studies. *Proceedings of the Workshop. Speech and the Dentofacial Complex: The State of the Art.* Washington, D.C.: ASHA Reports Number 5 (1970).

Hixon, T., Some new techniques for measuring the biomechanical events of speech production: One laboratory's experiences. *Proceedings of the Conference. Orofacial Function: Clinical Research in Dentistry and Speech Pathology.* Washington, D.C.: ASHA Reports Number 7 (1972).

Johnson, W., F. Darley, and D. Spriestersbach, *Diagnostic Methods in Speech Pathology.* New York: Harper & Row, (1963).

Kelsey, C., F. Minifie, and T. Hixon, Applications of ultrasound in speech research. *J. Speech Hearing Res.,* 12, 564-575 (1969).

Lubker, J., Aerodynamic and ultrasonic assessment techniques in speech-dentofacial research. *Proceedings of the Workshop. Speech and the Dentofacial Complex: The State of the Art.* Washington, D.C.: ASHA Reports Number 5 (1970).

Lubker, J., and K. Moll, Simultaneous oral-nasal air flow measurements and cinefluorographic observations during speech production. *Cleft Pal. J.,* 2, 257-272 (1965).

Minifie, F., C. Kelsey, and T. Hixon, Measurement of vocal fold motion using an ultrasonic Doppler velocity monitor. *J. Acoust. Soc. Amer.,* 43, 1165-1169 (1968).

Moll, K., Photographic and radiographic procedures in speech research. *Proceedings of the Conference: Communicative Problems in Cleft Palate.* Washington, D.C.: ASHA Reports Number 1 (1965).

Netsell, R., *Kineseology Studies of the Dysarthrias.* Madison, Wis.: University of Wisconsin, (1975).

Netsell, R., Evaluation of velopharyngeal function in dysarthria. *J. Speech Hearing Dis.,* 34, 113-122 (1969).

Netsell, R., and T. Hixon, A noninvasive method for clinically estimating subglottal air pressure. *J. Speech Hearing Dis.*, 43, 326-330 (1978).

Spriestersbach, D. C., K. L. Moll, and H. L. Morris, Subject classification and articulation of speakers with cleft palates. *J. Speech Hearing Res.*, 4, 362-372 (1961).

Strong, P., *Biophysical Measurements.* Beaverton, Oregon: Tektronix, Inc., (1970).

Subtelny, J. and others, Multidimensional analysis of bilabial stop and nasal consonants–cineradiographic and pressure-flow analysis. *Cleft Pal. J.*, 263-289 (1979).

Subtelny, J., J. Worth, and M. Sakuda, Intraoral pressure and rate of flow during speech. *J. Speech Hearing Res.*, 9, 498-518 (1966).

Sussman, H., and K. Smith, Transducer for measuring lip movements during speech. *J. Acoust. Soc. Amer.*, 48, 858-860 (1970a).

Sussman, H., and K. Smith, Transducer for measuring mandibular movements during speech. *J. Acous. Soc. Amer.*, 48, 857-858 (1970b).

Van Hattum, R., and J. Worth, Air flow rates in normal speakers. *Cleft Pal. J.*, 4, 137-147 (1967).

Wakita, H., Instrumentation for the study of speech acoustics, in *Contemporary Issues in Experimental Phonetics,* ed. N. Lass. New York: Academic Press, (1976).

Warren, D., Aerodynamics of speech production, in *Contemporary Issues in Experimental Phonetics,* ed. N. Lass. New York: Academic Press, (1976).

Watkin, K., and J. Zagzebski, On-line ultrasonic technique for monitoring tongue displacements. *J. Acous. Soc. Amer.*, 54, 544-547 (1973).

Evaluation of Fluency

IX

Nothing in nature is quite so separate as two mounds of expertise.

Marvin Harris
Cows, Pigs, Wars, and Witches: The Riddles of Culture

In many ways the evaluation of fluency and/or the diagnosis of stuttering may be a more difficult task than most of the speech and language problems we have discussed to this point. Part of the difficulty arises from the lack of objective measures of stuttering and norms to clearly separate "fluent" from "disfluent" speakers. Stuttering and disfluency are not equivalent terms. Fluency norms are not sufficient to designate a *problem* which the speaker may have—or which his listeners may perceive. We obviously need more than a description of speech per se. There are definitions, but there is no single agreed-upon definition. There are no tests for stuttering (Wingate 1978): evaluation is entirely a matter of observation, inquiry, and judgment. This does not mean that our task of appraisal is impossible; it means that we must be careful to be descriptive in our observations, and we must be chary in our assignment of a diagnostic label. Two types of judgmental errors are possible. The labelling of a normally disfluent child as a stutterer is the error which the stuttering literature seems to have been primarily concerned with, but misjudging the beginnings of stuttering as normal fluency would deny the need for therapy intervention—and this may also be a serious error (Adams 1977). What this means, in practical terms, is that to reduce the probability of an error in judgment, we must be concerned with more than just the child's speech.

Within an evaluational framework, a great many different aspects of the speaker, her behavior, and her environment may be considered grist for the diagnostician's mill, depending partly on the class of theories or explanations with which the clinician is comfortable. In no other communication disorder will it be more obvious that diagnostic evaluation and therapeutic intervention overlap in time. During the course of our therapy regime we will obviously continue to evaluate and chart behavioral responses, but equally obvious is that our preferred theories of causation and maintenance of stuttering will tend to influence the types of judgments we make during the diagnostic evaluation.

Necessary information for the evaluation of a stuttering problem (Williams 1974) must include background information in five major areas: (1) case history; (2) description of speaking behavior; (3) variability of stuttering; (4) reactions to stuttering; and (5) personality factors. Wingate (1978, p. 259) noted that although the details will vary somewhat depending on the point of view of the person conducting the evaluation, it may be assumed that the evaluation should nonetheless include: "(1) an adequate appraisal of the symptoms; (2) a history of the problem in the individual; and (3) inquiry into the person's attitude toward the problem."

Our concern as diagnosticians must include a complete speech and language appraisal as well as a description of stuttering, normal disfluencies, and associated behaviors which may indicate that a communication barrier exists, as well as a utilization of these findings to highlight danger signs by which the clinician may decide that there is a problem—and who has the problem. We need to know whether the problem is properly called stuttering, whether therapy is indicated, with whom therapy is indicated, the severity of the problem if one exists, and the probabilities of our accomplishing a positive therapeutic change.

WHEN STUTTERING IS STUTTERING

Most definitions of stuttering are not restricted to speech alone but also include references to a negative reaction on the part of the speaker and/or his listeners. Van Riper's (1978, p. 257) definition is quite succinct: "Stuttering occurs when the forward flow of speech is interrupted abnormally by repetitions or prolongations of a sound, syllable, or articulatory posture, or by avoidance and struggle behaviors." Wingate (1964, p. 488) proffered a more elaborate definition, but one which also placed the primary emphasis on speech and the speaker:

> The term "stuttering" means:
>
> 1. (a) Disruption in the fluency of verbal expression, which is (b) characterized by involuntary, audible or silent, repetitions or prolongations in the utterance of short speech elements, namely: sounds, syllables, and words of one syllable. These disruptions (c) usually occur frequently or are marked in character and (d) are not readily controllable.

2. Sometimes the disruptions are (e) accompanied by accessory activities involving the speech apparatus, related or unrelated body structures, or stereotyped speech utterances. These activities give the appearance of being speech related struggle.
3. Also, there are not infrequently (f) indications or report of the presence of an emotional state, ranging from a general condition of "excitement" or "tension" to more specific emotions of a negative nature such as fear, embarrassment, irritation, or the like. (g) The immediate source of stuttering is some incoordination expressed in the peripheral speech mechanism; the ultimate cause is presently unknown and may be complex or compound.

In terms of speech, those two definitions speak of stuttering disfluencies primarily as related to the production of sounds or syllables. A broader definition of "disfluencies" would include at least eight categories–as defined by Johnson and others (1959). The eight categories include:

1. Interjections of sounds, syllables, or phrases,
2. Part word repetitions–primarily syllables and sounds,
3. Word repetitions, including words of one syllable,
4. Phrase repetitions–two or more words,
5. Revisions–where the content of the phrase is modified,
6. Incomplete phrases–the thought or the content is not completed,
7. Broken words–the words are not completely pronounced (e.g., g–––oing home), and
8. Prolonged sounds–usually the initial sound in a word.

Table 9-1 displays mean numbers for each of the eight types of disfluencies for stuttering and nonstuttering children. These data are from the *Onset of*

Table 9-1 Mean number of disfluencies per 100 words observed in the speech of 89 stuttering and 89 matched nonstuttering children with a mean age of approximately five years.

Category of Disfluency	*Stutterers*		*Nonstutterers*	
	Male	*Female*	*Male*	*Female*
Interjections	3.62	4.44	3.13	3.45
Part-word repetitions	5.44	3.93	.61	.83
Word repetitions	4.28	3.65	1.07	1.14
Phrase repetitions	1.14	.84	.61	.58
Revisions	1.30	1.30	1.43	1.38
Incomplete phrases	.34	.22	.23	.28
Broken words	.12	.63	.04	.10
Prolonged sounds	1.67	1.24	.16	.14
Total	17.91	16.25	7.28	7.90

Adapted from The Onset of Stuttering, *Johnson and Associates, University of Minnesota Press, 1959. Used by permission.*

Stuttering studies (Johnson 1959) conducted over a period of more than 20 years and which included a total of 246 children judged by their parents to be stutterers and their parents (the experimental group) and 246 children judged by their parents to be nonstutterers and their parents (the control group).

From the data shown on Table 9-1 it is apparent that both children judged as stutterers and those judged to be nonstutterers displayed some degree of disfluency. The most frequently occurring disfluencies for the nonstuttering children were on interjections, revisions, and word repetitions in that order. Those same three categories of disfluencies were also relatively frequent in the children judged to be stutterers, but the greatest differences between groups occurred on syllable repetitions and sound prolongations. The differences between the two samples were statistically significant for only sound and word repetitions and prolongations, for both boys and girls.

It should also be noted that these are mean data. Considerable overlap was shown for individual children within the two groups. In fact, "... 20 to 30 percent of the children regarded by their parents as normal speakers spoke with more disfluencies than did 20 to 30 percent of the children who had been for an average of 18 months regarded by their parents as stutterers" (Johnson and others 1963, pp. 247-248). In other words, we obviously cannot consistently identify stuttering on the basis of disfluency alone—either frequency or type of disfluency. Partly as a function of the *Onset* studies, Johnson (1963, p. 241) emphasized that there was more to the stuttering problem than speech disfluencies. He proposed three general meanings for stuttering. They were:

1. a term to refer to what the speaker does;
2. a name for the category in which the listener classifies what the speaker does; and
3. the problem that ensues when the listeners classify what a speaker does as stuttering and evaluate it as undesirable, and the speaker senses their evaluation and reacts to them with tension and concern confirming and intensifying their evaluations, and in the bargain further deepening his own concern—in an ever-outreaching spiral of distress.

Note that Johnson's definition is of the *problem* of stuttering, and not disfluency per se. For purposes of illustration, he sketched three theoretical continua: one for the number of disfluencies in the speech sample; one for the listener's reaction to the speaker; and the third for the speaker's reaction to his perception of the listener's reaction.

(little or few)		(much or many)
	disfluencies	
	listener reaction	
	speaker reaction to listener	

Assume that the ends of the continua are labeled "little or few" and "much or many" as the range of possible judgments. While it is probable that the greater the total number of disfluencies in the speech, the more likely is the speaker to be aware and/or demonstrate some reaction, we cannot assume that a summation of the judgments on the three continua will indicate the severity of the problem for the speaker. We commented earlier that 20 to 30 percent of the five-year-old children judged as nonstutterers (in the *Onset* studies) were likely to be less fluent than the children judged as stutterers, and 20 to 30 percent of the stuttering children were more fluent than the children judged as normally fluent. The number of disfluencies does not necessarily indicate a problem, nor the severity of the problem if one exists.

Bloodstein (1975, p. 4) put it this way: "Unfortunately, we have no satisfactory *objective* means of differentiating moments of stuttering from other instances of disfluency. Consequently, the identification of moments of stuttering always involves the judgment of a listener." Johnson (1967, p. 238) suggested that "there are no 'natural' lines of demarcation between 'normal' and 'abnormal' disfluencies." We commented earlier that some types of disfluencies, notably sound or syllable repetitions or prolonged sounds, were more likely to elicit a judgment of stuttering than some other types of disfluencies. However, according to Bloodstein (1975, p. 9), this would still not be sufficient to define stuttering:

> (for) . . . the investigator who is anxious to define carefully what he means by stuttering the best definition we appear to be able to offer at present is: whatever is perceived as stuttering by a reliable observer who has relatively good agreement with others. If he wants to be guided by a more "objective" definition he must not ask questions about "stuttering" but about repetitions, prolongations, broken words, speech rate, and the like, and he must be content with answers that are not about stuttering, but about repetitions, prolongations, and so forth.

What the "reliable observer" was likely to respond to as part of her objective judgment (Bloodstein, 1975) may include "associated symptoms" of overt muscular activities, vocal abnormalities, evidence of avoidance, postponement, escape or release mechanisms, physiological concomitants such as tremors, eye movements, biochemical changes and other reflex activity—which may or may not be a part of the stutter or even of stuttering. Many of these same bodily changes have been observed to occur in normal speakers under conditions of excitement and tension. Introspective concomitants may also be part of the "associated symptoms," such as feelings of frustration in an effort to speak, feelings of muscular tension, affective reactions, such as apprehension, and so forth, but introspections are not operational definitions.

In other words, the number of disfluencies or the types of disfluencies are not of themselves sufficient to classify a speaker as stuttering rather than normally disfluent. More often the classification of "stuttering" is assigned to a speaker when we, as observers, note a set of concomitant activities with the act of speaking. But these concomitant activities, as well, may be observed in speakers who are ill at ease—especially children. There is likely to be more uncertainty in the mind of the listener if the speaker is a child and if the question is whether the speech heard is indicative of stuttering or normal-child disfluency. One of the recent publications of the Speech Foundation of America series concerned with stuttering (Ainsworth 1977), lists eight "danger signs" which indicate that the child has moved beyond the type or level of speech interruptions that are normal for his age and thereby reflect stuttering. Ainsworth (pp. 12-16) lists:

1. The use of multiple repetitions—more importantly, the repetitions are of parts of words, and sounds or syllables.
2. The schwa is used as a filler or starter. The child's production of repetitions such as "go-go-going" is likely to be viewed as normal, but "guh-guh-going" is more likely to be classed as stuttering.
3. The use of prolongations.

These first three are considered "danger" signs when they occur too frequently, in too many situations, and when they begin to affect the child's ability to communicate. They may occur occasionally in all children. The last five danger signs include speech attempts in which there are apparent:

4. tremors,
5. pitch and loudness rise,
6. struggle and tension.
7. moment of fear, and
8. avoidance.

The last five may occur together. According to Ainsworth, the eight danger signs differ from normal interruptions in two ways. The first three distort the speech patterns; the next five occur as the child reacts to interruptions in her speech. They represent behaviors that seriously inhibit the speech flow and disturb communication and indicate that the child is trying to do something about her interruptions. The presence of these "danger signs" does not necessarily mean that the child *is* stuttering, but that she *may* develop a stuttering problem unless something is done.

"STUTTERED WORD" COUNTS

The bulk of the discussion to now may seem to imply that the identification of stuttered speech is a simpler task than the identification of "stutterer." The identification of "what words are stuttered," however, is also subject to some variation. Williams and Kent (1958) reported that what the listeners were listening for was important. They asked a group of listeners to identify stutterings in tape-recorded samples of speech. A second group marked the normal interruptions in the same samples. A significantly greater number of stuttering instances was marked when the instructions were to note stuttering, and a greater number of normal disfluencies were marked when the listeners were asked to identify normal interruptions. When asked to note "stuttering interruptions" and "normal interruptions," the listeners commented that they were confused as to what was normal and what was stuttered.

MacDonald and Martin (1973), on the other hand, reported that their data showed stuttering and disfluency as two reliable and unambiguous response classes. The two sets of judges used for their study were college students who were not speech pathologists, and stuttering was not defined for them. The apparent assumption was that "anyone could identify stuttering." One set of judges listened to tape-recorded samples of speech and were asked to identify stuttering. From six to eleven days later, they were asked to listen to the same tapes but this time were asked to identify normal disfluency. The two listening instructions were reversed for the second group of judges. MacDonald and Martin reasoned that if a response were judged only as stuttering or only as disfluency, the judgments would be considered as not ambiguous. If a response were judged (by different listeners or at different times) as both stuttering and disfluency, it would be ambiguous. They reported that of all units judged as stutterings, 71 percent were identified unambiguously as stuttering; and of all disfluency judgments, 85 percent were identified unambiguously. However, only 13 percent of the judged instances of stuttering were agreed-upon by more than half the judges, and 65 percent were agreed-upon by less than 10 percent of the judges. Seven percent of the disfluencies were agreed-upon by more than half of the listeners, and 50 percent were agreed-upon by less than 10 percent of the judges. In other words, the lack of ambiguity did not mean that there was agreement among the listeners as to whether a word was stuttered or normally disfluent. A small group of responses were unambiguously identified as stuttering, and a small group were unambiguously identified as nonstuttering disfluency.

Young (1975) reported that a group of college student judges rated tape-recorded samples of speech as containing more severe examples of stuttering when the rating was done before lunch, than when the same samples were rated by a similar group of judges after lunch. It would seem that, not only are we likely to be affected by instructions as to what we are listening for (whether these instructions are given internally or externally), but we may even be affected by factors quite unrelated to the speaker's speech performance. High agreement among listeners for word-by-word disfluency judgments are unlikely (Young 1975).

In order to reduce the fallibility which appears to be built in to an attempt to count the number of stuttered words in a passage, some researchers (for example, Williams 1971) have used ten-second time periods. An automatic clock signals ten-second intervals with a buzzer. All the speech behaviors which occur within the ten-second interval are scored as if they were a single instance. If no disfluencies occurred within the ten-second unit, it would be scored as "fluent"; if one or more disfluencies occurred within the ten-second unit, regardless of the number or duration of such disfluencies, the unit would be scored as "disfluent." The advantage of ten-second scoring is that it is almost certain to be a more repeatable measure (greater agreement among listeners), and it still yields data for a measure of adaptation. However, this stability of measurement may also yield less exact consistency data and may not reveal the details of improvement or change as accurately as individual word scoring for one who stuttered more frequently.

Adaptation and Consistency

In terms of disfluency counts, two other phenomena are frequently tested with stuttering populations: adaptation and consistency. Adaptation is a group phenomenon probably first reported by Johnson and Knott (1937). The term was borrowed from learning psychology and refers to the reduction of performance errors with successive repetitions of a learning task. In reference to stuttering it refers to the reduction in moments of stuttering with repeated readings of the same material. An adaptation curve is usually charted over five successive readings, and the greatest reduction in stuttering usually occurs within the first three readings. It is a group phenomenon in that individuals may or may not reduce the instances of stuttering with successive readings. An adaptation effect in reading has been reported for both stuttering and nonstuttering children (Williams, Silverman, and Kools, 1968, 1969) and in at least one report of older children and adult nonstutterers (Silverman and Bloom 1973) in which the subjects did show an adaptation effect in reading on the first day but did not show the "spontaneous recovery"* the second day comparable to that reported for stutterers. Adaptation is greater in readings of the same material (about 50 percent) than in different material (about 20 percent) according to Wingate (1966).

Consistency is an individual phenomenon. Consistency is the tendency of the reader to stutter on the same words on successive readings. Taken together, adaptation and consistency probably indicate something about the severity of stuttering—or at least the speaker's reaction to certain word cues. The consistency of the words and the loci of the words on which the reader stuttered relate to his prediction of stuttered words (which words he expects to stutter

*The term "spontaneous recovery" is taken from the same learning paradigm as "adaptation" and "consistency." It refers to a return to the previous level of (stuttering) performance with the passage of time—commonly an interval of at least 24 hours.

on) and word fears. Adaptation theoretically relates to the speaker's situational reaction—that is, situational fears. The decelerating curve of frequency of stuttering with successive readings assumes that the speaker is progressively "more at ease" in the particular situation. If the situation changes between readings—for example, more listeners, the number of disfluencies may describe an accelerating or static curve rather than a decelerating curve. Adaptation can also be measured in terms of overall time of reading with an expected reduction in reading time, or an increase in words-per-minute with successive readings. Minifie and Cooker (1964) proposed a "disfluency index" as an expression of the efficiency of information transmission in speaking. Repetition of syllables and words may increase words-per-minute spoken without increasing information transmitted, and pauses and prolongations of sounds would reduce the number of words-per-minute spoken. With this reasoning, rather than a words-per-minute or syllables-per-minute count, Minifie and Cooker proposed a ratio of syllables (s) divided by words-per-minute (w/m). Their data demonstrated that this ratio was a more stable measure than either syllables- or words-per-minute counts. If we accept the premise of a more fluent speaker being a more efficient transmitter of verbal information, then an adaptation curve expressed in this way $(\frac{S}{W/M})$ would be a relative measure of verbal efficiency of the speaker.

Adaptation and consistency are both effected by the absolute frequency of stutterings or disfluencies (Tate, Cullinan, and Ahlstrand 1961). The more frequent are the occurrences of stuttering on initial reading of a passage, the greater the likelihood of a high consistency percentage, and the greater the probability of showing an adaptation effect. In order to eliminate the effect of frequency, Silverman and Williams (1968) proposed the adaptation curve be charted to show the proportion of total number of stutterings for all readings which occurred during each reading of a passage. These proportionate numbers would not be effected by frequency of stuttering instances and would therefore allow a comparison between individuals or groups.

RATING AND PERCEPTUAL SCALES OF STUTTERING SEVERITY

While a count of the frequency and category or types of disfluencies is obviously important in our description of speech behavior, the accuracy of this count may be questionable, and the number, by itself, is apparently not sufficient for our diagnostic (problem-no problem) decision. The descriptions and data reviewed to now would seem to agree on two important aspects:

1. a greater than "usual" number of disfluencies, especially syllable repetitions, and sound prolongations, and

2. apparent struggle behavior (facial grimaces, and the like) in speech activities, especially those which the listener perceives as demonstrating emotionality or concern for speaking on the part of the child.

In other words, in the designation of stuttering, a perceptual judgment is presumed to be operating both on the part of the speaker and on the part of the listener. One alternative to a straight "count" procedure is a severity-scale judgment based on frequency and duration of disfluencies.

Young (1961) used a nine-point scale for judging stuttering severity of tape-recorded samples. His judges were given explicit definitions of the values of each point from "1" as no stuttering, to "9" as very severe stuttering, with equal intervals of severity for the points between those two extremes. He also assumed that this elaborate scaling technique would not be practical in most clinical settings. Johnson, Darley, and Spriestersbach (1963) provide a less precise scale for rating severity (identified as the *Iowa Scale of Stuttering Behavior*) which includes frequency and duration of stuttered words plus facial movements and general bodily activity. Scale judgments (1963, p. 281) varied from "0" for no stuttering, "1" for *very mild* stuttering on less than 1 percent of words, little tension, simple disfluency patterns and disfluencies generally less than one second in duration, with no apparent associated bodily movements, to "7" for *very severe* with stuttering on more than 25 percent of words, very conspicuous tension and disfluencies averaging more than four seconds in duration, distracting sounds, and very conspicuous grimaces and other associated bodily movements. The agreement between listeners for the separations along this scale would depend on their perceptions of the frequency (1-2 percent, 2-5 percent, 5-8 percent, 8-12 percent, and 12-25 percent for the "2" through "6" or mild through severe categories) and duration of stuttered words as well as their connotative definitions of the extent or degree of distraction generated by facial or bodily movements. Because of the expected differences in judgments among listeners, the ratings obtained are expected to be gross measures only. It is expected, however, that a clinician's judgments will have some degree of uniformity and comparability with this, or some other set of judgments.

Wertheim (1972) approached the classification and measurement of stuttering with both quantitative and qualitative measures. She counted the frequency of the child's disfluencies (prolonged sounds, sound-syllable-word repetitions, broken words, and interjections), and "blocks" ("failure to vocalize in spite of efforts to do so") in answering questions put by the examiner and in conversation with his parents on a prearranged consensus task. The quantitative measure was the count of disfluencies and blocks in the talking situations; the qualitative aspect was what Wertheim defined as the situational stability of the stuttering pattern, that is, whether the child's stuttering was more severe, for example, in a school-like (two-person) situation or in a "family" situation where the child was interacting with his parents. The definition of these "stutterogenic" or sensitive areas had to do with the child's self-concept, and his perception of his relative role in school or in home situations. The report of this study does not include numerical data but describes the children as "High" (H) or "Low" (L) in frequency of disfluencies and blocks in the two talking situations. The consistency of the child's stuttering frequency (F) and block (B) scores for the two-person versus the family situation was the basis for her classifications of these stuttering subjects as "invariable," "variable," or "semi-variable." A child who was scored as "HH" in both two-person and family situations would be described as severe and of the invariable class; and "LL" in both situations would classify him as mild and invariable. If the pattern of stuttering was dependent on the situation, he was classed as variable.

Riley (1972) published a *Stuttering Severity Instrument* (SSI) in which she attempted to calibrate severity on the basis of frequency, duration, and physical concomitants. Her scale was designed to be applicable to children or adults by tallying frequency of stuttering in either reading and "job-task" descriptions or, for nonreaders, in their description of picture stories. For readers, a value of from 2 to 9 was assigned for the percentage of words stuttered in reading a 125-word passage. Reading material represented third-grade, fifth-grade, or adult reading levels, according to the capability of the reader. The first 25 words were disregarded and the next 100 were used to determine percentage of stuttered words. In addition to the reading passage, the stutterer was asked to talk about a job task–for school children the topic might be a school activity instead. The job task also was valued from 2 to 9 according to frequency of stuttering. For example, one percent of the words stuttered on either reading or job task is scored "2"; 29 percent or greater frequency of stuttering on the job task is rated as "9"; and 27 percent or greater frequency on the reading task is scored "9." These two scores are added and treated as the frequency score. For nonreaders (less than third-grade reading ability), frequency of stuttering in their description of picture stories is scored on a range from 4 to 18 points. Where the Iowa Scale utilized an estimate of average duration of stuttered word, Riley used an estimate of the three longest blocks in the reading or conversation. The score range was from "1" for "fleeting" to "7" for more than 60-second estimated duration. Physical concomitants were rated from 0 (none) to 5 (severe and painful looking) for each of four areas: distracting sounds, facial grimaces, head movements, extremity movements. In other words, a total of 18 points was possible for frequency, 7 points for duration, and 20 points for physical concomitants.

The total test score (range 0-45) is interpreted as a severity index. According to the 1972 publication, a percentile rank is also available to correspond to the SSI total score, but it is not clear from the published data whether or not these percentile rankings, the total score divisions, and the severity assignment (very mild, mild, moderate, and so forth) are arbitrarily applied. Validity was reported in terms of a ranking correlation between the SSI and the *Iowa Scale of Stuttering Severity*. It is interesting to note that the validity comparison between these two measures was slightly higher (0.89) than inter-examiner reliability (0.84) for the SSI. For comparison purposes to record the stutterer's progress in therapy, Riley suggested that the total score and/or scores on each of the three parameters (frequency, duration, and physical concomitants) be charted.

What is consistent among the various scales for stuttering is the inclusion of a judgment of "associated symptoms,"–whether separately identified or not, and approximate frequency counts of stuttered words. One other common feature is that the judgments are made by listeners, rather than by the speaker, and therefore may incorporate biases of unknown magnitude. For example, the nine-point scale ratings generated by Young (1961) were derived from 48 listeners who were categorized as stutterers, clinicians, and laymen. The mean rating for all listeners was 3.84, but stutterers were apparently most critical (mean rating 4.01), followed by clinicians (3.88), and laymen (3.68). What you know about stuttering apparently makes a difference in your judgment. What apparently is being measured is not *stuttering* per se, but the *perception* of stuttering.

Two examples of perceptual scales to be completed by the speakers are the *Iowa Scale of Attitude Toward Stuttering* (Ammons and Johnson 1944) and the *Perception of Stuttering Inventory* (Woolf 1967). The Iowa Scale consists of 45 statements (for example, If she stutters, a girl should not apply for a position as salesgirl in a department store. If a person stutters while answering a question in class, he should just stop and start over again. A barber who stutters should not stutter while giving haircuts.) which are to be marked on a five-point scale from "strongly agree" to "strongly disagree." The scale can be given to the stutterer, family members, or both to help determine attitudes held. Responses are weighted (strongly agree and agree = 4 and 3 points respectively, disagree and strongly disagree = 2 and 1 points respectively, undecided = 0 points). A mean score is derived by dividing the sum of the weights by the number of items completed, with undecided items omitted. Lower scores indicate a better attitude toward stuttering. The approximate divisions were given as:

1. from 1.0 to 1.4 represents a very good attitude with considerable tolerance of stuttering
2. from 1.4 to 2.2 indicates an average or moderate attitude and
3. above 2.2 represents a poor attitude with considerable intolerance of stuttering

Woolf's *Perceptions of Stuttering Inventory* (PSI) is a somewhat more descriptive scale designed to be administered to the one who stutters. The PSI consists of 60 statements–20 meant to indicate "struggle," 20 to indicate "avoidance," and 20 to indicate "expectancy." With the PSI scale the rater is asked to mark as many of the statements as he feels are characteristic of his speech (for example, Avoiding talking to people in authority. Feeling that interruptions in your speech will lead to stuttering. Having extra and unnecessary facial movements). The examiner can then total the number of struggle, avoidance, and expectancy items checked and to some extent, agree or disagree with the rater's check marks. Theoretically, both the attitude scale and the PSI can be used to evaluate changes with therapy, but the scores can also be used to reflect what the rater wishes to project and to that extent may or may not be valid.

Behavioral checklists also are available for the diagnostician's use in making observations. They may be viewed as having some intermediate evaluative position between observations of speech-sound productions and perceptual judgments of perceived difficulty. Behavioral checklists for speech and "associated" behaviors (for example, Luper and Mulder 1964; Johnson, Darley, and Spriestersbach 1963) typically may include type and loci of repetitions, associated tension of the respiratory mechanism, inhaling and exhaling irregularly, facial tension, movements of extremities, turning head sideways, use of avoidance and postponement devices, and the like.

DIAGNOSIS: THE PROBLEM OF STUTTERING–REACTIONS OF IMPORTANT LISTENERS

The bulk of our discussion to this point has been on the assessment of speech and speaking behavior. The intent of this chapter is to sketch an outline of suggested avenues by which the clinician may describe disfluent speech and associated behaviors which may frequently be categorized as stuttering, to separate between normally disfluent and stuttered speech, and to help define the *problem* of stuttering. Murphy (1962) lists six characteristics by which stuttering may be revealed:

1. Facial contortions, blockings, strugglings, prolongations, breaks in rhythm of speech or other signs of breakdown in the forward flow of speech to a degree that sets the speaker off from his associates.
2. An understanding between speaker and listener that stuttering actually has taken place—that is, that the speaker is trying to speak without these interferences, but often fails in the attempt.
3. Some feelings of frustration and helplessness brought on by the difficulty plus the fear of possible difficulty.
4. Some feelings of fearfulness or concern about the ability to speak at all.
5. Anxiety concerning uncertainties—not necessarily connected with speaking, and which interferes with speaking ability.
6. The speaker having a picture of himself as a stutterer, perhaps a troubled awareness that his way of talking is unnatural and is disturbing to the listener.

Note that in none of the listed six criteria is speech fluency the primary concern. The first criterion is not concerned with . . . "breaks in the rhythm of speech . . . ," but rather with the degree that such interruptions in the forward flow of speech "sets the speaker off from his associates." In other words, they are perceptions of a listener rather than observations or descriptions and are not necessarily subject to refutation or corroboration on the part of the speaker. What is assumed to be basic to the diagnosis of a problem of stuttering is an interaction between speaker and listener. A case history interview is one basic means of determining the interactive relationship. A second means, of course, is our observation of the interaction between the talker and one of his important listeners. In both cases perceptual judgments and biases may exist to distort the presenting picture. The attitude scales mentioned earlier can be an important contribution to the interactive relationship between speaker and listeners–and some of the expressed attitudes or perceptions are subject to our clinical review.

Case history forms for stuttering are not necessarily different from the general case history interview we discussed in Chapter II. That is, the forms contain suggested questions for the interview and not necessarily all of the important probes. Some forms are designed to be administered to parents (or guardian, or other knowledgeable adult) when the subject of concern is a child. With older children or adults many of the same questions may be asked of the speaker directly. Suggested interview items may frequently request descriptions of speech, when what is identified as stuttering began, signs of concern or embarrassment on the part of the speaker, judgments of the adequacy of speaking skills, listing of persons to whom the speaker talks easily and those with whom talking is more difficult, any recent change in speaking proficiency, and other similar questions which may alert the examiner to important interactions. One point bears repeating here from our earlier (Chapter II) discussion regarding case history information. The "facts" gathered are not necessarily real. The information being supplied, with the best and most honest of intentions, will have been filtered through a set of biases. For example, if you ask the child's mother when the stuttering began, her answer can only indicate when she identified her child's speech as stuttering. According to the *Onset of Stuttering* data, both parents would probably not agree as to the age, and date, when stuttering began and could probably not tell you how the speech was different on the week, or day, or month before stuttering was said to have begun. If, in the case interview, you ask the parent if the child was late in learning to talk, or late in learning to walk, you will get a judgment based on the parent's internal norms. A *judgment* of "late" may well be an important bit of information reflecting a concern with the child's speaking ability, but it may not be "real." Johnson and others (1959) reported (pp. 61-62) that more experimental (stuttering) than control (nonstuttering) group mothers rated their children much slower than the average (at the 0.01 level of confidence), but the differences in mean ages for first words and first sentences were not statistically different (at the 0.05 level of confidence):

> There were no statistically significant differences between the two groups of children with regard to the mean ages, as reported by the mothers, at which they met various specified criteria of development, including the ages at which they spoke their first words and sentences. They were essentially alike also in other aspects of speech development and speech behavior.
>
> The experimental group children were, however, rated somewhat less favorably than were the control group children by their respective parents, particularly with reference to social development. That is, there was a tendency for the experimental group parents to make ratings of their children that were somewhat less favorable than relevant objective data appeared to warrant. (p. 224)

In other words, we are seeking the evaluative judgment of the parent and as much description as possible of the speech in order to determine what that judgment was based on. We need to determine how much reeducation and re-evaluation our intervention regime must include.

With older children, or persons who have identified themselves as having a stuttering problem, questions about "when stuttering began," "age of onset," or "earliest memory of stuttering" may well be answered with other than first-hand knowledge. The most likely ages and descriptions quoted (for example, to questions as to what the speech was like at that time) will probably be what someone told them. It is also entirely logical to have a person say that a stuttering problem began in the second grade, or seventh grade, or some other milestone she remembers while her mother may say she was concerned about stuttering at the age of four or five. Wingate (1978, pp. 255-256) has reported that most stutterers are children.

> Stuttering is predominantly a disorder of early childhood. Several sources indicate that approximately 85 percent of cases of stuttering begin well before age five, and most of the remainder before age seven. . . . There is substantial evidence that over 40 percent of the youngsters identified as stuttering before five years of age will no longer be stuttering by the time they are about eight years old. . . . (There is also) ample evidence that recovery from stuttering continues to occur long after age eight.[1]

With persons who have identified themselves as stuttering, or with younger children for whom the parents supply the answers, it is pertinent to ask what, in their opinion, causes stuttering and how the stuttering is maintained. What they believe is the cause can be important to the planning of a therapy regime. It

[1]Quote from M. E. Wingate, in P. H. Skinner and R. L. Shelton, *Speech, Language, and Hearing* (Reading, Mass.: Addison-Wesley, 1979), p. 13. Reprinted by permission.

is also important to know whether the answer given denoted *the* theory or *a* theory–in other words, how important is that theoretical base to the client in question. In this and other ways it can be helpful to find out what the person knows about stuttering and what he thinks can be done about it. "Who else do you know who stutters?" can yield quite different interpretations from the same question. If Uncle Harry stuttered, "but he got over it," the evaluative reaction to the child's speech may be much less negative than if Uncle Harry stuttered, "and I sure don't want my child to have to go through that."

Especially with older children or adults, it may be important to know what, if any, previous therapy has accomplished, or what has been done about the stuttering. If therapy had been previously scheduled, you might ask how long it was continued, what was done in therapy, and why the therapy was terminated. If previous therapy was judged to be unsuccessful, as the new clinician you must either plan to do something different from what was done before or at least explain it differently, if you wish the patient to predict a different outcome from last time. When interviewing the parent of a young child, the question more likely would be phrased as "Have any special means been taken by you or anyone else to help him change his speech?" or "Have any changes occurred in his speech recently?" (and if so) "Do you have any idea what those changes may be attributed to?" With either children or adults, it may be pertinent to ask what has been done (by the speaker) to stop the stuttering, what things have helped the most, and what have helped least. The point of these questions, again, is the informational and theoretical base from which the informant or the speaker is operating.

DEGREE OF STUTTERING

We have discussed definitions of stuttering and types of disfluencies which may help separate between normal disfluency and stuttering disfluency. We have also discussed fluency counts, attitude scales, behavioral checklists, and case history information to help determine the speaker-listener interaction. We want both general and specific information to help plan the intervention regime. The questions of intervention and the type of intervention (if that is the decision) are based, not only on the information gathered in the previous methods, but on the clinician's definition of degree of stuttering and what that entails. Several categories or degrees of stuttering have been proposed. The following discussion will serve as an example.

Earlier divisions (circa 1930-1940) were usually confined to primary and secondary stuttering.*

*The words "primary" and "secondary" were usually paired with "symptom," therefore, *primary symptoms* or *secondary symptoms* of stuttering. Since the word *symptom* denotes some superficial evidence of a basic underlying fault, usually medical or psychological in

Robinson (1964) used three categories or divisions: beginning stuttering, advanced stuttering, and secondary stuttering. Bloodstein (1960a, 1960b, 1961) defined four stages or phases, which Luper and Mulder (1964) named incipient, transitional, confirmed, and advanced. The three terms of "primary," "beginning," and "incipient" refer approximately to the same group of children. The most common age of onset of stuttering (specifically, Bloodstein's Phase I) is given as preschool age, and it is for this age group that our most important diagnostic interpretation is whether or not a problem exists–and whether the problem is the child's fluency or her listener's evaluation. Phase II, the transitional stage, usually begins in early elementary school; Phase III, (Confirmed) commonly begins in Junior High or High school; and Phase IV (Advanced) commonly has its onset in High school or older, according to Bloodstein.

The diagnostic determination of phase of development of stuttering is one base for the choice of intervention techniques. For example, Bloodstein's Phase I child's speech may show episodic periods of fluctuating fluency. Repetitions of syllables and monosyllables are the characteristic speech pattern. He does not react emotionally to himself as a stutterer; stuttered words are frequently the first words in sentences or are conjunctions, prepositions, and pronouns. The child tends to speak freely in all situations with essentially no fear or embarrassment. With many clinicians, the therapy for this phase may be indirect–working more with the important persons in the child's environment than directly with the child on fluency. The distinguishing characteristic of Phase II (Transitional) is the appearance of stuttering primarily when the child talks fast and gets excited. She stutters equally frequently at home, at school, or with friends. She thinks of herself as a stutterer but talks freely in all situations with little or no concern about stuttering except in special cases or moments of unusual difficulty. The outstanding characteristic of Phase III (Confirmed) stuttering is that stuttering is fully developed but without avoidance of speech. The stuttering is essentially chronic although the child will distinctly show more difficulty in some situations than in others. The child in this phase will have developed "secondary symptoms" of postponement, starting and releasing tricks or devices. She is likely to become exasperated, annoyed or disgusted when she stutters severely, but there is generally no tendency to avoid speaking nor any outward appearance of fear or deep embarrassment. The Phase IV stutterer (Advanced) views herself as having a serious personal problem. Avoidance, postponement, starting and release

---

nature, one of the theoretical differences of opinion was whether "primary stuttering" was basically different from normal childhood disfluency. If it was, children were first primary and then secondary stutterers. If it was not, then children became stutterers from a normal disfluency stage because of the negative evaluative reaction on the part of important listeners–which the speaker internalized.

From a different frame of reference, Wingate (1978) refers to stuttering as a "primary" speech disorder (fluency) in contrast to neurological disorders, such as Parkinsonism or cerebral palsy in which there may be fluency disorders which are secondary or result from a more basic problem.

devices are highly developed, and she shows a definite emotional reaction to stuttering, complete with the avoidance of some speaking situations, and obvious fear and embarrassment.

Fluency—Developmental and Judgmental

This text is not concerned with therapy except incidentally, but it is obvious that a diagnostic evaluation should also supply information relative to an intervention plan. Fluency, like articulation or language skill, is a dimension of speech that is developmental (Gregory 1973). One of the important aspects of an evaluation for a child referred for professional advice because of a concern with fluency is therefore a thorough evaluation of his speech and language skill. Just as we need to know about his disfluency patterns, his reactions to his speech, his general health, and his history of speech and language development, we need to know how he copes with his world in general. It has been mentioned previously that a diagnosis of a stuttering problem is not made purely on the basis of what comes out of the child's mouth. The "problem" may be an evaluative reaction or just lack of "normative" information on the part of the parent. It is not enough for you as an examiner merely to determine to your own satisfaction whether or not the child is normally fluent. The important question to ask yourself, when concerned with a young child, is "What are the likely consequences of the diagnostic judgment?" If the parent were seeking reassurance, your decision that the child was displaying normal speech, language, and fluency may be a welcome corroboration. If the parent were seeking help for a problem she was sure existed, your reassurance of "normal" may or may not be sufficient. One of the important implications of Johnson's definition of the *problem* of stuttering–which we discussed with the three continua–is that in our therapeutic intervention we should work with the one who has the problem. It may be helpful to schedule the child with a group of others who have near-normal language skills for the sake of definition and comparison. In response to the Williams and Kent (1958) data which suggested that their listeners heard more stuttering when asked to identify stuttering, and more normal disfluencies when they were asked to mark normal interruptions, one of the objectives in counseling parents who consider their child to be stuttering is to help them re-evaluate some of the child's speech interruptions.

Disfluency as an Index of Language Skill

The basic reason for the child's speech disfluency may be inadequately developed language skills. From somewhat different bases, Weiss (1964), Luchsinger and Arnold (1965), Berry (1938), Froeschels (1958), Wyatt (1969), and Luper (1970) have all postulated interactions between language skills and stuttering. Many reporters have noted a difference in the fluency of young children depending on the linguistic complexity of the utterance. Muma (1971) reported that more disfluencies occurred in the speech of young children in the production of double-base sentences than on sentences with a single-base structure. That study did not answer whether the greater amount of disfluency was a function of the language the child used or of the child who used the language. Daughtry (1976) attempted to find a partial answer to that question. She separated a group of first-grade children on the basis of more or fewer disfluencies of all types in their repetition of sentences. These two groups of children were then asked to perceptually locate clicks embedded in tape-recorded sentences. On the assumption that children with greater linguistic skill would tend to displace the click to a syntactic boundry, (for example, Ladefoged and Broadbent 1960; Fodor and Bever 1965; Garrett, Bever, and Fodor 1965), a difference in linguistic skill should be reflected in the perceptual accuracy of the click placement. Keeping in mind that the validity of this technique has not been unambiguously established (Olson and Clark 1976), the data from this study indicated that the children in the disfluent group tended to place the clicks more veridically and the more fluent children tended to displace the click toward a syntactic boundary, thus implying greater language skill for the fluent children.

It should be noted that neither the Muma study nor the Daughtry study was concerned with stuttering per se, and we have assumed earlier that stuttering and disfluency are not the same thing, although they may be difficult to separate in young children. The specific purpose in commenting on these studies at this point is to stress the importance of language testing with young children referred with a question of stuttering or normal disfluency and the frequent logic of therapy to improve language proficiency with these children as a means of improving fluency.

Differentiation between Normal and Abnormal Disfluencies

The differentiation between stuttering and normal disfluencies is not at all difficult when the disorder is severe or in more advanced stages. The difficulty is greatest when the disorder is very mild or in earliest stages of development. One of the reasons for this difficulty, it may be assumed, is the relative subjectivity of the judgments we are asked to make. There are, however, some objective comparisons that can be made. In the decade of the 1970s there was a considerable interest in acoustic description of stuttered speech and stuttering speakers. Two such measures are Voice Onset Time (VOT) and Reaction Time (RT). As used here, VOT is the latency between a speaker's assumption of an articulatory gesture and the initiation of voicing, or the transition between unvoiced and voiced phonemes. RT is the latency between a signal, such as a pure-tone delivered through earphones, and the speaker's response, for example in producing a vowel or tapping a key. There is some evidence that more stuttering occurs when the manner of vocalization (voiced or unvoiced) is changed (Wingate 1976), and that less stuttering occurs when voiceless sounds are removed from a specially constructed passage (Adams and Reis 1971, 1974). Starkweather and others (1976), Adams and Hayden (1976), Cross and Luper (1979) and others have shown that stuttering adults and children are generally slower in reaction time than are nonstutterers, and that the stuttering subjects are slower in the transition from unvoiced to voiced sound productions.

Stuttering and nonstuttering speakers have been shown to differ also in vowel duration and transition times (Zimmerman 1980; Hand 1979) which may be a function of what Cooper and Allen (1977) define as a "timing control" problem. The differences between groups are slight, usually ranging under 15 msec, and individual speaker variations are reported in most studies having to do with these types of measures. One point bears repeating in our concern with differentiating between normal disfluency and beginning stuttering. The small, but relatively consistent, differences between groups of stutterers and nonstutterers have been with adults and with "confirmed" samples of children who stutter. We implied earlier in this chapter that there was little difficulty in identifying stuttering adults, but that the separation between normal disfluency and stuttering in young children was more difficult and may have different consequences. It should also be remembered that these types of acoustic measures may be made from a sound spectograph but cannot be made reliably without the aid of such instrumentation.

The instrumental measures were mentioned here to give credence to the statement which frequently appears in clinical reporting that the stuttering child's speech is "jerky." For example, Van Riper (1971) defines stuttering behavior as ". . . a word improperly patterned in time. . . ." (p. 15), and that the differentiation of normal from abnormal disfluency is made partly on the basis of irregularity of syllable repetitions.

> The few syllabic repetitions which normal speakers show not only occur at the same tempos as the rest of their syllables, but they occur evenly, regularly. When we find a person repeating syllables jerkily rather then smoothly, we tend to diagnose abnormality. (Van Riper 1971, p. 23)

and further, (p. 25):

> The airflow in stuttering repetitions is usually interrupted whereas in the normal speakers it usually continues during disfluencies. Moreover the interruption in stuttering repetitions is usually sudden while in contrast, the syllable of normal nonfluency shows a gradual termination before it

is repeated. And there is another characteristic that seems to distinguish the abnormal from the normal syllabic repetitions: the pauses between syllables are much shorter in stuttered repetitions.

Lest we appear to have made it too simple or too precise—lest we appear to have suddenly resolved the distinction between a judgment of normal and abnormal disfluency, remember that the Van Riper descriptions listed here are still subjective. Table 9-2 is a set of relative guideline statements where many of the behaviors are qualified as "may be present," "often apparent," "usually absent," and so forth.

Along the same lines as the Van Riper checklist is the clinical strategy published by Adams (1977). The five behavioral characteristics utilized by Adams for differentiating normal from abnormal disfluencies include:

(1) the number of disfluencies per 100 words. Stuttering children are expected to average 10 or more disfluencies per 100 words; their normally disfluent peers average five to six disfluencies per 100 words.

(2) The proportion of the disfluencies which are part-word repetitions and sound prolongations differ. Adams reported that "young stutterers evinced more than four times as many part-word repetitions, and 10 times as many sound prolongations, as normal nonfluent control group children."

(3) Part-word repetitions will consist of one to five productions of the unit being repeated with probably more than three iterations ("b-b-b-b-ball"). The nonstuttering children's repetitions will range from one to three productions.

(4) "The part-word repetitions and sound prolongations of young stutterers seem to be marked by the abrupt, abnormal cessation of voice or air flow through the vocal tract."

(5) In their part-word repetitions the stuttering children are likely to substitute the schwa for the vowel expected* ("puh-puh-puh-paper").

If all five of the behavioral characteristics appear to fall on one side or the other of the stuttering-normal disfluency choice, the child can be characterized with relative assurance (according to Adams). The observational results may also be equivocal, with three judgments on one side of the coin and two on the other. If that were the case, the interpretation of choice would probably be conservative. If, as the diagnostician, you were unsure whether the behavior presented was normal disfluency or "incipient" stuttering, Adams's advice is to view the child as normally disfluent but to maintain weekly contacts with the parents and monthly contacts with the child. The child's variations in fluency can be monitored in that way until the diagnostic decision can be made with more confidence.

*Montgomery and Cooke (1976) question the prevalence of the schwa vowel in stuttered speech. They played CV segments of stuttered speech to a panel of five judges who were asked to transcribe the vowels they heard. Less than 25 percent were perceived as schwas with the vast majority of the schwa confusions occurring when either /ɝ/ or /aI/ were intended.

Table 9-2 Guidelines for Differentiating Normal from Abnormal Disfluency

Behavior	*Stuttering*	*Normal Disfluency*
Syllable Repetitions:		
a. Frequency per word	More than two	Less than two
b. Frequency per 100 words	More than two	Less than two
c. Tempo	Faster than normal	Normal tempo
d. Regularity	Irregular	Regular
e. Schwa vowel	Often present	Absent or rare
f. Airflow	Often interrupted	Rarely interrupted
g. Vocal tension	Often apparent	Absent
Prolongations:		
h. Duration	Longer than one second	Less than one second
i. Frequency	More than one per 100 words	Less than one per 100 words
j. Regularity	Uneven or interrupted	Smooth
k. Tension	Important when present	Absent
l. When voiced (sonant)	May show rise in pitch	No pitch rise
m. When unvoiced (surd)	Interrupted airflow	Airflow present
n. Termination	Sudden	Gradual
Gaps (silent pauses):		
o. Within the word boundary	May be present	Absent
p. Prior to speech attempt	Unusually long	Not marked
q. After the disfluency	May be present	Absent
Phonation:		
r. Inflections	Restricted; monotone	Normal
s. Phonatory arrest	May be present	Absent
t. Vocal fry	May be present	Usually absent
Articulating Postures:		
u. Appropriateness	May be inappropriate	Appropriate
Reactions to Stress:		
v. Type	More broken words	Normal disfluencies
Evidence of Awareness:		
w. Phonemic consistency	May be present	Absent
x. Frustration	May be present	Absent
y. Postponements (stallers)	May be present	Absent
z. Eye contact	May waver	Normal

From C. Van Riper, The Nature of Stuttering, *Englewood Cliffs N.J.: Prentice-Hall, Inc., 1971. Used by permission.*

Whether Child Stuttering Is Chronic

There are a number of reports in the literature concerning children who once stuttered but who no longer stutter–some hopefully because of therapy, some probably in spite of therapy, and some who had no exposure to speech therapy. Cooper (1973) summarized these reports with the assumption that two out of every three stutterers speech clinicians meet in the schools will recover spontaneously. It is possible that at least some of these "recovered stutterers" were misclassified, but it is also possible that there may be predictive variables concerning the chronicity of stuttering. In his review of the literature, Cooper discussed some of the variables. Briefly summarized, there does not appear to be a consistency of relationship between chronic stuttering and family history of stuttering. There is general agreement that, at least to a degree, the more severe the initial stuttering the more likely it will be maintained and require therapeutic intervention. The duration or length of time the stuttering is reported to have existed does not appear to be related to chronicity. There was no apparent sex bias in the literature–both boys and girls were equally likely to maintain stuttering or to spontaneously recover. It has also been reported–and it is an empirically logical statement–that those who had incorporated stuttering into their self-concept were much more likely to have remained stutterers (Sheehan and Martyn 1966). There is one other general agreement in the literature regarding chronicity–recovery from stuttering is a gradual process.

For our diagnostic purposes, it is important to note three items from that list: (1) the more severe the stuttering, the more likely it will be maintained, (2) the more the speaker's self-concept includes an identification of "stutterer" the more likely stuttering will be maintained, and (3) the recovery from stuttering is a gradual process. The severity variable is important because although there may be disagreement among listeners as to the exact frequency of disfluencies in a child's speech, disagreement is much less likely when a severe stuttering problem exists. The self-concept statement highlights the importance of background information and perceptual judgments on the part of the speaker and/or her concerned listeners; and the "gradual recovery" statement is important to remember for all who are concerned with the therapeutic process–on both sides of the table. Therapeutic change is a process, and change occurs by degree not by decree.

One other very important point relative to the "diagnosis" of stuttering is highlighted in the following quote from Luper and Ford (1980):

> The experienced clinician recognizes also that it is wise to avoid jumping to conclusions on the basis of initial evaluation data. The variability of the occurrence of stuttering and of the conditions which appear to set it off is so great that frequent reevaluation is considered highly important.

SUMMARY

There is a considerable body of literature available on stuttering. Van Riper collected a bibliography (see Sheehan, 1970) of nearly 900 entries for the period from 1950 to 1970. Bloodstein (1975) included more than 950 citations on stuttering in a single text. Much is known about stuttering, but there are no objective tests of this speech disorder. There is little that the stutterer does, of a sort that can be conveyed by available descriptions of nonfluent speech behavior, that the nonstutterer does not also do to some extent and in some instances in equivalent measure (Johnson and others, 1959). In spite of the divergent views held on stuttering, it is doubtful that there would be any disagreement that the fundamental observable characteristic of stuttering is a disruption in the flow of speech. There is general agreement that stuttering most often includes specific types of disfluencies–but the presence, the frequency, or the articulatory effort with which these disfluencies are produced does not consistently separate between normally disfluent and stuttering speakers. Stuttering always involves a perceptual judgment on the part of a listener (who may also be the talker), and an important variable in the problem of stuttering involves the interaction between the talker and his listener (or listeners).

The bulk of our discussion on stuttering has had to do with a description of disfluency indices and the ubiquitous implication that it may be difficult to separate between beginning stuttering and normal disfluency. The distinction has therapeutic as well as theoretical implications. Luper and Mulder (1964) have stated that the examiner's task is to collect the information, summarize the findings, draw conclusions, and make recommendations concerning treatment. Planning for therapy begins with the evaluation. It is the clinician's task to arrive at a reasonable understanding of the child so that therapy can be fitted to the child rather than the child fitted to the therapy. Among the questions to be answered is whether therapy intervention will be direct or indirect. "Even if it is found that a child's speech is normal, it is not enough simply to tell his parents or teacher this." (Luper and Mulder 1964).

We have made relatively few specific comments about what stuttering is and what it is not–and little about separating between early stuttering and normal disfluency. In that lack of specificity, we are in concert with most of the authorities on stuttering. Bloodstein (1977), in a state-of-the-art comment, has written:

> The principal questions about stuttering 25 to 50 years ago were: What is it?; What causes it?; How should we treat it? Those were the big questions then, and of course they are still unanswered now . . . A very large amount of information about stuttering has accumulated. But the basic questions remain. (p. 148):

> What relationships, if any, does early stuttering have to normal childhood disfluency? There are at least three possible answers to this question. First, there may be no relationship whatever. If that is the answer, we will not be very fortunate, because it will leave us in the dark. Second, early stuttering may be the child's effort to avoid normal disfluency. This was Johnson's answer. If it is correct we will be moderately lucky. It is an illuminating hypothesis, but it has proved difficult to verify. Third, early stuttering and normal speech repetitions may be merely the same thing in different degrees. If this is the case we will probably be very fortunate, because it should be relatively easy to verify it by careful comparative studies of early stuttering and normal disfluency. (p. 149)

With or without an apparent agreement among the scientific community as to the distinguishing characteristics between early stuttering and normal disfluency, it is the clinician's obligation to observe carefully, to operationally describe the speech behavior and the associated mannerisms accompanying the act of speech, to carefully interpret reactions and perceptions of the speaker and her important audience (being aware that these are *interpretations* and not necessarily facts), and to make a judgment concerning any necessary intervention. With older children or adults who stutter, the description of the stuttering behavior and a judgment concerning therapy may be a relatively easy task. With younger children, especially preschoolers, the task is complicated because there is more at stake. One of the concerns the clinician must have has to do with the consequences of the judgment to be pronounced. If a parent is seeking reassurance, it may be sufficient that you describe the speech behaviors observed in terms of what is to be expected of a child in the process of speech and language development. If the parent is seeking intervention and correction of what she perceives as a problem, reassurance may not be adequate. As a diagnostician you must make a judgment of the consequences of the child being placed in therapy—and the consequences of his not being placed in therapy. Is there a problem? What is the problem? Who has the problem? What can be done about it?

REFERENCES

Adams, M. R., A clinical strategy for differentiating the normally nonfluent child and the incipient stutterer. *J. Fluency Dis.,* 2, 141-148 (1977).

Adams, M. R., and R. Reis, The influence of the onset of phonation on the frequency of stuttering. *J. Speech Hearing Res.,* 14, 639-644 (1971).

Adams, M. R., and R. Reis. The influence of the onset of phonation on the frequency of stuttering: A replication and reevaluation. *J. Speech Hearing Res.,* 17, 752-754 (1974).

Adams, M. R., and P. Hayden, The ability of stutterers and non-stutterers to initiate and terminate phonation during production of an isolated vowel. *J. Speech Hearing Res.,* 19, 290-296 (1976).

Ainsworth, S., ed., *If Your Child Stutters: A Guide for Parents.* Memphis, Tennessee: Speech Foundation of America, (1977).

Ammons, R., and W. Johnson, The construction and application of a test of attitude toward stuttering. *J. Speech Dis.,* 9, 39-49 (1944).

Berry, M. F., The developmental history of stuttering children. *J. Pediatrics,* 12, 209-217 (1938).

Bloodstein, O., Stuttering. *J. Speech Hearing Dis.,* 42, 148-151 (1977).

Bloodstein, O., *A Handbook on Stuttering.* Chicago: The National Easter Seal Society for Crippled Children and Adults, (1975).

Bloodstein, O., The development of stuttering: III. Theoretical and clinical implications. *J. Speech Hearing Dis.,* 26, 67-82 (1961).

Bloodstein, O., The development of stuttering: I. Changes in nine basic features. *J. Speech Hearing Dis.* 25, 219-237 (1960a).

Bloodstein, O., The development of stuttering: II. Developmental phases. *J. Speech Hearing Dis.* 25, 366-376 (1960b).

Cooper, E. B., The development of a stuttering chronicity prediction checklist: A preliminary report. *J. Speech Hearing Dis.,* 38, 2, 215-223 (1973).

Cooper, M. H., and G. D. Allen, Timing control accuracy in normal speakers and stutterers. *J. Speech Hearing Res.,* 20, 55-71 (1977).

Cross, D. E., and H. L. Luper, Voice reaction time of stuttering and nonstuttering children and adults. *J. Fluency Dis.,* 4, 59-77 (1979).

Daughtry, G. H., The performance of fluent and disfluent seven-year-old males in locating clicks superimposed on sentences. Unpublished paper, University of Tennessee, Knoxville, (1976).

Fodor, J., and T. Bever, The psychological reality of linguistic segments. *J. Verb. Learn. Verb. Behav.,* 4, 414-420 (1965).

Froeschels, E., Summary statement written in 1955. *Stuttering: Significant Theories and Therapies,* ed. E. F. Hahn. Stanford: Stanford University Press, (1958).

Garrett, M., T. Bever, and J. Fodor, The active use of grammar in speech perception. *Percep. Psychophysics,* 1, 30-32 (1965).

Gregory, H., *Stuttering: Differential Evaluation and Therapy.* Indianapolis: Bobbs-Merrill, (1973).

Hand, R., An acoustical study of fluent speech in stutterers and nonstutterers. Unpublished Doctoral dissertation, University of Tennessee, Knoxville, (1979).

Johnson, W., Stuttering, in *Speech Handicapped School Children,* eds. W. Johnson and D. Moeller. New York: Harper & Row, (1967).

Johnson, W. and Associates, *The Onset of Stuttering.* Minneapolis: University of Minnesota Press, (1959).

Johnson, W., F. L. Darley, and D. C. Spriestersbach, *Diagnostic Methods in Speech Pathology.* New York: Harper & Row, (1963).

Johnson, W., and J. R. Knott, The distribution of moments of stuttering in successive readings of the same material. *J. Speech Dis.,* 2, 17-19 (1937).

Ladefoged, P., and D. Broadbent, Perception of sequence in auditory events. *Quart. J. Exper. Psych.,* 12, 162-170 (1960).

Luchsinger, R., and G. E. Arnold, *Voice-Speech-Language.* Belmont, Calif.: Wadsworth, (1965).

Luper, H. L., Some speculations on the nature of stuttering in children. *Annual Postgraduate Symposium on Hearing and Speech, University of Kansas Medical School,* Kansas City, 23-27 (1970).

Luper, H. L., and S. C. Ford, Disorders of fluency, in *Communication Disorders: An Introduction,* ed. R. Van Hattum. New York: Macmillan, (1980).

Luper, H. L., and R. L. Mulder, *Stuttering: Therapy for Children.* Englewood Cliffs, N.J.: Prentice-Hall, Inc., (1964).

MacDonald, J. D., and R. R. Martin, Stuttering and disfluency as two reliable and unambiguous response classes. *J. Speech Hearing Res.,* 16, 691-699 (1973).

Minifie, F. D., and H. S. Cooker, A disfluency index. *J. Speech Hearing Dis.,* 29, 189-192 (1964).

Montgomery, A. A., and P. A. Cooke, Perceptual and acoustic analysis of repetitions in stuttered speech. *J. Comm. Dis.,* 9, 317-330 (1976).

Muma, J., Syntax of preschool fluent and disfluent speech: A transformational analysis. *J. Speech Hearing Res.,* 14, 428-441 (1971).

Murphy, A., ed., *Stuttering, Its Prevention.* Memphis, Tenn.: Speech Foundation of America, (1962).

Olson, G., and H. Clark, Research methods in psycholinguistics, in *Handbook of Perception: Vol. VII Language and Speech,* eds. E. Carterette and M. Friedman. New York: Academic Press (1976).

Riley, G. D., A stuttering severity instrument for children and adults. *J. Speech Hearing Dis.,* 37, 314-322 (1972).

Robinson, F. B., *Introduction to Stuttering.* Englewood Cliffs, N.J.: Prentice-Hall, Inc., (1964).

Sheehan, J., *Stuttering: Research and Therapy.* New York: Harper & Row. (1970).

Sheehan, J. G., and M. M. Martyn, Spontaneous recovery from stuttering. *J. Speech Hearing Res.,* 9, 121-155 (1966).

Silverman, F. H., and C. M. Bloom, Spontaneous recovery of nonstutterers' disfluency following adaptation. *J. Speech Hearing Res.,* 16, 452-455 (1973).

Silverman, F. H., and D. E. Williams, A proportional measure of stuttering adaptation. *J. Speech Hearing Res.,* 11, 444-446 (1968).

Starkweather, C. W., P. Hirschman, and R. S. Tannenbaum, Latency of vocalization: Stutterers vs. nonstutterers. *J. Speech Hearing Res.,* 19, 481-492 (1976).

Tate, M., W. Cullinan, and A. Ahlstrand, Measurement of adaptation in stuttering. *J. Speech Hearing Res.,* 4, 321-339 (1961).

Van Riper, C., Bibliography, 1950-1970, in J. G. Sheehan, *Stuttering: Research and Therapy.* New York: Harper & Row, (1970).

Van Riper, C., *The Nature of Stuttering.* Englewood Cliffs, N.J.: Prentice-Hall, Inc., (1971).

Van Riper, C., *Speech Correction: Principles and Methods.* 6th ed. Englewood Cliffs, N.J.: Prentice-Hall, Inc., (1978).

Weiss, D. A., *Cluttering.* Englewood Cliffs, N.J.: Prentice-Hall, Inc., (1964).

Wertheim, E. S., A new approach to the classification and measurement of stuttering. *J. Speech Hearing Dis.,* 37, 2, 242-251 (1972).

Williams, D., Evaluation, in *Therapy for Stutterers,* ed. C. W. Starkweather. Memphis, Tenn.: Speech Foundation of America, (1974).

Williams, D. E., and L. R. Kent, Listener evaluations of speech interruption. *J. Speech Hearing Res.,* 1, 124-131 (1958).

Williams, D. E., F. H. Silverman, and J. A. Kools, Disfluency behavior of elementary school stutterers and nonstutterers: The adaptation effect. *J. Speech Hearing Res.,* 11, 622-630 (1968).

Williams, D. E., F. H. Silverman, and J. A. Kools, Disfluency behavior of elementary school stutterers and nonstutterers: The consistency effect. *J. Speech Hearing Res.,* 12, 301-307 (1969).

Williams, J. G., A study concerning the relationship of disfluencies to selected linguistic skills. Unpublished Master's thesis, University of Tennessee, Knoxville (1974).

Wingate, M. E., Disorders of fluency, in *Speech, Language, and Hearing: Normal Processes and Disorders,* eds. P. H. Skinner and P. Shelton. Reading, Mass.: Addison-Wesley, (1978).

Wingate, M. E., *Stuttering: Theory and Treatment,* New York: Irvington Publishers, (1976).

Wingate, M. E., Stuttering adaptations and learning: I. The relevance of adaptation studies to stuttering as "learned behavior." *J. Speech Hearing Dis.,* 31, 148-156 (1966).

Wingate, M. E., A standard definition of stuttering. *J. Speech Hearing Dis.,* 29, 484-489 (1964).

Woolf, C., The assessment of stuttering as struggle, avoidance and expectancy. *Brit. J. Dis. Comm.,* 2, 158-171 (1967).

Wyatt, G. L., *Language Learning and Communication Disorders in Children.* New York: The Free Press, (1969).

Young, M. A., Observer agreement for marking moments of stuttering. *J. Speech Hearing Res.,* 18, 530-540 (1975).

Young, M. A., Predicting ratings of severity of stuttering, *J. Speech Hearing Dis.,* Monogr. Sup. 7, 31-54 (1961).

Zimmerman, G., Articulatory Dynamics of fluent utterances of stutterers and nonstutterers. *J. Speech Hearing Res.,* 23, 95-105 (1980).

Evaluation of Adult Neurological Disorders

X

. . . if the patient doesn't agree with the book, throw away the book, not the patient. The patient cannot be wrong.

Kurt Goldstein to Aaron Smith

A host of speech and language disorders result from damage to the brain after communicative skills have been acquired. These disorders are termed *acquired* to contrast them with *congenital* deficits which develop from brain damage incurred before the acquisition of communicative skills. Perhaps no other group of disorders, with the possible exception of stuttering, has been as controversial, as rich in history, or as burdened with a confusing nomenclature.

The controversies that have resulted from attempts to model the functional landscape of the brain and to describe syndromes of impairment associated with particular sites of lesion stem from its complex architecture and operation. The brain is characterized by a dense anatomic connectivity and a continuous activity such that no part is isolated functionally from all other parts. Consequently, a lesion does not destroy a particular cortical area and its corresponding function but deforms the normal patterns of interaction of a whole network of activities. This conceptualization of the nervous system by Lenneberg (1975) may serve as a partial explanation for two conundrums he has eloquently described. First, studies of brain lesions and brain stimulation affects do not agree; that is, cognitive and/or motor activities that are lost due to a lesion are not necessarily the activities observed during stimulation of the same area. Secondly, patients with widespread cortical damage frequently exhibit

similar speech-language deficits while patients with very similar cortical damage can often exhibit very different symptoms.

Given that Lenneberg's conceptualization of neural activity is valid, it is not surprising that early attempts to localize specific functions to circumscribed areas of the brain, as if it were a functional mosaic that only needed to be mapped to be understood and attempts to describe the brain as equipotential in terms of its ability to subserve a multitude of functions have led to controversy. At the same time we, as clinicians, must be cognizant of the fact that these early efforts to impose theoretical constructs on a mechanism of great complexity have been the source for our test models and terminology.

The terms that have evolved to serve as abbreviations for constellations of deficits resulting from brain damage are confusing and serve to obstruct, rather than facilitate, communication. Consequently, for purposes of discussion and clarification, we will define the major categories of communication disorders to be considered.

DEFINITIONS AND DESCRIPTIONS OF NEUROGENIC DISORDERS

At birth, both hemispheres of the brain are capable of establishing activity patterns that constitute verbal processes, but as the organism matures, there is a genetically predetermined displacement of verbal functions to the left hemisphere and nonverbal functions to the right hemisphere (Krashen 1976; Gates and Bradshaw 1977). The dominance is functional rather than anatomical although there are some differences between the left and right hemispheres (LeMay and Geschwind 1978). Consequently, almost all right-handed and most left-handed individuals will have left-hemisphere dominance for speech and language representation.

Damage to the dominant hemisphere will produce disturbances on a variety of tasks, usually affecting some more than others, depending on the site and extent of lesion. *Aphasia* is a multimodality language disorder characterized by reduced ability to encode and decode linguistic elements. Reading, writing, speaking, and comprehension abilities are involved; and the impairment affects semantic, syntactic, lexical, and phonological aspects of the linguistic process. Considerable difference of opinion exists as to whether aphasia is best viewed as a singular disorder or as a disorder with a number of identifiable syndromes of impairment. *Apraxia* is an inability to program movements or sequences of movements for speech production (Darley, Aronson, and Brown 1975). The disorder is considered to be independent of linguistic deficits and neuromuscular impairment, although these disorders may be frequent concomitants. *Agnosia* is a disorder characterized by an inability to recognize stimuli even though the sensory pathway to the brain is intact. We have chosen to define this disorder because it is a primary diagnostic label on several test batteries. We wish to

quickly point out, however, that there seems to be less and less support for its use. For example, Penfield and Roberts (1959) observed that "terms such as those of agnosia . . . do nothing but confuse us. There is not a single case in the literature of . . . agnosia without other defects."

Damage to the right hemisphere, which typically is dominant for performance activities, produces a syndrome of communication-related deficits. These patients demonstrate poor judgment, inability to follow through on a task which requires several steps for its completion, verbosity, difficulty recognizing familiar faces, and poor locational and directional skills (Brookshire 1978; Joynt and Goldstein 1975). No specific term has been developed for this syndrome.

Acute and chronic bihemispheric structural changes or interference with neural activity produce disorders which have been termed by Darley (1964) as the *language of confusion* and the *language of generalized intellectual deterioration,* respectively. The language of confusion is characterized by reduced recognition and understanding of and responsiveness to the environment, faulty short-term memory, mistaken reasoning, disorientation in time and space, and behavior which is less adaptive and less appropriate than normal (Darley 1964). The language of generalized intellectual deterioration includes a prominent impairment of memory, particularly for recent events; impoverished, concrete thinking which may lead to difficulty in coping with simple tasks; emotional and personality changes, and word-finding problems (Darley 1964; Miller 1977).

Dysarthrias are neuromuscular speech disorders. They may affect the entire speech-production mechanism including respiratory, phonatory, and articulatory processes or be limited to more specific musculature, such as in laryngeal paralysis. The type of dysarthria demonstrated by the patient will depend upon the site of lesion within the motor pathways.

It is important to note that none of the acquired neuropathological disorders are mutually exclusive. In fact, it is more common to find a patient demonstrating more than one of the disorders described since the anatomical connectivity of the nervous system seldom produces as isolated deficit. Our consideration of appraisal procedures for these patients will include an examination of aphasia batteries and related assessment tools, a description of language categories useful in differentiating among disorders, and a short procedural guide for evaluating the patient.

TESTS FOR APHASIA AND RELATED DISORDERS

Numerous test batteries have been developed to evaluate communicative disabilities arising from injury to the dominant hemisphere for verbal skills. In general, they include a number of subtests which evaluate specific subskills of the communicative process, rather than a single estimate of a skill such as

writing. One simplistic model of the communicative skills evaluated by these batteries and described by Brookshire is provided in Figure 10-1.

This model separates language processes into three sections: an input or reception stage, a central or processing stage, and an output or expression stage. Within these sections, three types of input are identified: auditory, visual, and tactile and three types of output: verbal, graphic, and gestural.

During testing one or more input modalities are combined in the presentation of a stimulus and one or more output modalities are utilized for the response. Inferences regarding the integrity of the processing mechanism are then drawn, based on the output responses to stimuli presented through one or more of the input modalities at various complexity levels. For example, the patient may be presented auditorally with the name of a tool and asked to demonstrate its use. This is an example of an auditory input and a gestural response. Alternatively, the patient may be handed a pencil and asked to name it—here a visual and tactile input are coupled to a verbal response. Similar examples can be developed for all combinations of input and output. Other models of language processing in aphasia can be found in Osgood and Miron (1963).

The aphasia battery you choose to evaluate these processes will, as mentioned earlier, be based on your purposes in testing and your biases. However, Brookshire (1978) has provided some criteria based on suggestions by Weisenburg and McBride (1935); Schuell (1965) and Porch (1967, 1971) as to what constitutes an adequate test for the evaluation of these disorders (see list on p. 248):

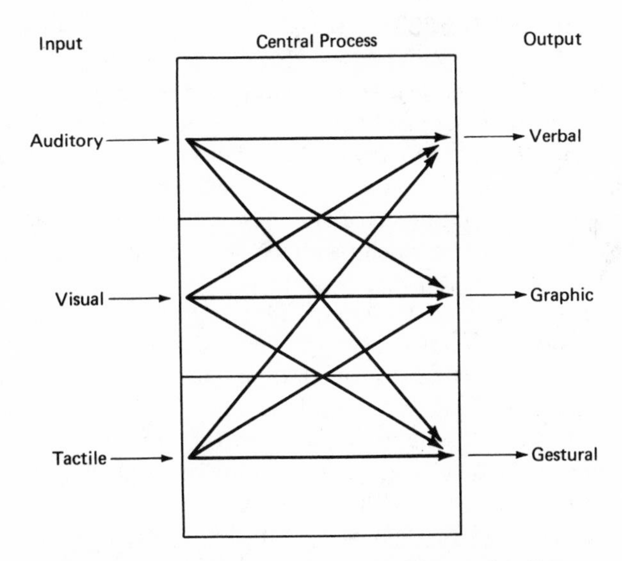

Figure 10-1 Model of the Language Processing System

(Adapted from R. Brookshire, ***An Introduction to Aphasia,*** 2nd ed. Minneapolis: BRK Publishers, 1978. By permission.)

a. The examination should measure the patient's performance with stimuli and responses in all language modalities.
b. The examination should provide for measurement of nonlanguage abilities which may influence speech and language functioning.
c. The examination should be qualitative. It should provide information regarding *how* and *why* performance is deficient.
d. The examination should minimize the effects of intelligence and education on test performance.
e. The examination should be reliable, so that different examiners, and the same examiner on different occasions, obtain comparable results.
f. The examination should include tests of graduated difficulty in each modality.
g. The examination should include a sufficient number of items in each subtest so that unsystematic variability in responding will not dramatically alter the test results.
h. The examination should provide information which will make possible predictions regarding the course and extent of potential recovery.
i. The examination should provide information which will be useable in planning and implementing treatment programs.

Not all tests meet these criteria. You will have to decide which of the criteria are the most important for your purposes. A review of some batteries for the evaluation of aphasia and related disorders may help provide a basis for your judgment.

TEST BATTERIES FOR APHASIA AND RELATED DISORDERS

Aphasia test batteries can be viewed along a number of dimensions: for example, the qualitative nature of the scoring, the number of test items and subtests, the prognostic value of quantified behaviors, and the ease of administration and interpretation. The tack used here will be a historical perspective because it serves as the best means of interlocking theoretical assumptions about neurogenic communication deficits and the tests constructed to assess these disorders.

Examining for Aphasia (Eisenson 1954) was developed on the premise that aphasic disturbances are impairments in the ability of the patient to handle situations involving significant symbolization manifested in internal symbol processes (thinking) and external symbol processes (speaking, reading, writing). The battery contains 16 subtests divided into two main parts: items used to evaluate abilities to deal with simple recognition or evaluation (predominantly receptive) and items used to evaluate expressive verbal and nonverbal skills (predominantly expressive). The approach of the test follows from the work of Weisenburg and McBride (1935) who classified aphasia on the basis of receptive and expressive functioning.

The items in each subtest are arranged in order of difficulty and the test attempts to obtain a maximal performance from the patient under ideal conditions. Specific procedures are provided for administering each item, but on several subtests only general directions are provided because the examiner may have to determine the optimal means of presentation. Scoring is primarily dichotomous, but space is provided on the record form for noting behavior, response times, and modifications of procedure used by the examiner.

The examiner may accept a variety of possible responses so long as the response signifies understanding of the item. The test has not been standardized in terms of normative data, stimulus presentation, or scoring responses. No scale or percentage scores or other weighting is provided. Rather, an estimate of the patient's degree of deficit relative to each symbol-function area is made and categorized as complete, severe, moderate, little, or none. Symbol-function areas include subtests used to determine the presence and severity of aphasic, apractic, and agnosic disturbances. The test can be shortened by administering only every other item, and presentation of only the first item of each subtest constitutes a screening test.

The *Language Modalities Test of Aphasia* (Wepman and Jones 1961) was constructed on the basis of the performance of over 200 adult aphasic patients. Factor analysis of the data from these subjects (Jones and Wepman 1961) led the authors to posit two roles for language in the central nervous system: transmissive functions, producing nonsymbolic language processes, and integrative functions, producing symbolic comprehension and formulation processes. They suggested that dysfunction of the transmissive functions results in agnosias and apraxias and integration dysfunctions produce aphasias.

The test consists of two forms comparable in difficulty which are presented on film strips 120 frames in length. The two forms of the test allow test-retest evaluations as a means of measuring the stability of the performance of the patient. The initial items on each form of the test are identical and constitute a screening section. Five different types of responses are elicited from the patient: oral, graphic, and three types of matching. Dichotomous scoring is utilized for the screening section and the standardized visual and auditory matching items. For the standardized oral and graphic responses and story-telling sections, the response is scored on a six-point scale and identified as normal, syntactic, semantic, pragmatic, jargon, and global. The results of testing are summarized, and the subject is classified according to one of the available categories: pragmatic, semantic, syntactic, jargon, or global aphasia, apraxia, and/or agnosia. Interscorer reliability has been reported to range from 0.88 to 0.96. Alternate form reliability and stability of subject performance also are reported to be high.

The *Minnesota Test for the Differential Diagnosis of Aphasia* (Schuell 1965) contains 47 subtests divided into five areas: auditory disturbances, visual and reading disturbances; speech and language disturbances; visuo-motor and writing disturbances, and disturbances of numerical relations and arithmetic processes. Dichotomous scoring is used for most subtests. Scores are summarized on the front sheet of the test form by subtest and area. Schuell has suggested that the subtests can be used to assign a patient to one of five major or two minor categories based on the *pattern of impairment.* The five major groups include: simple aphasia, aphasia with visual involvement, aphasia with sensorimotor involvement, aphasia with scattered findings compatible with generalized brain damage, and irreversible aphasic syndrome. The two minor syndromes are aphasia with partial auditory imperception, and aphasia with persisting dysarthria. The prognosis for recovery for each of these groups is provided.

Factor analysis of the scores from 157 aphasic subjects and means, standard deviations, median scores, and percentage of subjects making errors are provided for each subtest. However, no standard scores or numerical indices of severity are provided because Schuell rejected them as ". . . meaningless when dealing with aphasic populations which are heterogeneous in age, intelligence, cultural milieu, medical history, locus and extent of brain damage, and severity and duration of aphasia." Additionally, she stated that ". . . the most effective way of interpreting test data is in terms of clinical signs and total test pattern." Test-retest reliability and interscorer agreement for the test have not been determined.

It should be noted that the battery does not include any gestural subtests and appears from the instructions to have a strong auditory emphasis in testing. A short version, intended for screening, has been developed (Schuell 1957) and reevaluated (Schuell 1966). Diagnostic and severity rating scales also are included in the complete test battery.

The *Minnesota Test for the Differential Diagnosis of Aphasia* does not arise from clear-cut theroretical notions. Rather, it is clearly premised on the need to be descriptive in clinical testing because description forms the structure for determining both prognosis and treatment in aphasia.

The *Neurosensory Center Comprehensive Examination of Aphasia* (Spreen and Benton 1969) consists of twenty tests of language performance and four tests of visual and tactile function. The twenty language tests assess language comprehension and production, retention of verbal information, and reading and writing. The four visual and tactile function tests are designed to detect deficits in these skills and are administered whenever the patient's performance on tests such as visual or tactile naming are subnormal.

Eleven of the tests use sets of common objects with the items in each set sequenced in order of increasing difficulty. Four of the tests are presented on recorded tape; two use materials from the Token Test. One uses block letters; four require the use of a small box with a drop curtain so that items can be presented out of the view of the patient. Printed cards and unruled paper are required for reading and copying tasks. Dichotomous scoring is used (correct and incorrect). The examiner also should record incorrect and/or mispronounced correct responses and note any unusual features of performance.

This battery is unique in that there is a provision for construction of a profile of directly comparable percentile scores corrected for age and educational level. Two profile sheets have been developed for this purpose. The first profile is based on the performance of normal adults on the battery. The raw scores are computed for each of the twenty language tests, corrected for age and educational level (where appropriate), and transformed into the corresponding percentile rank of a normal population. The developers suggest that patients without language deficits will perform at the 40th percentile or above. Performance from the 30th to 40th percentile suggests minimal difficulty; from the 20th to 30th percentile suggests mild impairment, and below the 20th percentile indicates more severe dysfunction. The second profile allows comparison of the patient's performance with a reference group of aphasic patients. This permits the determination of the patient's strengths and weaknesses relative to the "average" performance of this reference group. Validity and reliability indices have not been reported for this battery.

The *Porch Index of Communicative Ability* (Porch 1971) was designed to assess verbal, gestural, and graphic abilities and was based on the premise that two major requirements of an aphasia examination are high reliability and a scoring system which specifies the nature of the patient's response in terms of multiple dimensions. The test contains 18 subtests (four verbal, eight gestural, and six graphic), each of ten items. The responses to the 180 items of the test are scored according to a 16-point binary choice system which considers the accuracy, responsiveness, completeness, promptness, and efficiency of the response. A mean score for each subtest, each modality, and the entire battery are computed from the 180 scored responses. The mean subtest scores can be examined on a Modality Response Summary which plots subtest scores by modality (verbal, gestural, graphic) and a Ranked Response Summary which plots the means in order of decreasing subtest difficulty.

The Porch Index was standardized on 280 left-hemisphere damaged patients and 100 bilaterally damaged patients. The test manual includes percentiles for the test as a whole, for each modality, and for the mean of the nine high and nine low subtests. The means of the nine low and nine high subtests and the overall mean are used to plot a recovery curve for the patient. The recovery curve is used to make predictions regarding the patient's eventual communicative functioning based on his performance one month post-onset. At six months post-onset, the mean of the patient's nine high subtests is considered the best estimate of his eventual maximal level of recovery. The test manual also provides some general guidelines for treatment. Five types of profiles are identified based on test results: (1) aphasia without complications, (2) aphasia complicated by verbal formulation or verbal expression problems, (3) aphasia patterns with accompanying illiteracy, (4) bilateral brain damage, and (5) aberrant patterns suggesting that the communicative disorder is not aphasia. Test-retest reliability has been established at 0.98, although interscorer agreement is somewhat lower.

A large data base has been developed for the Porch Index since its standardization. For example, Duffy and others (1976) provided subtest, modality, and overall test scores for 130 normal nonbrain-injured adults, and Watson and Records (1978) investigated the effectiveness of the test in assessing specific behaviors in senile dementia. The test also has been criticized on the basis of its ordinality (McNeil, Prescott, and Chang 1975) and its lack of specification of the response, neglect of factors related to communication, distortions in modality scoring, inadequacies of the response categories, statistical treatment of scores, and conceptual limits (Martin 1977).

The *Boston Diagnostic Aphasia Examination* (Goodglass and Kaplan 1972) is based on the assumption that the aphasia deficit is determined by "(a) the anatomical organization of language in the brain, (b) the location of the causative lesion, and (c) the functional interactions (e.g., inhibitory, regulatory, selective) of various parts of the language system." Accordingly, the test battery is geared toward determining the type of aphasic syndrome so that inferences can be made regarding localization of the cerebral lesion; measurement of communicative and related skills over a wide range for initial description and for detecting change in performance over time; and comprehensive assessment of abilities and deficits which may serve as a guide to therapy.

The battery contains 23 subtests and rating scales designed to assess articulation, loss of verbal fluency, word-finding difficulty, repetition, serial speech, loss of grammar, syntax, auditory comprehension, reading, and writing. Scoring includes plus-minus scores, longhand notation, and rating of conversational and expository speech. The test was standardized on 207 aphasic patients. Based on the range, mean and standard deviation of their performances, Z-scores were computed which allow the patient's performance on each subtest to be compared with the normative population scores in standard deviation units. The patient may be assigned to one of several diagnostic categories including Broca's aphasia, Wernicke's aphasia, Anomic aphasia, Conduction aphasia, and Transcortical Sensory or Motor aphasia based on the rating-scale profile of speech characteristics and Z-scores. The battery also contains supplementary language tests to explore both comprehension and expression skills and supplementary nonlanguage tests, such as reproducing three-dimensional block designs, drawing to command, and so forth. Although test-retest data have not been obtained for this instrument, reliability coefficients based on profiles from 34 patients were from 0.68 to 0.98 which suggests good internal consistency with respect to what the items were measuring. This instrument is unique in that results of testing are used to estimate the site of brain damage responsible for the communicative deficits.

The *Aphasia Language Performance Scales* (Keenan and Brassel 1975) was developed because the authors believed that existing aphasia tests had several unsatisfactory conditions: they were time consuming, were limited by space and environmental restrictions, tended to break down rapport, and gave little help in planning for therapy. This test is composed of four scales (listening, talking, reading, writing), each containing ten items. The items on each scale are graded in difficulty and range in linguistic complexity from virtual absence of function to near normal function. The four scales are purported to be independent of one another; that is, performance on items of one scale is not affected by deficits tested on items from another scale.

Each item is scored one point if the response is correct or self-corrected, one-half point if the response is correct following a prompt, and zero points for an incorrect response. The score on each scale is computed and plotted on a summary form which can be used to illustrate the patient's pattern of impairment, severity of the deficit in each modality, and rate of improvement. The numerical scores also can be related to the degree of impairment as follows:

Numerical Score	*Impairment Rating*
0-1.0	Profound
1.5-3.0	Severe
3.5-5.0	Moderate-Severe
5.5-7.0	Mild-Moderate
7.5-9.0	Mild
9.5-10.0	Insignificant

The Talking Scale was administered to 90 patients by eight speech pathologists to determine internal reliability using the Kuder-Richardson Formula 20 (Keenan and Brassel 1974). This procedure yielded a reliability coefficient of 0.90. In a related study, Basili and others (1974) administered the Aphasia Language Performance Scales and subtests of the *Porch Index of Communicative Abilities* to 50 aphasic patients. Spearman rank-order correlation coefficients for scale scores and comparable Porch subtest scores ranged from 0.84 to 0.93, which suggested adequate concurrent validity.

The *Functional Communication Profile* (Sarno 1969) begins from an entirely different perspective. Sarno suggested that most clinical tests of aphasia do not take into account the fact that many aphasic patients use gestures to communicate, respond accurately but inconsistently, require a longer period of time to respond even when vocabulary and syntax are intact, and have more difficulty with highly specific tasks. Moreover, she indicated that many of the more standard aphasia batteries are relatively insensitive to minimal impairments and may contain many items to which the severely involved patient cannot respond.

The test consists of 45 integrated communicative behaviors divided into five areas including: movement, speaking, understanding, reading, and miscellaneous (including writing and calculation). Ratings of each behavior are made on a continuum along a nine-point scale from zero to normal and take into account ". . . speed, accuracy, consistency, voluntary control without benefit of external cues and compensatory function of the behavior." The ratings are made following informal interaction with the patient in conversational situations and, when necessary, are supplemented with other reports of the patient's abilities. The ratings for each of the five sections and for the entire profile are converted to percentages which reflect the percent of premorbid functioning. A patient functioning at the 60th percentile, for example, would be functioning at 60 percent of his premorbid level. Premorbid capacity consequently serves as a reference against which the performance of the patient is measured. The profile of the patient also can be used to visually differentiate between types of verbal impairment. For example, if a patient demonstrates severely impaired speaking skill compared to rated performances on the other sections of the test, she might be described as demonstrating verbal apraxia.

Sarno reported that Taylor and Sands (1965) investigated the inter-rater reliability of the Profile. Three observers rated the performance of twenty aphasic adults. Agreement of the raters, when expressed as Spearman rank-order correlations, ranged from 0.87 to 0.95 for the five sections of the Profile. A related study by Greenberg (1969), reported by Sarno, indicated further that investigations have demonstrated that the Profile has concurrent and predictive validity; the convergence of these findings suggesting construct validity.

Communicative Abilities in Daily Life (Holland 1979, 1980) is a 68-item test instrument which emphasizes a functional approach to assessing the patient's communicative impairment. The primary focus according to Holland is not on whether the message was communicated by verbal or nonverbal means, but that it was completed, regardless of the means. Consequently, the test is not modality specific. The Communicative Abilities scale has a three-point scoring system. If the patient's response is successful, whether it has been accomplished by verbal, gestural, or graphic means, it is considered correct and scored 2. If it was failed, it is scored as 0, and if it is not totally correct, but signifies a communicative relationship to the task item, it is scored as 1. Tasks on the test are everyday activities "ranging from responding to and giving social greetings, to differentiating nonverbal signs on restroom doors, to comprehending metaphors, to recognizing statements which are contextually absurd and unpredictable." The items are encompassed within simulated, real-world activities, including going to the doctor's office, riding in a car, shopping, using the telephone, and being interviewed by a stranger. The total score is simply the cumulative sum of the item scores.

ADDITIONAL CONSIDERATIONS IN THE SELECTION OF APHASIA TESTS

Earlier we presented criteria for evaluating the adequacy of aphasia test batteries. Although these may be important variables in your selection of a test, other considerations may enter into your decision.

First, the administration time of the test may influence your choice. The Aphasia Language Performance Scales require less than 30 minutes to administer and the screening tests of the Minnesota, Examining for Aphasia, and Language Modalities Test offer a quick means of determining the primary deficits of the patient. Conversely, if time is not a factor and a comprehensive assessment of abilities is required, then the Boston Examination, which includes supplementary tests for nonlanguage skills and in-depth exploration of expressive and receptive psycholinguistic skills, or the Minnesota Test, which contain more items than any other battery, may be your choice.

Second, if you wish to aid in localizing the site of lesion, then you may chose the Boston Test because the results allow the clinician to determine a syndrome of aphasia symptomology consistent with a specific area of brain damage. Other aphasia tests do not purport to localize the site of lesion.

Third, standardization of the test to aid in the interpretation of test results may influence your decision. The Neurosensory Center Examination, the Boston Test, and the Porch Index provide for a comparison of the patient's results with scores from normal and/or aphasic patients. No standardization data is available for several other tests we have reviewed such as the Language Modalities Test or Examining for Aphasia.

Obviously, other criteria may dictate your choice of test, such as the degree of auditory or visual emphasis of the battery and the inclusion or noninclusion of gestural subtests. Ultimately your decision on a test battery will depend on the weight of many if not all of these factors.

Clinical Example

A clinical example may serve to make the interpretations available for different test batteries more apparent. Ms. ET (for English Teacher) suffered an occlusion of the left internal carotid artery with resultant aphasia and right hemiplegia following an automobile accident. Two months after discharge from the hospital, she was seen for a speech and language evaluation. Three tests were administered: the *Boston Diagnostic Aphasia Examination, the Minnesota Test for the Differential Diagnosis of Aphasia,* and the *Functional Communication Profile.* The Boston and Minnesota tests typically would not both be administered during the course of an evaluation, but we have done so for purposes of comparison. On the Boston test, the Rating Scale Profile of Speech Characteristics was most consistent with a classification of Broca's aphasia. Minnesota test results were as follows: 9 percent errors on the Auditory Comprehension tests, 19 percent errors on Visual and Reading tests, 34 percent errors on Speech and Language tests, 18 percent errors on Visuomotor and Writing tests, and 13 percent errors on Numerical Relations and Arithmetic Processes tests. On the Functional Communication Profile, ET received a 77 percent rating on Movement, 87 percent on Understanding, 57 percent on Speaking, 81 percent on Reading, and 79 percent on Other (telling time, handling money, calculation ability, and the like). The total rating was 77.2 percent. The results of these tests would be expected to reveal some consistencies, and they are evident: The patient demonstrates speaking skills that are more impaired than other aspects of communication.

The finding of a Boston profile consistent with Broca's aphasia suggests that the primary site of lesion is the foot of the third frontal gyrus and surrounding tissue of the left frontal lobe. Results of the Minnesota test are consistent with a Group III-type patient; that is, aphasia with sensorimotor involvement or aphasia with persisting dysfluency (Jenkins and others 1975). The prognosis for recovery for this type of patient is excellent. Finally, results of the Functional Communication Profile suggest that ET's residual communicative abilities in everyday situations are approximately 77 percent of premorbid functioning. Based on these test findings, the best description of the patient's condition would be mild aphasia with verbal apraxia due to damage to the left frontal lobe. The patient functions adequately in everyday communicative situations, and the prognosis for additional recovery is excellent.

OTHER TESTS FOR NEUROGENIC DISORDERS

While aphasia batteries serve as reasonably comprehensive assessment instruments for aphasia and to a more limited extent, apraxia and dysarthria, they are insufficient for differential diagnosis of other neurogenic disorders. Darley (1979) observed that a ". . . curious failure in aphasia test development relates to the general absence of built-in ways of distinguishing aphasic patients from patients with language disorders that might be confused with aphasia" and "Test makers have not demonstrated that aphasia can be differentiated from syndromes of confusion, dementia, or psychosis through the use of their tests." Therefore, other tests must be used to allow the examiner to differentially diagnose disorders that may superficially resemble aphasia but which are neurologically different. Moreover, other tests and assessment protocols may be needed to evaluate particular neurogenically based linguistic disorders in more detail. Several tests and test protocols will be reviewed, not to serve as an exhaustive listing, but to provide examples of tools available.

The *Token Test* (DeRenzi and Vignolo 1962) was developed to assess high-level auditory comprehension deficits associated with brain damage. The tokens used are large and small squares and circles, blue, green, red, white, and yellow in color. The patient's task is to manipulate the tokens in response to instructions of increasing length and complexity on the five levels of the test. Identification of the different sizes, colors, and shapes of the tokens is required before administration of the test items. Part I includes items such as "Touch the yellow circle"; Part II requires responses such as "Touch the little green circle"; Part III asks the patient, for example, to "Touch the blue square and the yellow square"; Part IV requires the patient to "Touch the little blue square and the little yellow circle"; and Part V asks the patient, for example, to "Put the green square beside the red circle." The test purports to test auditory comprehension, but it is apparent that it also places a considerable burden on the memory skills of the patient.

The test has undergone a number of modifications since its development. There have been changes in the shape of the tokens (Spreen and Benton 1969), the commands (Boller and Vignolo 1966; Orgass and Poeck 1966; Spreen and Benton 1969), and the number of test items (Boller and Vignolo 1966; Orgass and Poeck 1966; Spellacy and Spreen 1969). The test has been proven useful for testing a wide range of patients including: left-brain-damaged with aphasia, brain-damaged without aphasia, and nonbrain-damaged subjects (Swisher and Sarno 1969; Orgass and Poeck 1966), patients with cerebral commissurotomy and hemispherectomy (Zaidel 1977), and children (Cartwright and Lass 1974; Lass and Golden 1975; Lass and others 1975; Robb and Lass 1976; Trimboli and Lass 1976). Reliability using pass-fail scoring has been established at 0.92. The test has been found to reliably discriminate aphasic from nonaphasic patients (Orgass and Poeck 1966; Boller and Vignolo 1966; Spellacy and Spreen 1969), which is an index of its criterion validity, and to correlate positively with the severity of the aphasic disturbance (Orgass and Poeck 1966) and with scores from the Funtional Communication Profile (Swisher and Sarno 1969). A method of correcting Part V scores for age and educational level has been developed (Flowers 1973), and a short form of the test is available. (Spellacy and Spreen 1969).

The Revised Token Test (RTT) (McNeil and Prescott 1978) is the result of a major effort to standardize the original test which had undergone numerous modifications. It was standardized in terms of:

> (1) a pretest designed to assess the subject's basic knowledge of colors, shapes, and sizes, as well as balanced representation for each; (2) specific colors (shades), materials, and sizes of the tokens; (3) specific placement of the tokens (designed to reduce the visual search aspect of the subject's performance); (4) a consistent order of presentation for each subtest and commands within subtests; (5) a procedure for scoring each linguistic element, each stimulus, each subtest and an overall test mean; and (6) specific rules for applying each of the 15 categories in the evaluative system.

The RTT contains ten subtests, and responses are scored by means of a 15-point multidimensional scoring system similar to the one used in the *Porch Index of Communicative Ability*. The test was standardized on 90 neurologically normal, 30 left-brain-damaged, and 30 right-brain-damaged adults. Percentiles for overall, subtest, and linguistic element means are provided for the three subject types of the standardization population. Test-retest reliability has been reported at 0.90, intrascorer reliability at 0.97, and interscorer reliability from 0.97 to 0.98. The test appears to be a sensitive instrument for detecting brain damage, and the severity levels obtained appear efficient at differentiating between auditory performance in normal, right-brain-damaged and left-brain-damaged patients.

The *Wechsler Memory Scale* (Wechsler and Stone 1948) contains seven subtests which explore various aspects of visual and auditory memory. The subtests include: personal and current information (How old are you? Who is President of the United States?); general orientation (What year is this? What month is this? What day is this?); mental control (Count by threes, Say the letters of the alphabet); logical memory (recall of ideas from two short paragraphs presented auditorially); digits forward and backward (recall of digit series of increasing length); visual reproduction (recall of geometric designs presented for ten seconds); and associative learning (recall of the second word of word pairs presented over three trials). The patient's subtest scores are added, corrected for age, and used to determine an equivalent Mental Quotient.

The scale was standardized on more than 200 normal adult men and women from 25 to 50 years of age. A score correction for age is provided for patients from 20 to 64 years at five-year intervals. The scale contains two equivalent forms. The authors estimated reliability to be greater than 0.83. The scale requires relatively intact receptive and expressive skills and therefore is probably more appropriate for patients with right-brain-damage or bihemispheric involvement than for most patients with aphasia.

Only two tests that serve to aid in appraising neurogenic linguistic disorders have been reviewed. There are many others that may be used. For example, the *Peabody Picture Vocabulary Test* (Dunn 1965), *Gates Primary Reading Test* (Gates 1958), *Benton Visual Retention Test* (Benton 1974), *Word Fluency Measure* (Borkowski, Benton, and Spreen 1967) and the *Coloured Progressive Matrices* (Raven 1963). The purpose in selecting these tests for administration is to expand the range of testing for particular deficits when they are insufficiently explored by aphasia batteries or to appraise areas of dysfunction not included on the batteries. The initial statement of this section must be reemphasized: There are no tests specifically constructed to investigate communicative deficits associated with dementia, confusion, or psychoses. Therefore, an array of measures may need to be chosen from existent diagnostic materials created for evaluating aphasia and related disorders.

PROCEDURES FOR ASSESSING NEUROMOTOR DISORDERS

A number of less formalized tests have been applied to the assessment of acquired neuromotor disorders. In general, they are outgrowths of pragmatic clinical procedures frequently associated with the neurological examination.

DeRenzi, Pieczuro, and Vignolo (1966) developed procedures to evaluate oral and limb apraxia. The test included ten oral and ten limb items in which subjects were asked to perform gestures following verbal command, and if necessary, on imitation. Oral gestures included the following: (1) Stick out your tongue, (2) Whistle, (3) Yawn, (4) Try to touch the tip of your nose with your tongue, (5) Give a "Bronx cheer" or "raspberry," (6) Show how you would kiss someone, (7) Show how your teeth chatter when you are cold, (8) Click your tongue, imitating the sound of a horse galloping, (9) Puff or blow, and (10) Clear your throat. Limb gestures are as follows: (1) Make the sign of the cross, (2) Salute, (3) Wave goodbye, (4) Threaten somebody with your hand, (5) Show that you are hungry, (6) Thumb your nose, (7) Snap your fingers, (8) Make the sign of the horns to designate a cuckold, (9) Indicate that someone is crazy, and (10) Make the letter 0 with your fingers. Five categories of response were determined, and each response was scored as 2 (correct); 1 (accurate performance preceded by pause or acceptable performance with defective movements); or 0 (important part of gesture absent, perseveration of preceding item, incorrect oral performance, no response). Determination of the presence and severity of oral and limb apraxia was based on the performance of 40 control subjects, 40 patients with lesions of the right hemisphere, and 134 patients with lesions of the left hemisphere. None of the control or right-brain-damaged subjects received a score of less than 16 on either the oral or limb tests. Therefore, 16 was used as the cut-off point; that is, patients with scores of 15 or less were classified as apractic. The cut-off score for separating mild and severe involvement was set at 11.

Darley, Aronson, and Brown (1975) modified the oral apraxia portion of the test by increasing the number of items to twenty and by providing eleven categories for grading the response. They also presented 18 test words and phrases useful for eliciting verbal apractic errors, such as "gingerbread," "statistical analysis," "zip-zipper-zippering," and "The shipwreck washed up on the shore." Rosenbek and Wertz (1976) developed a battery of apraxia measures which included verbal, oral, and limb items. The verbal portion requires the patient to prolong vowels, imitate syllable sequences, and produce words and phrases. Responses are transcribed, scored, and analyzed to determine the type and frequency of phonemic and prosodic errors. The oral apraxia section is identical to the twenty items of the Darley and others test, and the limb apraxia test is a modification of the DeRenzi and others test. The oral and limb apraxia responses are graded on an 11-point system similar to Darley and others.

We have taken the time to present in detail these procedures for evaluating apraxia because they demonstrate the evolution of a test battery to fulfill the need for an instrument to measure specific deficits. With standardization, the battery may prove to be an excellent tool in the assessment of motor-programming disturbances, but like many other tests, it owes its origins to earlier testmakers.

Other assessment procedures have been developed which might better be termed protocols than tests. Larsen (1972) described a protocol for evaluating swallowing problems (dysphagia) due to neuromuscular disorders. Included within the evaluation were a history (patient complaint, eating habits, food preferred, incidence of choking); examination of the speech mechanism (muscle strength and structural range of motion); evaluation of swallowing (volitional and reflexive); determination of the integrity of taste sensation (sweet, sour, salty); and ability of the patient to masticate and swallow various nutritional substances (liquids, solids, dry, moist). A similar protocol was developed for deglutition deficits in patients with head and neck cancer by Bell and Goepfert (1977). Rosenbek and Wertz (1976) integrated a series of examinations for systematically evaluating cranial-nerve function in dysarthria, utilizing speech and nonspeech tasks. Only time will tell if these protocols will develop from their current embryonic stage into reliable and objective indices of dysfunction.

CLINICAL PROCEDURES

Differential diagnosis of communicative disorders due to neurological deficits may be difficult. For example, Table 10-1 compares the performance of patients with aphasia, apraxia, generalized intellectual impairment, and the language of confusion (Halpern, Darley, and Brown 1973) with that of schizophrenic patients (DiSimoni, Darley, and Aronson 1977). Examination of the categories (auditory retention, adequacy, arithmetic, auditory comprehension, fluency, naming, syntax, reading comprehension, writing, and relevance) reveals that all five groups were impaired on at least seven of the ten task classifications. Even though five of the categories may help to differentiate the five groups (DiSimoni and others, 1977), the overlap of communicative deficits among the groups suggests that the acquisition of biographical and medical information in addition to the behavioral testing may be paramount in establishing the diagnosis. A brief procedural guide to the acquisition of the necessary information is provided to facilitate this process.

The History. In the chapter on case history, we discussed some aspects of information gathering. For patients who have suffered brain damage, a great deal of information can be gleaned from the patient's medical records to supplement information gained from the standard interview which will include information on education level, occupation, family history, and so forth. For patients still in the hospital, information from the medical chart will include reports of the medical history, the results of the medical and neurological examination, results of laboratory tests, and nurses and doctor's notes. The medical history should be reviewed carefully for information regarding earlier incidences of brain damage, periods of confusion or disorientation, and complicating conditions, such as metabolic diseases, cardiac disease, or seizures.

The results of the neurological examination will provide information on the site, size, and nature of the lesion and possible progression of the disorder.

Table 10-1 Rank order of percentage of impairment of the 10 language categories for each of Halpern and associates' (1973) four groups with cerebral impairment and for the schizophrenic patients. Categories in italics tend to differentiate the five groups.

Rank Order	*Aphasia (%)*	*General Intellectual Impairment (%)*	*Apraxia of Speech (%)*	*Confused Language (%)*	*Schizophrenia (%)*
1	Adequacy, 43	Adequacy, 45	Adequacy, 30	Arithmetic, 54	Relevance, 45
2	*Auditory Retention*, 42	*Reading Comprehension*, 41	*Fluency*, 22	*Reading Comprehension*, 47	Arithmetic, 42
3	Arithmetic, 36	Arithmetic, 40	Arithmetic, 21	*Writing to Dictation*, 44	*Reading Comprehension*, 22
4		Auditory Comprehension, 29	Syntax, 20	*Relevance*, 40	*Fluency*, 17
4½	Auditory Comprehension, 33 *Fluency*, 33				
5		*Auditory Retention*, 18		Adequacy, 28	Auditory Comprehension, 13
5½			Auditory Comprehension, 13 *Writing to Dictation*, 13		

Table 10-1 Rank order of percentage of impairment of the 10 language categories for each of Halpern and associates' (1973) four groups with cerebral impairment and for the schizophrenic patients. Categories in italics tend to differentiate the five groups. (continued)

Rank Order	*Aphasia (%)*	*General Intellectual Impairment (%)*	*Apraxia of Speech (%)*	*Confused Language (%)*	*Schizophrenia (%)*
6	Naming, 31	Naming, 16		Auditory Comprehension, 24	*Auditory Retention*, 10
7	Syntax, 27	Syntax, 11	*Auditory Retention*, 11	Syntax, 21	*Writing to Dictation*, 9
8	*Reading Comprehension*, 24		Naming, 7	Naming, 19	*Adequacy*,* 6
8½		*Relevance*, 10 *Writing to Dictation*, 10			
9	*Writing to Dictation*, 21		*Reading Comprehension*, 6	*Auditory Retention*, 17	Naming, 3
10	*Relevance*, 18	*Fluency*, 9	*Relevance*, 2	*Fluency*, 14	Syntax, 2
Mean	31	22	14	28	17

*Adequacy is capitalized in this group as it differentiates schizophrenia from the other four disorders.

(From DiSimoni, Darley, and Aronson 1977).

Specifically, the neurological examination performed by the physician includes evaluation of mental state, cranial nerves, motor and reflex systems, the cerebellar apparatus, sensory modalities, and the autonomic nervous system. Evaluation of mental state will include assessment of intellectual facility and fund of knowledge; orientation for time, place, and person; memory; attention span; understanding of simple and complex commands; general information; calculation; abstract thinking; and judgment. The cranial nerves are assessed by testing the sensory and motor functions of the areas of the body that they subserve. For example, the integrity of the facial nerve is assessed by evaluating facial movement and the reaction of the face to sensory stimulation such as a pin prick.

Examination of the motor systems will provide information on muscle power, bulk and tone, active and passive movements, involuntary movements, cerebellar functioning, and status of the reflexes. Evaluation of sensory function includes investigation of touch, pain, heat, cold, position, vibration, and a variety of discriminatory senses. An attempt is made to determine what elements of sensation are effected, the degree of involvement, and the areas of sensory impairment or loss. The history may also contain information on past cerebrovascular accidents or disease, associated problems, and medications which may affect behavior. The nurses' notes may offer information on the alertness of the patient, his orientation to time, place, and person, and his adjustment to the problem. The physician's orders should provide information on the current status of the patient and the treatment program that has been proposed and is being carried out.

Review of all the case history and medical information should provide you with knowledge of the deficits exhibited by the patient, his adjustment to the problem, and the proposed course of treatment and should be reviewed carefully before the patient is seen. The amount and type of information already available may be helpful in your determination of the type of aphasia instrument and related evaluations you wish to make.

Evaluation of the Patient. Before administering a test battery, it is always helpful to observe the patient in an informal situation. In a hospital, you may visit the patient in his room; in a speech and hearing center you may visit with him before the formal evaluation begins. This time should be used to assess informally the patient's communicative functioning; to note any significant sensory or motor impairment (visual deficits, hearing loss, hemiplegia); and to determine how closely the patient's condition matches with the available medical information. Determination of sensory and motor problems is crucial because they may suggest ways in which the standard test procedures will need to be modified in the assessment of the patient.

In the formal examination of the patient, the test selected will depend on the type of problems exhibited, the severity of the problems, and complicating conditions, such as sensory or motor impairment. Choose tests and procedures that fulfill your needs (see Table 10-2).

Table 10-2 Summary of aphasia test batteries

Test	*Description*	*Scoring*	*Norms*	*Interpretation*
EXAMINING FOR APHASIA (Eisenson 1954)	Subtests dichotomized into primarily receptive and primarily expressive portions. Within each section, subtests divided into those designed to test for subsymbolic or low symbolic function (agnosias, apraxias) and those designed to evaluate high symbolic function (aphasias).	Plus-minus with some long-hand notation.	None.	Rating of presence and severity of aphasia, apraxia, and agnosia as revealed by subtest performance.
THE LANGUAGE MODALITIES TEST FOR APHASIA (Wepman and Jones 1961)	Eleven screening items and two sets of 23 items presented on filmstrips 120 frames in length designed to assess auditory comprehension, verbal expression, reading and writing skills, plus calculation.	Plus-minus for screening and auditory and visual matching items. Oral and graphic and story-telling sections rated on a six-point scale according to predominant characteristics of the response.	Factor analysis of the responses of 168 aphasic patients.	Results used to assign patient to categories based upon predominant characteristics of the disorder; pragmatic, semantic, syntactic, jargon or global aphasia, and/or apraxia and/or agnosia.
MINNESOTA TEST FOR DIFFERENTIAL DIAGNOSIS OF APHASIA (Schuell 1965)	Fifty-seven subtests divided into five major sections: auditory disturbances, visual and reading disturbances, speech and language	Plus-minus with some long-hand notation.	Means, standard deviations, median scores, percentages of 157 subjects making errors on each subtest.	Test score summarization and lists of signs and most discriminating tests used to assign patient to one of five major and two minor prognostic

Table 10-2 Summary of aphasia test batteries (continued)

Test	*Description*	*Scoring*	*Norms*	*Interpretation*
	disturbances; visuomotor and writing disturbances; disturbances of numerical relations and arithmetic processes. Also includes clinical and severity rating scales and screening version.			categories based on pattern of impairment.
FUNCTIONAL COMMUNICATION PROFILE (Sarno 1969)	Forty-five integrated behaviors divided into movement, speaking, understanding, reading and miscellaneous sections.	Behaviors rated on a nine-point rating scale,	None. However sample profiles presented.	Ratings converted to percentages for each section and test as a whole. Percentage purported to reflect residual communicative abilities compared to premorbid functioning.
NEUROSENSORY CENTER COMPREHENSIVE EXAMINATION OF APHASIA (Spreen and Benton 1969)	Twenty tests of language production and comprehension, retention of verbal information, reading, writing. Four tests of visual and tactile function.	Primarily plus-minus; some long-hand notation.	Percentiles for each subtest from performance of neurologically normal and aphasic subjects. Number of subjects unspecified.	Some subtests corrected for age and education. Construction of subtest performance profile to compare patient performance to that of normal and aphasic standardization populations.

Table 10-2 Summary of aphasia test batteries (continued)

Test	*Description*	*Scoring*	*Norms*	*Interpretation*
PORCH INDEX OF COMMUNICATIVE ABILITY (Porch 1967; 1971)	Four verbal, 2 auditory, 2 reading, 2 gestural, 2 visual matching subtests, and 6 graphic subtests with 10 items per subtest.	Responses scored according to 16-point binary choice system on the basis of accuracy, responsiveness, completeness, promptness, and efficiency.	Percentiles for the test as a whole, for each subtest, and for combinations of subtests by modality for 280 left-hemisphere brain-damaged and 100 bilaterally brain-damaged subjects. Also percentiles for nine high, nine low and overall scores. Examples of 5 basic performance patterns provided.	Overall and gestural, verbal and graphic modality means compared to standardization population. Subtest scores plotted as a function of subtest difficulty. Also recovery curves determined by computation of nine high, nine low and overall test means.
BOSTON DIAGNOSTIC APHASIA EXAMINATION (Goodglass and Kaplan 1972)	Twenty-three subtests used to assess auditory comprehension, oral expression, reading, writing. Ratings of conversational and expository speech on 6 parameters and rating of severity. Also includes 13 language and 14 nonlanguage tests.	Primarily plus-minus with some long-hand notation.	Z-score profiles based on the range, mean and standard deviation of scores from 207 aphasic subjects. Intercorrelation analyses, factor analyses and reliability coefficients among subtests also provided.	Overall severity on a six point scale, speech characteristics rating on 7 factors and Z-score profiles used to assign patient to classical aphasic syndromes: Broca's aphasia, Wernicke's aphasia, anomic aphasia, conduction aphasia,

Table 10-2 Summary of aphasia test batteries (continued)

Test	*Description*	*Scoring*	*Norms*	*Interpretation*
				transcortical sensory aphasia, transcortical motor aphasia, alexia with graphia.
APHASIA LANGUAGE PERFORMANCE SCALES (Keenan and Brassel 1975)	Four scales: listening talking, reading, writing each comprised of 10 items.	One point per item if correct or self-corrected, one-half point if correct following prompt. No points if incorrect.	None.	Arbitrary assignments of scores from scales to degree of language impairment. 0-1.0 profound 1.5-3.0 severe 3.5-5.0 moderate-severe 5.5-7.0 mild-moderate 7.5-9.0 mild 9.5-10.0 insignificant
COMMUNICATIVE ABILITIES IN DAILY LIFE (Holland 1979)	Sixty-eight items encompassed within simulated, real-world activities.	Two points if correct, one point if not totally correct but signifies a communicative realtionship to the task item. No points if incorrect.	Means and standard deviations of scores from 130 neurologically normal and 130 aphasic subjects as a function of age, sex, institutionalization and type of aphasia.	Total score is indication of communicative abilities during the course of everyday activities.

SUMMARY

A large variety of communicative disorders result from damage to the brain after speech and language have been acquired. The problems demonstrated by the patient depend on the site and extent of the brain damage. A number of formal and informal tests to measure these disorders are available, but they vary significantly in the way they view the problem and the means they use to assess deficits. The tests selected for assessing these disorders depend on the type of problem, its severity and your purposes in testing.

REFERENCES

Basili, A. and others, The comparisons between the Aphasia Language Performance Scales and two established tests of aphasic impairment. Paper presented at the American Speech and Hearing Association Convention, Las Vegas, (1974).

Bell, K., and H. Goepfert, Rehabilitation of head and neck cancer patients to deglutinate. *Tejas,* 2, 3-5 (1977).

Benton, A., *Benton Revised Visual Retenton Test.* New York: The Psychological Corporation, (1974).

Boller, F., and L. Vignolo, Latent sensory aphasia in hemisphere-damaged patients: An experimental study with the Token Test. *Brain,* 89, 815-830 (1966).

Borkowski, J., A. Benton, and O. Spreen, Word fluency and brain damage. *Neuropsychologia,* 5, 135-140 (1967).

Brookshire, R. H., *An Introduction to Aphasia,* 2nd ed. Minneapolis: BRK Publishers, (1978).

Cartwright, L., and N. Lass, Comparative study of children's performance on the Token Test, Northwestern Syntax Screening Test, and Peabody Picture Vocabulary Test. *Acta Symbolica,* 5, 19-29 (1974).

Darley, F. L., *Diagnosis and Appraisal of Communication Disorders.* Englewood Cliffs, N.J.: Prentice-Hall, Inc., (1964).

Darley, F., *Evaluation of Appraisal Techniques in Speech and Language Pathology.* Reading, Mass.: Addison-Wesley, (1979).

Darley, F., A. Aronson, and J. Brown, *Motor Speech Disorders.* Philadelphia: W. B. Saunders, (1975).

DeRenzi, E., A. Pieczuro, and L. Vignolo, Oral apraxia and aphasia. *Cortex,* 2, 50-73 (1966).

DeRenzi, E., and L. Vignolo, The Token Test: A sensitive test to detect receptive disturbances in aphasics. *Brain,* 85, 655-678 (1962).

DiSimoni, F., F. Darley, and A. Aronson, Patterns of dysfunction in schizophrenic patients on an aphasia test battery. *J. Speech Hearing Dis.,* 42, 498-513 (1977).

Duffy, J. and others, Performance of normal (non-brain injured) adults on the Porch Index of Communicative Ability, in *Clinical Aphasiology: Confer-*

ence Proceedings 1976, ed. R. Brookshire. Minneapolis: BRK Publishers, (1976).

Dunn, L., *Peabody Picture Vocabulary Test.* Circle Pines, Minn.: American Guidance Service, Inc., (1965).

Eisenson, J., *Examining for Aphasia.* New York: Psychological Corporation, (1954).

Flowers, C., A method of correcting Part V Token Test scores for age and educational level. Mayo Graduate School of Medicine. Unpublished paper, (1973).

Gates, A., and J. Bradshaw, The role of the cerebral hemispheres in music. *Brain Lang.,* 4, 403-431 (1977).

Gates, A., *Gates Advanced Primary Reading Test.* New York: Columbia University, Teachers College Press, (1958).

Goodglass, H., and E. Kaplan, *The Assessment of Aphasia and Related Disorders.* Philadelphia: Lea and Febiger, (1972).

Greenberg, F., Measurements of improvement in completed stroke. *Proceedings of Conference on Stroke Predictors.* Chicago, (1969).

Halpern, H., F. Darley, and J. Brown, Differential language and neurologic characteristics in cerebral involvement. *J. Speech Hearing Dis.,* 38, 162-173 (1973).

Holland, A., *Communicative Abilities in Daily Living.* Baltimore: University Park Press, (1980).

Holland, A., Estimates of Aphasic Patients' Communicative Performance in Daily Life. NINCDS 75-05 (N01-NS-5-2317) (1979).

Jenkins, J. and others, *Schuell's Aphasia in Adults.* New York: Harper & Row, (1975).

Jones, L., and J. Wepman, Dimensions of language performance in aphasia. *J. Speech Hearing Res.,* 4, 220-232 (1961).

Joynt, R., and M. Goldstein, Minor cerebral hemisphere, in *Advances in Neurology, Vol. 7,* ed. W. Friedlander. New York: Raven Press, (1975).

Keenan, J., and E. Brassel, *Aphasia Language Performance Scales.* Murfreesboro, Tenn.: Pinnacle Press, (1975).

Keenan, J., and E. Brassel, Development of a scale of aphasic speech impairment. Paper presented at the American Speech and Hearing Association Convention, Las Vegas, (1974).

Krashen, S., Cerebral Asymmetry. In *Studies in Neurolinguistics, Vol. 2,* eds. H. Whitaker and H. Whitaker. New York: Academic Press, (1976).

Larsen, G., Rehabilitation of dysphagia paralytica. *J. Speech Hearing Dis.,* 37, 187-194 (1972).

Lass, N. and others, A normative study of children's performance on the short form of the Token Test. *J. Comm. Dis.,* 8, 193-198 (1975).

Lass, N., and S. Golden, A correlational study of children's performance on three tests for receptive language abilities. *J. Auditory Res.,* 15, 177-182 (1975).

LeMay, M., and N. Geschwind, Asymmetries of the human cerebral hemisphere, in *Language Acquisition and Language Breakdown,* eds. A. Caramazza and E. Zurif. Baltimore: Johns Hopkins Press, (1978).

Lenneberg, E., In search of a dynamic theory of aphasia, in *Foundation of Language Development,* eds. *Vol. II,* E. Lenneberg, and E. Lenneberg. New York: Academic Press, (1975).

McNeil, M., and T. Prescott, *Revised Token Test.* Baltimore: University Park Press, (1978).

McNeil, M., T. Prescott, and E. Chang, A measure of PICA ordinality, in *Clinical Aphasiology Conference Proceedings,* ed. R. Brookshire. Minneapolis: BRK Publishers, 113-124 (1975).

Martin, A., Aphasia testing: A second look at the Porch Index of Communicative Ability. *J. Speech Hearing Dis.,* 42, 536-546 (1977).

Miller, E., *Abnormal Aging.* London: Wiley, (1977).

Orgass, B., and K. Poeck, Clinical validation of a new test for aphasia: An experimental study of the Token Test. *Cortex,* 2, 222-243 (1966).

Osgood, C., and M. Miron, *Approaches to the Study of Aphasia.* Urbana, Ill.: University of Illinois Press, (1963).

Penfield, W., and L. Roberts, *Speech and Brain Mechanisms.* Princeton, N.J.: Princeton University Press, (1959).

Porch, B., *The Porch Index of Communicative Ability.* Palo Alto, Calif.: Consulting Psychologists Press, (1967, 1971).

Raven, J., *Guide to Using the Coloured Progressive Matrices.* London: H. K. Lewis, (1963).

Robb, E., and N. Lass, A correlational investigation of children's performance on the Token Test, the Brenner Developmental Gestalt Test of School Readiness, and a basic grammatical concepts test. *J. Auditory Res.,* 16, 64-67 (1976).

Rosenbek, J., and R. Wertz, Veterans Administration Workshop on Motor Speech Disorders. Madison, Wis., (1976).

Sarno, M. T., *The Functional Communication Profile.* New York: New York University Medical Center Rehabilitation Monograph 42 (1969).

Schuell, H., *Minnesota Test for Differential Diagnosis of Aphasia.* Minneapolis: University of Minnesota Press, (1965).

Schuell, H., A short examination for aphasia. *Neurology,* 7, 615-634 (1957).

Schuell, H., A re-evaluation of the short examination for aphasia. *J. Speech Hearing Dis.,* 31, 137-147 (1966).

Spellacy, F., and O. Spreen, A short form of the Token Test. *Cortex,* 5, 390-397 (1969).

Spreen, O., and A. Benton, *Neurosensory Center Comprehensive Examination for Aphasia.* Victoria, B.C.: Neuropsychology Laboratory, University of Victoria, (1969).

Swisher, L., and M. Sarno, Token Test scores of three matched patient groups: Left brain-damaged with aphasia; right brain-damaged without aphasia; nonbrain-damaged. *Cortex,* 5, 264-273 (1969).

Taylor, M., and E. Sands, Reliability measures of the Functional Communication Profile. Paper presented at the American Speech and Hearing Association Convention, Chicago (1965).

Trimboli, B., and N. Lass, A comparative study of the performance of middle class and economically deprived children on the short form of the Token Test. *J. Auditory Res.,* 6, 59-63 (1976).

Watson, J., and L. Records, The effectiveness of the Porch Index of Communicative Ability as a diagnostic tool in assessing specific behaviors of senile dementia, in *Clinical Aphasiology: Conference Proceedings 1978,* ed. R. Brookshire. Minneapolis: BRK Publishers, (1978).

Wechsler, D., and C. P. Stone, *Wechsler Memory Scale.* New York: The Psychological Corporation, (1948).

Weisenberg, T., and K. McBride, *Aphasia.* New York: The Commonwealth Fund, (1935).

Wepman, J., and L. Jones, *The Language Modalities Test for Aphasia.* Chicago: Education-Industry Service, (1961).

Zaidel, E., Unilateral auditory language comprehension on the Token Test following cerebral commissurotomy and hemispherectomy. *Neuropsychologia,* 15, 1-15 (1977).

PART IV

Assessment Formats for Structural Disorders

XI

Structural deviations are not synonomous with functional differences.

Several disorders, such as laryngectomee, cleft palate, glossectomee, and cerebral palsy, result from structural and/or neuromuscular abnormalities. The assessment strategies for these disorders have some procedures in common with problem areas previously discussed, but specialized appraisal tools also may be used. The assessment formats for these disorders will be considered because they exemplify the eclectic derivation of evaluative instruments and because they demonstrate the wide range of behaviors that need to be quantified in order to determine the communicative disorder to be addressed in treatment.

EVALUATION OF LARYNGECTOMEE

There is general agreement (Berlin and Virden 1971; Boone 1977; Warner 1971; Gardner 1971; Martin and Hoops 1974) that a diagnostic evaluation of the laryngectomee should include consideration of factors concerning the surgery; the patient's physical condition, auditory functioning, emotional status, vocation, and articulation and language abilities; the familial attitude toward the patient with esophageal speech; and the use of this information for determining a prognosis for esophageal speech development. The information obtained clearly is prognostic in nature. Since some of the information is acquired before surgery, we will consider preoperative as well as postoperative assessment procedures.

Preoperative Assessment. Preoperative assessment will include a detailed medical, social, and educational history. The medical history will provide information on conditions that may have a significant bearing on the ability to develop esophageal speech. For example, a history of hernia, abdominal surgery, cleft palate or palatal paresis, pulmonary disease, and colostomy are negative prognostic indicators (Diedrich and Youngstrom 1966). Job duties, leisure-time activities, and the emotional status of the patient should be explored. Patients employed in highly communicative positions and with a history of vocational success are more likely to develop functional esophageal speech. Family attitudes also are important. A supportive encouraging family accepting of esophageal speech development will have a positive effect on rehabilitation efforts.

Surgical removal of the larynx has a marked impact on oral-peripheral structures. Nevertheless, an examination of the speech-production mechanism should be completed preoperatively. Hearing acuity also is assessed because it is prognostically significant. Berlin (1963) found that 40 percent of the laryngectomees who were poor esophageal speakers had a significant hearing loss. Kahane and Irwin (1975) noted that hearing sensitivity is a critical element in esophageal-voice rehabilitation and may have adverse affects on the control of stoma noise, voice quality, and length of rehabilitation. The audiological battery should include speech discrimination, speech reception threshold, and pure-tone testing.

Other preoperative appraisals may be used. Berlin and Virden (1971) suggested that a preoperative recording of a standard speech passage and plosive production in consonant-vowel or vowel-consonant-vowel contexts be recorded and later compared to esophageal speech. Logemann (1975) recommended that articulatory patterns and rate of speech production be evaluated preoperatively. Finally, an attempt *may* be made to determine the ability of the patient to produce esophageal phonation. This is of limited value, however, since the structural integrity of the esophagus and oral structures is frequently altered by surgery.

Postoperative Assessment. Following surgery, a careful review of the surgical report is in order. This is important because it will provide information on the integrity of the apparatus that will be used for esophageal speech. Important information includes reports of denervation of muscular structures of the head and neck, postradiation fibrosis, stenosis of the esophagus, and the extension of the surgery, particularly to excision of the pharynx, base of the tongue, and floor of the mouth.

Attention should be paid to examination of labial, palatal, and lingual structures since they are of primary importance to insufflation of the esophagus. The lips, if there is facial weakness, may not be able to effectively seal air within the intraoral cavity. Likewise, partial removal of the tongue or interruption of the neural supply to the tongue or velopharyngeal mechanism will reduce or prevent insufflation. If the patient has dentures, they should be examined because, if not fit properly, oral structural movements will be impeded during attempts to force air into the esophagus. Finally, hearing should be reassessed since edema or metastasis of the carcinoma to the auditory nerve may produce hearing impairment.

Instruments for appraising esophageal speech are primarily scaling devices that estimate the proficiency of the patient or monitor the acquisition of alaryngeal speech skills. Perhaps the earliest scale was developed by Wepman, MacGahan, Richard, and Shelton (1953). The seven-point rating scale extends from Level 7, no esophageal speech production, to Level 1, automatic esophageal speech. Wepman and his associates proposed that the scale be used for self-evaluation and for observation since it serves the dual role of monitoring the progression of esophageal-sound production and providing an estimate of speech proficiency.

Berlin and Virden (1971) developed assessment tasks which have at least face validity in relation to adequate esophageal speech. The four skills evaluated include the reliability of phonation on demand, the maintenance of a short latency between insufflation of the esophagus and vocalization, the maintenance of an optimal duration of phonation, and the ability to sustain phonation during articulation. In order to assess these skills, the patient is asked to perform two tasks: to phonate as long as possible on the vowel /a/ over twenty trials and to repeat the syllable /da/ as many times as possible, without consciously reinflating the esophagus, over ten trials. The ability to phonate on demand is determined by the percentage of successful vocalizations in 20 trials; any vocalization exceeding 0.4 seconds is considered successful. Maintenance of short latency is measured by finding the mean time between insufflation and production of /a/. Optimal duration is determined by the mean duration of /a/ over 20 trials, and sustaining phonation during articulation is evaluated by recording the mean number of syllables articulated with a single overt insufflation. Berlin and Virden indicated that a good esophageal speaker could phonate reliably on demand with a short latency, sustain a vowel for approximately two seconds, and produce approximately ten syllables per insufflation.

Similar appraisal devices were proposed by Weinberg (1975). He suggested that assessment should be divided into two areas: skill building and speech building. Examples of skill building included determining mean latency, mean duration of phonation, and number of syllables produced on one insufflation. Speech-building assessment included evaluating the patient's ability to produce syllables or words, estimating the intelligibility of speech in conversational settings, and determining the rate of speech production in words per minute.

In summary, assessment of the laryngectomized patient is eclectic. Much of the information gained is biographical in nature and used for determining prognosis. Appraisal tools are limited almost entirely to determining the esophageal speech proficiency of the patient on the basis of clinical judgment, rather than through standardized appraisal tools.

EVALUATION OF GLOSSECTOMEE

Although there are several clinical case reports and small sample studies of patients who have undergone partial or complete removal of the tongue (Goldstein 1940; Herberman 1958; Massengill, Maxwell, and Pickrell 1970), there has been only one major study of glossectomized patients (Skelly and others 1971; Skelly and others 1972; Skelly, 1973). Skelly and others studied the articulatory and phonatory deficits of 25 partial and complete glossectomee patients and their assessment instruments serve as the primary source for appraisal procedures.

Glossectomees are performed as a life-saving surgical procedure for cancer of the tongue. The amount of tissue removed is dependent on the site of lesion and metastasis of the disease, and the degree of communicative impairment and dysphagia is dependent upon the amount of tissue resected and the degree of interruption of innervation to the musculature of the head and neck. Partial removal, especially of either the right or left half of the tongue, has far less marked an affect on speech production than complete removal. As would be expected, total removal produces marked deficits in the ability to produce lingual consonants, semivowels, and vowels since the egressive airstream cannot be valved by the tongue, and the tongue is no longer available to alter the resonant characteristics of the vocal tract. Due to the critical role of the tongue in deglutition, drooling and dysphagia are concomitant problems.

There are no standardized tests for the glossectomee. Assessment procedures derive almost wholly from the work of Skelly and others and include consideration of case history and phonatory and articulatory functioning. The case history information and medical and surgical reports provide a social context from which to view the patient and a detailed summary of the anatomical and innervation effects of surgery. Responses to biographical questions and the reading of a standard passage (for example, Arthur the Rat) are tape recorded to establish base-line performance. The patient then is asked to produce five vowels which are judged by the examiner to determine if they are *distinguishable* from one another and not to determine if they are *identifiable.* This procedure is followed by the patient's production of a vowel (one he produces easily) and the voiced and voiceless labiodental fricatives /v/ and /f/ which are maintained for a maximal duration. Skelly noted that normal duration is approximately 18 seconds, and durations of 14 seconds or less are indicative or laryngeal and/or respiratory problems that should be evaluated further by determining mean duration for each of the three phonemes over three trials.

The next task is for the patient to produce an open vowel at his highest and then lowest pitch followed by glides from highest to lowest and lowest to highest pitch. This procedure, when coupled to the patient's productions of a vowel at the highest pitch and lowest pitch with intervening pauses, provides an estimate of pitch range and additional information regarding the integrity of the respiratory-laryngeal mechanism.

Articulatory abilities are appraised by asking the patient to produce syllables, words, and sentences containing glossal and nonglossal consonants. The glossal and nonglossal consonant productions then are compared and serve as an estimate of residual articulatory facility.

The next task is for the patient to produce words without glossal consonants such as *pave* under a number of conditions: with greater labial compression, with greater jaw excursion, at faster and slower rates, at a higher pitch, with the jaw "thrust forward," with vowel prolongation, and with increased intensity. It is evident that the purpose of these tasks is to assess the patient's compensatory abilities following major structural changes of the oral cavity.

Skelly (1973) suggests that a speech sample be used to determine what substitutions are used for glossal consonants, to assess the patient's ability to communicate information, and to provide estimates of intelligibility based upon ratings by the patient, the clinician, and naive listeners. She also recommends that the patient be administered a complete audiological battery, a test for short-term auditory memory, and the *Leiter International Performance Scale.*

In the aggregate, the procedures we have reviewed include primarily non-standardized instruments, the function of which is to evaluate the residual and compensatory abilities of the speech-production apparatus. These procedures appear intuitively to be adequate for the assessment of the glossectomee, but in the absence of validity and reliability statements their comparative value cannot be determined. In the end, the value of the information obtained will be at least as much determined by the experience and expertise of the examiner as by the procedures used to obtain the information.

With a few rare exceptions (Backus 1940; Peterson 1973), laryngectomees and glossectomees are adults. We now turn our attention to appraisal procedures for two disorders, cleft palate and cerebral palsy, that are most often associated with childhood.

ASSESSMENT OF CLEFT PALATE

Articulation and resonance disorders are the primary communicative deficits associated with cleft palate and arise from the congenital structural abnormalities of the speech-production apparatus. There may be associated deficits in language and auditory acuity, but these problems are secondary and typically are mild. The evaluation of the cleft-palate patient includes a case history; articulation, resonance, and nasal emission testing; audiological assessment; and determination of linguistic abilities. We earlier provided information on procedures for acquiring case history information and the steps to be followed in completing an oral-peripheral examination of the speech mechanism. Likewise, we previously considered articulation testing, language assessment, some aspects of testing resonance, and instrumentation useful for evaluating structural disorders. The focus here will be to evaluate measures that were developed specifically with cleft-palate patients in mind but which are appropriate for other patients with comparable communicative deficits.

Articulation Tests

One effect of velopharyngeal incompetence is to produce compensations at other constrictions in the vocal tract. Consequently, some of the articulation behaviors of cleft-palate children are different from those normally encountered in noncleft children. Behaviors which demonstrate compensatory efforts are attempts to constrict the nares to gain or maintain intraoral pressure and the substitution of pharyngeal and velar fricatives and glottal stops. The production of these articulatory substitutions exemplify the efforts made by the cleft-palate speaker to constrict the egressive airstream posterior to the insufficient velopharyngeal valve. Fricatives, affricates, and plosives are most frequently in error because they require the highest intraoral pressure for their production. This is not to say that children with cleft palate will not use substitutions associated with normal phonological development, but rather to point out that the substitutions are conditioned by a structurally inadequate speech-production apparatus. It also is noteworthy that the substitutions used by the cleft-palate patient may persist after surgical and/or prosthetic management have restored velopharyngeal competency since they have become habituated. Finally, even if correctly produced, the consonants may be distorted by nasal emission of air.

One articulation measure already reviewed is the *Iowa Pressure Articulation Test* (Morris, Spriestersbach, and Darley 1961). The test is composed of 43 items selected from the *Templin-Darley Tests of Articulation* (Templin and Darley 1960). Included are fricatives, affricates, and plosives which best discriminate between adequate and inadequate velopharyngeal closure. The errors on the test can be compared to norms from the Templin-Darley test. The sounds in error also are stimulated to determine a prognosis for correction and to separate errors due to physiological inadequacy from those due to delayed phonological development. *The Iowa Pressure Articulation Test* also has been found to be of predictive value in determining the need for secondary management of cleft-palate patients (Van Demark and Morris 1977).

Another articulatory measure developed to assess velopharyngeal function is the *Miami Imitative Ability Test* (Jacobs, Phillips, and Harrison 1970). The test evaluates the ability to imitate acoustic production and articulatory placement for consonants. The measure includes 24 consonants presented in consonant-vowel contexts using the neutral vowel /ʌ/. The patient is instructed to watch and listen as the examiner repeats each syllable three times. The patient then is asked to repeat the syllable. Articulatory placement and acoustic production are scored separately. Responses are assigned one point if produced correctly, one-half point if questionable, or no point if incorrect. Both placement and acoustic scores can range from zero to 24 points. For visible sounds, placement is scored by direct observation. If the placement is not readily visible, the examiner must base her judgment on the visual assessment supplemented by the acoustic production. Since acoustic information must be used to determine placement accuracy, the two evaluational procedures are not independent of one another.

Administration of the test to 129 children with cleft palate and 154 children without orofacial anomalies between 30 and 72 months of age revealed that the cleft-palate children were inferior to the normal group on both evaluations. In fact, at 72 months, cleft-palate children did not have the proficiency on the test of 30-month-old normal children.

The *Bzoch Error Pattern Diagnostic Articulation Test* (described by Bzoch 1979) is based on the articulation characteristics of cleft palate and matched normal control subjects from three to six years of age (Bzoch 1956). The test contains 100 elements (67 single consonants and 33 blends). The single consonants are tested in the initial, medial, and final positions of words and are grouped by manner of production (plosives, fricatives, affrictives, aspirates, glides, nasals). Within each manner grouping, the most peripheral articulations are tested first followed by evaluation of anterior to posterior placements.

Sounds are tested first in the initial position followed by medial and then final positions. Cognate pairs are listed together for the plosive and fricative categories, and the testing of an unvoiced consonant precedes testing of its voiced cognate.

Words with the test element correctly produced are scored as correct whether other elements are correct or not. If the consonant element was produced correctly but was distorted by nasal emission alone, it is scored accordingly. If the test element is produced incorrectly, the child is asked to repeat it two more times, and the most severe error is recorded according to an ascending order of error severity: distortion (due to imprecise articulation), simple substitution (use of another phoneme for the target phoneme), gross substitution (use of velar fricative, pharyngeal fricative, or glottal stop), or omission of the phoneme. Blends are considered, for the purposes of recording and scoring, as single elements. If one or more of the elements of the blend are distorted but all are present, it is scored as a distortion; if part of the blend is missing but some of the sounds are used in place of it (for example, /th/ for /thr/ in *thread*), it is scored as a simple substitution. Any gross substitution of a blend element is recorded as a gross substitution for the entire blend, and an omission is defined as omission of all blend elements.

The Bzoch Test is not particularly unusual. It follows the more traditional format of assessing single elements in the initial, medial, and final positions of words and includes items typically found on many of the articulation tests we reviewed earlier. It is clearly different, however, in its scoring system because it provides error categories that are anticipated for patients with inadequate velopharyngeal closure.

Articulation errors of cleft-palate speakers may vary between single words and connected speech. Van Demark (1964) constructed thirteen test sentences containing 149 consonant sounds: 56 plosives, 33 fricatives, 31 nasal semi-vowels, and 29 glides. The sentences contain 21 consonant blends in various combinations. The sentences are constructed to approximate the frequency of occurrence of the various consonant sounds found in the English language. Scoring is accomplished by evaluating the correctness of production of the 149 test consonants. If a consonant is produced incorrectly, the response is categorized according to the manner of production (fricative, plosive, glide, nasal semi-vowel) and the type of error (distortion-oral, distortion-nasal, glottal stop substitution, substitution, and omission). The test sentences therefore provide an estimate of consonant-production accuracy in connected speech.

Clinical Methods of Estimating Velopharyngeal Competence

Nasal emission of air and hypernasality are not the same phenomenon. Both typically result from inadequate velopharyngeal closure, but emission is the audible flow of air through the nasal passages during the production of consonants requiring high intraoral pressure while hypernasality is the acoustic endproduct of an abnormal coupling of the nasal and oral cavities during voiced segments.

Bzoch (1979) has suggested several clinical tests that yield estimates of nasal emission, hypernasality, and hyponasality. Hyponasality is evaluated because it may be characteristic of patients with overly broad pharyngeal flaps or obturators that effectively valve the velopharyngeal port during the production of nasals. Each test is based on the performance of the patient on ten items. For the hypernasality test, the patient produces ten words initiated with /b/ and terminated with /t/. Each word is produced by the patient with the nostrils open and with the nares manually closed. A ratio is determined by counting the number of productions of the ten on which there is a perceived change of tone. Ten words initiated with /m/ and ended with /t/ are produced with the nares open and occluded on the hyponasality test. Here the number of words that sound the same with the nares open and occluded is used to determine the clinical index of abnormal hyponasality. A nasal-emission clinical index is determined, according to Bzoch, by placing a small paddle wheel in front of the nares during production of ten bisyllabic words containing /p/ and /b/ in initial and medial word positions. The examiner counts the number of productions on which nasal emission occurs out of the ten words to determine a ratio.

There are no norms for these clinical tests. However, it can be assumed that a patient with high clinical index ratios on the three measures has abnormal velopharyngeal closure while low ratios are indicative of normal or near normal expected performance.

Another means of evaluating cleft-palate speakers is by scaling attributes of their speech production. Subtelny, Van Hattum, and Myers (1972) suggested that this be accomplished by assessing separately the nasality, articulation, and intelligibility of speech samples. The attributes may be rated on a seven-point, equal-interval scale or by other preset criteria. The reliability of the estimates will vary significantly depending on the nature of the speech sample and the procedures used to make the ratings. For example, Counihan and Cullinan (1970) found that the reliability of nasality ratings increased and the degree of ambiguity decreased from vowels to syllables to connected speech rated during backward play to connected speech rated during forward play. Hess (1971) noted that articulatory proficiency was significantly affected by the phoneme type and the stress of the consonant vowel environment. Moore and Sommers (1973) and Lintz and Sherman (1961) noted that context significantly affected ratings of nasality. Ratings may provide information on nasality and other attributes of speech production, but it must be remembered that the interpretation of these data must be cautious in light of contextual and procedural affects that reduce reliability.

Instrumentation

A mainstay in the assessment of velopharyngeal competence is instrumentation. The most frequently used clinical device is the oral manometer which provides an estimate of velopharyngeal competence by allowing a determination of an intraoral pressure ratio. The ratio is computed by comparing the intraoral pressure obtained with the nares occluded and unoccluded (Morris 1966). However, research findings have called into question the reliability of oral manometer ratios. Noll, Hawkins, and Weinberg (1977) obtained readings of maximum, sustained, positive and negative pressures from forty normal six- and seven-year-old children. They found that the majority of the subjects had difficulty generating and maintaining stable positive and negative pressures with the nostrils occluded and unoccluded. They concluded that the oral manometric ratio may be of questionable value in predicting velopharyngeal adequacy for speech, particularly if ratio data must be interpreted dichotomously.

Other instruments which we discussed earlier are available for estimating velopharyngeal competence including ultrasound, cinefluorography, air pressure, air flow, and acoustic measurements (Hollein 1976). However, none is infallible and capable of estimating velopharyngeal functioning under all context and prosodic conditions.

In conclusion, hypernasality is a complex acoustical phenomenon not easily quantified. Estimates of velopharyngeal closure from instrumental analyses and clinical ratings of nasality will be expected to be correlated. However, the relationship is not a linear one.

Other Tests

Children with cleft palate frequently have hearing disorders (Hayes 1965) and language deficits (Smith and McWilliams 1968; Philips and Harrison 1969). Tests for assessing language skills have been presented in an earlier chapter. Choose tests that meet your needs in assessing the linguistic skills of these patients.

EVALUATION IN CEREBRAL PALSY

A practical definition of cerebral palsy: a brain damage syndrome comprised of neuromuscular, sensory, psychological, intellectual, and behavioral disorders, quickly points out the large number of behaviors that may need to be assessed with these patients. If these deficits are viewed from a macroscopic vantagepoint, it would be expected that a large number of professionals–medical, allied health, and educational, all will contribute assessment data at one time or another if a full description of the cerebral-palsied child is to be obtained.

If we take a more restricted view of the appraisal process by delimiting the areas of concern which are the province of the speech-language pathologist, many of the tests we have discussed previously in this text would also be appropriate to determine communication deficits of cerebral-palsied children, depending partly on the severity of the disorder. The lines of demarcation as to which instruments and which areas of assessment are the province of the speech clinician are not entirely clear–nor should they necessarily be restricted in the context of a team evaluation of the patient. In general, the speech-language pathologist's role in the evaluation process will be dictated by the clinical situation in which she works, the neurophysiological rationale that serves as the basis for the process, and the problems of the patient to be addressed. These somewhat different formats and focuses are seen in assessment approaches proposed by several clinicians.

Crickmay (1966) indicated that an assessment in cerebral palsy should entail evaluation of (1) the ability to move body parts associated with the speech mechanism, such as the head, neck, and shoulders; (2) vegetative activities such as sucking, swallowing, biting, and chewing; (3) the ability to manipulate the jaw, lips, and tongue; and (4) the ability to vocalize and speak. She notes further:

> In making this speech assessment, it is necessary to find out which of the patient's reactions are normal, which are pathological and which are primitive but normal . . . with each reaction tested it is necessary to find out which movements the patient is able to do voluntarily, both with and without emotional stimulation, and which he can only do involuntarily, or merely as a reflex movement in response to a stimulus. (p. 77)

Certainly Crickmay would not view the language, auditory acuity, and other communication-related deficits to be unimportant since they are included in her therapy regime, but clearly the strategy she proposes focuses squarely on neuromuscular deficits as the primary area of concern.

A more comprehensive view of the areas in need of assessment is provided by Westlake and Rutherford (1961). They suggest that appraisal procedures, in addition to case history, will include consideration of expressive and receptive language, conceptualization, and vegetative and volitional functioning of the speech-production apparatus. There is some correspondence between Westlake and Rutherford and Crickmay as to the areas to be evaluated; that is the importance of appraising vegetative and voluntary functioning of the speech-production mechanism. There are similarities in the instruments selected (or not selected); neither Westlake and Rutherford nor Crickmay cite standardized instruments to be used as part of the evaluation. Does this mean that they do not see value in using standardized tests and age-referenced norms? Certainly not. Crickmay points out that "In treating him (the cerebral-palsied child) it is essential at all stages to measure his performance against that of the normal child and to follow the normal developmental pattern as closely as possible," and Westlake and Rutherford observe that two important pieces of information sought in the assessment of expressive behavior are "How does the child's level of oral language usage compare with that of other children of the same chronological age" and "In what ways are his oral language patterns different from those of other children his age?"

McDonald and Chance (1964) provide a format of evaluation in which the same areas as those cited by Westlake and Rutherford are proposed along with a de-emphasis on standardized instruments and an emphasis on age-referenced norms. Lencione (1966) and Mecham, Berko, and Berko (1960), on the other hand, see greater value in standardized tests for appraisal, although the areas of concern as to what is to be assessed are the same. The point to be made is that the instruments and procedures used, the areas to be assessed, and the weight and time afforded each of these areas will be determined in part by the problems demonstrated by the child and in part by the theroretical framework and clinical environment in which the clinician is operating.

Assessment Instruments for Cerebral Palsy

The instruments and procedures you choose for evaluating the cerebral-palsied child typically will include measures of articulation and language. Additionally, a case history will be secured, instrumental data may be obtained to enhance description of speech production adequacy, and examination of the speech-production mechanism will be performed in an expanded format that considers vegetative, nonverbal, and verbal performance tasks. The exact areas of assessment will depend on the problems demonstrated by the child, the focus and rationale of the assessment, and the availability of information from other professionals. Quite obviously, the appraisal process is not complete, in most cases, without appraisal data from the physician, audiologist, psychologist, occupational and physical therapists, and perhaps educational diagnostician.

Depending on the severity of the disorder, standardized tests may have to be adapted to fit the clinical situation. We cannot provide exact guidelines as to when the test procedures have been sufficiently altered to bring into question the validity and reliability of the test findings. This will depend on the tests and the adaptations made. The important thing to remember is that when assessing the child, there is no substitute for careful observation, detailed description, and clinical judgment when the findings are to be interpreted in light of normative data that serve as the reference for making statements about "normal" and "abnormal" performance.

Several measures have been developed for cerebral-palsied children that may serve to enhance descriptions of their communicative functioning. Denhoff and Holden (1951) studied 100 cerebral-palsied children and compared their performance to that of normal children on ten motor and communication items from the Gesell scales. Results of the study are displayed as histograms which show average, late normal, and abnormal late development based on the Gesell studies data and the mean performance of the cerebral-palsied children. As would be expected, the cerebral-palsied children were later than the ranges provided for the Gesell children. For example, on "walks alone," the average normal Gesell child accomplished this activity no later than 16 months while the average cerebral-palsied child did not accomplish this skill until 34 months. On "speech—single words," the average normal child would be expected, according to the Gesell data, to have reached this developmental milestone by 11 months while the average cerebral-palsied child did not begin using single words until 28 months. This scale may be helpful because it provides, in addition to normal and late performance in normal children, average development for cerebral-palsied children so that the patient can be compared to a normative reference group and to children with the same diagnosis. Unfortunately, no range is included for the cerebral-palsied children on each task. Denhoff and Holden did report, however, that the performances of the cerebral-palsied children were heterogeneous and that there was overlap with the performance of the Gesell children.

We would like to consider two tests which were developed specifically for cerebral-palsied children; one of articulation and the other of auditory discrimination developed by Irwin. O. C. Irwin, in a large number of studies published in the 1950s and 1960s, evaluated the communicative abilities of cerebral-palsied children in an effort to develop test instruments standardized specifically for these patients. An *Integrated Test for Use with Children with Cerebral Palsy* (Irwin 1961) is composed of five "short" tests which had been individually standardized on 1,155 cerebral-palsied children. Four of the tests were developed to evaluate consonants; the fifth, to evaluate vowels. The Integrated Test is a restandardization of the "short" tests on a group of 147 cerebral-palsied children from three to 16 years of age.

The test contains 24 consonants tested in initial, medial, and final word positions (where appropriate) and 11 vowels tested in initial and medial positions. Items are administered by imitation, and the entire test need not be administered at one time since it would be expected that the cerebral-palsied child will fatigue quickly. Items are scored as correct, substituted, omitted, distorted, no response, and neutral (defined as a response that bears no resemblance to the stimulus word). The number of errors of each type on each short test are then tabulated. An alternative list of stimulus words are provided for each of the short tests.

Results of the standardization of the Integrated Test are reported as means and variances for boys and girls; for initial, medial, and final word positions for consonants and initial and medial positions for vowels; for spastics and athetoids; for extent of involvement (quadriplegia, hemiplegia, and paraplegia); for left and right hemiplegics; for severity (mild, moderate, and severe); and for severity as a function of extent of involvement. Split-half reliability was found to be 0.98; Kuder-Richardson reliability coefficients were from 0.65 to 0.97 and inter-observer agreement was estimated at 90 percent. The validity of the test was reportedly demonstrated to be adequate by means of the method of extreme groups using both articulation scores and ratings of intelligibility.

Given the time and effort expended to develop and standardize the five short tests and the integrated test composed thereof, it might be expected that the test would be on the top of the list when appraising the articulatory development of cerebral-palsied children. However, this has not been the case, and the reasons are apparent. First, no data are available for normal children. Consequently, the performance of the cerebral-palsied child cannot be compared to a normative reference to make statements about the adequacy of his articulatory development. Moreover, even though the performance of cerebral-palsied children is reported on the basis of many factors as listed above, no mean and variance data are provided as a function of age. These weaknesses preclude the use of the test for making direct comparisons with normal or cerebral-palsied children. The test may serve as a descriptive device that provides a means of quantifying the articulatory behaviors of these children, but it appears to be of less value than articulation tests we discussed in an earlier chapter that were standardized on normal children.

Irwin and Jensen (1963a, b) developed two tests of sound discrimination for cerebral-palsied children. Since they are similar in format and design, we will examine only the first. The test is composed of thirty word-pairs. Twenty-five of the pairs differ by a single phoneme (pig-big) or by the presence of a blend versus a singleton consonant (brisket-biscuit). Ten are different in the initial position; ten, in the final position; and five, in the medial position. Five word-pairs are identical and serve as foils. The words are monosyllabic (tin-thin), bisyllabic (frisking-whisking), or multisyllabic (convergent-conversant). It should be noted that many of the stimulus words of the test (cytology-psychology; habitat-habitant) are not found in the vocabulary of young children.

The test was standardized on 153 cerebral-palsied children six to sixteen years of age with a mean of 10.3 years. Means and standard deviations are provided by two-year intervals except for the first level which includes only six year olds; by mental age; by severity of involvement; and by ratings of speech and language ability. Reliability of the test using a Kuder-Richardson formula was reported to be 0.87. Using the method of extreme groups, significant differences were found in discrimination scores for chronological age, mental age, and ratings of speech and language ability which Irwin and Jensen considered supportive of the validity of the test.

In light of our earlier stated reservations about the use of auditory discrimination tests, we would not expect this test to be administered to the cerebral-palsied child. However, it serves as another example of a test devised specifically for a group of communicatively handicapped patients but which appears to be of no more worth than comparable tests of the same functions standardized on normal subjects.

In summary, the evaluation format for the cerebral-palsied child is similar to that for other communicatively handicapped patients. There may be small differences depending on the theoretical bases from which the examiner is operating, the age of child, and the severity and type of disorder demonstrated, but the task remains the same—observations are made and quantified so that comparisons with normal performance will allow a determination of communicative ability.

SUMMARY

There are no strong strings that bind the diagnostic procedures and disorders presented in this chapter. We have discussed disorders typically associated with childhood and those acquired later in life; we have provided reasonably complete assessment protocols as well as abbreviated descriptions of procedures; and we have examined informal methods of evaluation as well as tests developed for particular groups of patients. The strings that bind, however, are those which emphasize the need to observe carefully, to quantify completely, and to use clinical judgment when statements regarding "abnormal" performance are to be made.

REFERENCES

Backus, O., Speech rehabilitation following excision of the tip of the tongue. *Amer. J. Disabled Child,* 60, 368-370 (1940).

Berlin, C., Clinical measurement of esophageal speech: I. Methodology and curves of skill acquisition. *J. Speech Hearing Dis.,* 28, 42-51 (1963).

Berlin, C., and V. Virden, Diagnostic techniques for determining methods and potential for teaching alaryngeal speech, in *Therapy for the Laryngectomized Patient,* eds. S. Rigrodsky, J. Lerman, and E. Morrison. New York: Teachers College Press, (1971).

Boone, D., *The Voice and Voice Therapy,* 2nd ed. Englewood Cliffs, N.J.: Prentice-Hall, Inc., (1977).

Bzoch, K., An investigation of the speech of pre-school cleft palate children. Doctoral dissertation, Northwestern University, Evanston, (1956).

Bzoch, K., Measurement and assessment of categorical aspects of cleft palate speech, in *Communicative Disorders Related to Cleft Lip and Palate,* 2nd ed., ed. K. Bzoch. Boston: Little, Brown, (1975).

Counihan, D., and W. Cullinan, Reliability and dispersion of nasality ratings. *Cleft Pal. J.,* 7, 261-270 (1970).

Crickmay, M., *Speech Therapy and the Bobath Approach to Cerebral Palsy.* Springfield, Ill.: Charles C Thomas, (1966).

Denhoff, E., and R. Holden, The developmental ladder in cerebral palsy. Reprinted by National Society for Crippled Children and Adults, Inc., Chicago, Illinois, (1951).

Diedrich, W., and K. Youngstrom, *Alaryngeal Speech.* Springfield, Ill.: Charles C Thomas, (1966).

Gardner, W., *Laryngectomee Speech and Rehabilitation.* Springfield, Ill.: Charles C Thomas, (1971).

Goldstein, M., Speech without a tongue. *J. Speech Dis.,* 5, 65-69 (1940).

Hayes, C., Audiological problems associated with cleft palate. *Proceedings of the Conference: Communicative Problems in Cleft Palate.* Washington, D.C.: ASHA Reports No. 1 (1965).

Herberman, M., Rehabilitation of patients following glossectomy. *Arch. Otolaryng.,* 67, 182-183 (1958).

Hess, D., Effects of certain variables on speech of cleft palate persons. *Cleft Pal. J.,* 8, 387-398 (1971).

Hollein, H., Status report on instrumentation useful for craniofacial research. *Cleft. Pal. J.,* 13, 138-155 (1976).

Irwin, O., A manual of articulation testing for use with children with cerebral palsy. *Cerebral Pal. Rev.,* 22, May-June, 1-20 (1961).

Irwin, O., and P. Jensen, A test of sound discrimination for use with cerebral palsied children. *Cerebral Pal. Rev.,* 24, March-April, 5-11 (1963a).

Irwin, O., and P. Jensen, A parallel test of sound discrimination for use with cerebral palsied children. *Cerebral Pal. Rev.,* 24, September-October, 3-10 (1963b).

Jacobs, R., B. Phillips, and R. Harrison, A stimulability test for cleft palate children. *J. Speech Hearing Dis.,* 35, 354-360 (1970).

Kahane, J., and J. Irwin, Comparison of hearing sensitivity, stoma noise and speech ratings and duration in therapy in ninety esophageal speakers. Paper presented at the Convention of the American Speech and Hearing Association, Washington, D.C., (1975).

Lencione, R., Speech and language problems in cerebral palsy, in *Cerebral Palsy: Its Individual and Community Problems,* ed. W. Cruickshank. Syracuse, N.Y.: Syracuse University Press, (1966).

Lintz, L., and D. Sherman, Phonetic elements and perception of nasality. *J. Speech Hearing Res.,* 4, 381-396 (1961).

Logemann, J., Assessing alaryngeal voice mechanisms. Paper presented to the 15th Annual Meeting of the International Association of Laryngectomees, (1975).

McDonald, E., and B. Chance, *Cerebral Palsy.* Englewood Cliffs, N.J.: Prentice-Hall, Inc., (1964).

Martin, D., and H. Hoops, The relationships between esophageal speech proficiency and selected measures of auditory function. *J. Speech Hearing Res.,* 17, 30-85 (1974).

Massengill, R., S. Maxwell, and K. Pickrell, An analysis of articulation following partial and total glossectomy. *J. Speech Hearing Dis.,* 35, 170-173 (1970).

Mecham, M., M. Berko, and F. Berko, *Speech Therapy in Cerebral Palsy.* Springfield, Ill.: Charles C Thomas, (1960).

Moore, W., and R. Sommers, Phonetic contexts: Their effects on perceived nasality in cleft palate speakers. *Cleft Pal. J.,* 10, 72-83 (1973).

Morris, H., The oral manometer as a diagnostic tool in clinical speech pathology. *J. Speech Hearing Dis.,* 31, 362-369 (1966).

Morris, H., D. Spriestersbach, and F. Darley, An articulation test for assessing competency of velopharyngeal closure. *J. Speech Hearing Res.,* 4, 48-55 (1961).

Noll, J., M. Hawkins, and B. Weinberg, Performance of normal six- and seven-year-old males on oral manometer tasks. *Cleft Pal. J.,* 14, 200-205 (1977).

Peterson, H. A., A case report of speech and language training for a two-year-old laryngectomized child. *J. Speech Hearing Dis.,* 38, 275-278 (1973).

Philips, B., and R. Harrison, Language skills of preschool cleft palate children. *Cleft Pal. J.,* 108-119 (1969).

Skelly, M., *Glossectomee Speech Rehabilitation.* Springfield, Ill.: Charles C Thomas, (1973).

Skelly, M. and others, Changes in phonatory aspects of glossectomee intelligibility through vocal parameter manipulation. *J. Speech Hearing Dis.,* 37, 379-389 (1972).

Skelly, M. and others, Compensatory physiologic phonetics for the glossectomee. *J. Speech Hearing Dis.,* 36, 101-114 (1971).

Smith, R., and B. McWilliams, Psycholinguistic abilities of children with clefts. *Cleft Pal. J.,* 5, 238-249 (1968).

Subtelny, J., R. Van Hattum, and B. Myers, Ratings and measures of cleft palate speech. *Cleft Pal. J.,* 9, 18-27 (1972).

Templin, M., and F. Darley, *The Templin-Darley Tests of Articulation.* Bureau of Education Research and Service, Extension Division, Univ. of Iowa, Iowa City, Iowa, (1960).

Van Demark, D., Misarticulations and listener judgments of the speech of children with cleft palate. *Cleft Pal. J.,* 1, 232-245 (1964).

Van Demark, D., and H. Morris, A preliminary study of the predictive value of the IPAT. *Cleft Pal. J.,* 14, 125-130 (1977).

Warner, J., Vocal rehabilitation following total laryngectomy. *J. Laryng. Otol.,* 85, 577-582 (1971).

Weinberg, B., Assessing esophageal speech. Paper presented at the Fifteenth Annual Meeting of the International Association of Laryngectomees, (1975).

Wepman, J. and others, The objective measurement of progressive esophageal speech development. *J. Speech Hearing Dis.,* 18, 247-251 (1953).

Westlake, H., and D. Rutherford, *Speech Therapy for the Cerebral Palsied.* Chicago: National Society for Crippled Children and Adults, Inc., (1961).

Psychological Assessment in Communication Disorders*

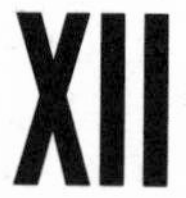

Examinations are formidable, even to the best prepared, for the greatest fool may ask more than the wisest man can answer.

C. Colton
Lacon (Revised Edition), 1836

Many psychological tests yield information useful for differential diagnosis of communication disorders. While most of these tests are restricted to administration by a psychologist, it is important for the diagnostician to know: (1) which tests are appropriate for patients with communicative disorders, (2) what information may be obtained from psychological test instruments, and (3) how communication disorders effect psychological test results. We will review tests of both intelligence and emotional status. The focus clearly will be on the information derived from the tests, the age groups the tests are designed for, and the rationale for their construction. To a lesser extent, specific information regarding standardization will be considered.

TESTS OF INTELLIGENCE

Intelligence is a general ability composed of a large number of interrelated mental functions. The functions or factors include verbal skills, numerical facility, reasoning, memory, spatial relations, and visual perception. Tests of

*Coauthored with Betty J. Hancock, M.A., Clinical Psychologist.

intelligence are geared toward testing one or more of these factors to assess the intellectual ability or capability of the child or adult. In other chapters we have presented tests which assess some of these functions but never in the context of intelligence testing.

Typically, tests of intelligence are divided into performance and verbal scales. Nunnally (1970) has noted, however, that:

> It has been the custom to call instruments "performance" tests if they de-emphasize language requirements, employ three-dimensional materials, and require manipulative responses. Because of these components, the performance tests usually measure motor coordination, speed, perceptual factors and spatial factors. Instruments are usually referred to as "verbal" tests if they are printed forms, emphasize verbal comprehension, and require symbolic responses. Because of the ease with which certain kinds of test materials can be placed on printed forms, the verbal tests tend to measure verbal comprehension, numerical computation, and the reasoning factors. There is no clear-cut separation between the factors found in verbal and performance tests, but there is a tendency for different factors to arise in the two kinds of materials. (p. 281)

We will review two types of intelligence tests: performance scales and instruments that evaluate performance and verbal factors.

MEASURES OF INTELLECTUAL POTENTIAL: PERFORMANCE SCALES

Performance tests require an overt nonverbal manipulative response. Judgments of intelligence are made based upon what the child can demonstrate with his hands, point to, arrange, insert, or put together (Horrocks 1964). They were developed because many individuals demonstrate deficits in hearing, language, and/or speech and consequently will be handicapped on test instruments which are verbally demanding. Performance scales, therefore, are particularly important in the evaluation of communicatively handicapped patients. These scales may not be completely nonverbal in that the patient may engage in verbal behavior during the course of completing manipulative tasks. However, the instructions and the tasks require no overt verbalizations to the extent that instructions are pantomimed or acted out.

Performance tests serve the important function of helping to rule out mental retardation in a patient with limited verbal abilities since these measures estimate the patient's nonverbal cognitive abilities. They also are important because they provide information on the content of language. Bloom and Lahey (1978) note that tests of this type fit into a content of language category:

> . . . (1) the test gives information about the child's capacities for representational thought and ability to act on represented information (in the

mind) as opposed to empirical information (in the context); (2) the test does not require that the child respond to much verbal instruction nor that the child interact verbally with the examiner in order to complete the task; and (3) completion of the tasks does not require that the child verbalize the answers but instead, the scoring reflects nonverbal solutions. If most of these tasks are successfully completed by the child, then it is possible to conclude that the child is able mentally to represent aspects of the world that are not perceptually present in the situation, and to perform actions that are contingent on these mental representations. Although the tasks in such tests are not direct measures of the content coded by language, age appropriate scores with these measures can suggest that the child's concepts of the world, and the ideas that are coded by language are most likely intact.

We will review several performance tests with the purpose of providing information on their format, design, standardization, and information obtained.

The *Merrill-Palmer Scale of Mental Tests* (Stutsman 1948) is primarily a performance test but also contains several verbal items. The test was designed for children 24 to 48 months of age and is composed of 93 items arranged in ascending order of difficulty with three to fourteen items at each three-month interval. The speed and accuracy with which the tasks are completed determines the age level credited to the child on many of the items. Timed items include pegboards, a form board, picture puzzles, tower building, picture matching, buttoning, and pyramid building with cubes. Nontimed items are the verbal and copying tasks. Language tests include repetition of words and phrases, answering questions, and an action-agent test with items such as "What cries?", "What runs?" The copying tasks include reproduction of a circle, cross, and asterisk.

A child is tested to a base level where all items are passed and upward to a level where more than one-half of the test items are failed. The test was standardized on 300 boys and 311 girls from 18 to 77 months at six-month intervals with 41 to 81 children at each level. The raw score is used to determine a mental age, percentile, and standard score. Computation of an intelligence quotient is not recommended since the I.Q. deviations are not the same size at various age levels. The reliability of the test has not been determined, but Stutsman (1948) reported that the test differentiates between bright and dull children, and a correlation of 0.92 between chronological age and the total score on the test has been reported (Horrocks 1964).

The Merrill-Palmer Scale is frequently the test of choice with the reluctant low-verbal two- to four-year-old child. Its colorful, age-graded, toy-like items appeal to most children. Verbal instructions used with the performance items are simple and are usually accompanied by pantomime. The test affords a unique opportunity for observing personal behavior that may be clinically significant, such as the child's persistence, frustration level, and dependency. However, it tends to overestimate the intellectual capacity of the language-impaired child and underestimates the ability of the motorically awkward child due to the many timed items.

The *Leiter International Performance Scale* (Leiter 1969) is a nonverbal mental age scale for assessing the intelligence of patients between two and eighteen years of age. Its primary use is with children with speech, hearing, and language disorders. Materials include blocks with pictures, colors, or designs which the child places in slots of an adjustable frame containing a stimulus card. The child is given three-months credits for each of the 54 tasks passed after the establishment of a basal age. Basal age is defined as correct completion of all four tests at an age level. Above ten years, six-months credit is provided for each correct completion of a task. The test is terminated when all items are failed for two consecutive age levels.

The total score on the test is converted to a mental age which can be used to establish an intelligence quotient. The first or Hawaiian standardization of the scale was later found to overestimate the mental age of the child by approximately 18 months. A second standardization of the scale was completed to alleviate this problem but was found to underestimate the performance of the child by approximately six months. Therefore, the intelligence quotient is corrected by the addition of five points to the derived score. The mean at each age level with the quotient correction is 100 with a standard deviation of 16.

The *Arthur Adaptation of the Leiter International Performance Scale* (Arthur 1952) is a restandardization and not a revision of the Leiter International Scale. It was restandardized because the norms of the first standardization by Leiter were too high. The test was reorganized to remove tasks demanding acquired skills such as telling time and to eliminate the timing of any of the test items to facilitate use of the instrument with motorically impaired patients. Some of the items at the upper age levels were omitted.

The test is designed for children from three to eight years of age and for other patients whose intellectual capacity would be expected to fall within this range. The lowest items on the test are determiners of the patient's ability to learn, rather than tests of acquired knowledge or skill. The child is given credit if she is able to successfully complete the task without demonstration or help during a trial, no matter how many previous opportunities were given. There are four items at each twelve-month age level for which the child can receive three-months credit. The exception is the four-year level where the child receives 2.25-months credit per item.

The test was standardized on 289 children from three to 7.99 years of age with 58 to 64 children at each age level. The mean intelligence quotient is 100 at each age level, and although not reported by Arthur, the standard deviation is estimated to be 16 (Leiter 1969).

The major asset of the test is in ruling out mental retardation and identifying the child with superior or above average intelligence. If the nonverbal child scores above his chronological age on the test, it is recommended that teaching be through the visual modality.

The *Hiskey-Nebraska Test of Learning Aptitude* (Hiskey 1966) is a unique performance scale in that separate instructions and norms are provided for deaf and normal hearing children from three to 17 years of age. The scale is composed of 163 items of increasing difficulty on twelve subtests. For children three to ten years old, eight subtests are presented. Instructions are pantomimed for the deaf and presented orally for the normal hearing child. Four of the subtests, bead patterns, memory for color, visual attention span, and paper folding, evaluate memory. For example, the bead patterns subtest requires the child to copy a design at the earlier age levels, while at older age levels he must reproduce the design from memory following a short exposure. Similarly, on the memory for color subtest, the child must match colored sticks following a short exposure by the examiner. Tasks not having a memory component are picture association, pictorial identification, block patterns, and completion of drawings. In general these four subtests tap concept formation, spatial relationships, reasoning ability, and visual closure and attention.

Seven subtests are administered to children from 11 to 16 years of age. Visual attention span, block patterns, and completion of drawings are identical to those administered to younger children. The tests specific to this age group include memory for digits, puzzle books, pictorial analogies, and spatial reasoning. The memory for digits test requires the child to remember numbers on a card and to reproduce them from a set of digits provided by the examiner. Puzzle blocks are a set of eight colored blocks cut into parts. Each must be combined to make a cube. Pictorial analogies requires the child to select a correct picture from a series of choices to complete a pictorial analogy. Spatial reasoning contains ten geometric designs presented one at a time followed by the presentation of a set of four fragmented geometric designs from which the child must choose the correct form that could be assembled from the original design.

An age score is derived from each subtest. A learning age for deaf children and a mental age for hearing children is determined from the median of the subtests. A learning age, rather than a mental age, is used with deaf children to reduce the possibility of comparing the two groups. A learning age of five years, for example, is interpreted to mean that the child is able to do those tasks that an average deaf child of five can perform. A learning quotient can be determined for the hearing-impaired child by dividing the learning age by chronological age. However, age improvement gradually reduces from twelve to sixteen years, and learning ages and learning quotients have less significance at older than at younger age levels. One out of every four months of chronological age is dropped out above twelve years, and a constant chronological age is used for computations above 16 years. For the normal-hearing child, an intelligence quotient is determined by dividing mental age by chronological age. The intelligence quotients have been set with a mean of 100 and an arbitrary standard deviation of 16 at each age level.

The test was standardized on 1,079 deaf children and 1,074 hearing children from 2-6 years to 17-5 years at one-year intervals. Children from 2-6 years to 3-5 years were grouped as three year olds, children from 3-6 years to 4-5 years were considered in the four-year group and so forth. The three-year group was very limited in size, and the norms for the upper limits are based on extrapolations. Therefore, the extremes of age must be considered reduced in reliability. The test has adequate concurrent validity as revealed by correlations with the Stanford-Binet (L-M) for normally hearing children. Moreover, reliability is high as judged by coefficients from 0.947 to 0.904 on split-half and Spearman-Brown statistical procedures.

The Hiskey-Nebraska offers a wide array of untimed performance tasks but is somewhat arduous for the young child. A deaf child must be at least four years of age before test administration is not difficult. It is also problematical as to which instructions—verbal or nonverbal, and which norms—hearing or deaf, to use with the hard-of-hearing child who is administered verbal instructions accompanied by demonstration.

The *Raven Progressive Matrices* (1960; 1963; 1965) is a nonverbal test which determines intellectual functioning by means of a single factor, visual perception. It is a:

> Test of the ability to apprehend meaningless figures presented for observation, see the relations between them, conceive the nature of the figure completing each system of relations presented, and by doing so, develop a systematic method of reasoning. (Raven 1960).

The *Standard Progressive Matrices* (1960) are composed of 60 items divided into five sets (A, B, C, D, E) of 12 each. On each set, the problems become more difficult. Stimuli are black and white drawings from which a part has been removed, and there are six possible choices to complete the design. The patient chooses the one which successfully completes the design. The test is typically untimed and can be individually or group administered. The individual administration format was designed for children from six to thirteen and one-half years of age although the test may be administered at any age; the same items are administered no matter what the age of the patient.

The test was standardized on subjects from 6 to 65 years of age. The total score is the number right which can be compared to the percentiles of the normative population which included 735 children from 6 to 13.5 years of age, 1,407 children from 8 to 14 years and 5,857 adults. By definition, the test requires intact visual perceptual skills for successful completion.

The *Coloured Progressive Matrices* (Raven 1963) were designed for children from 5 to 11, for old people, and for communication-impaired, intellectually subnormal, and intellectually deteriorated patients. It is composed of three sets of twelve items. Sets A and B are identical to the first two sets of the Standard Matrices except they are colored. Test Ab is a new set. The score is the total number correct which can be compared to percentile norms for children from 5 to 11.5 years of age or to norms for healthy old people from 65 to 85 years of age. If the Coloured Matrices are found to be too easy, Sets C, D, and E are administered, the results of Set Ab are discarded, and the total score is compared to norms for the Standard Matrices.

The *Advanced Progressive Matrices* (1965) were derived from the *Standard Progressive Matrices* and were designed for people of more than average intellectual ability. Set I is composed of 12 problems which tap the same intellectual processes encompassed in the Standard Matrices and is used to introduce the method of working. Set II contains 48 items similar to Sets C, D, and E of the Standard Matrices. Percentile norms are provided for children from 11.5 to 14 years of age at half-year intervals and for adults from 20 to 40 years old at decades.

The Matrices are most useful for identifying mental retardation in low-verbal and nonverbal adults and older children. The test is unique in that the Coloured Matrices have percentile norms for the normally aged and appears to be an appealing instrument for evaluating the patient with senile dementia. However, the test will not be typically used as the sole estimate of intellectual functioning, and its reliability is in doubt for young children and the severely retarded.

In summary, performance scales are specifically designed for patients with speech, hearing, and language deficits who typically would be penalized on tests requiring communicative abilities. The scales offer an estimate of intellectual potential without confounding by language impairment. We will now turn our attention to scales of general or global intelligence which assess both performance and verbal skills.

TESTS OF GENERAL OR GLOBAL INTELLIGENCE

Tests of general intelligence contain both verbal and performance items. Nunnally (1970) has reviewed the most pertinent findings from use of these tests.

> 1. Intelligence cannot at present be measured in children below the age of two years and not very well below the age of five or six.
>
> 2. The concept of general intelligence is more meaningful with children than with adults. It makes more sense to use tests of general intelligence with children than with adults.
>
> 3. Intelligence as measured by current "verbal" tests is due partly to heredity and partly to environment.
>
> 4. After the age of about six years, the individual's intelligence tends to remain stable with respect to his age group. That is, the superior people at one age level tend to be the superior people at other age levels.
>
> 5. There are definite group differences in intelligence test scores. Lower scores on the average are made by people of low socioeconomic status,

> people living in rural areas, people living in the Southern or Southwestern part of the United States, immigrants from southern Europe, and Indians and Negroes. The interpretation of differences of this kind places a large strain on the logical foundation of intelligence tests . . . the traditional measures of intelligence are constructed in such a way as to favor certain groups.
>
> 6. Many different kinds of attainment involve intelligence as measured by traditional "verbal" instruments. The individual's ability to succeed is determined by his intelligence and by a host of other things as well: abilities not measured by intelligence tests, interests, personality traits and just plain luck.

With these considerations in mind, we will review several tests of general intelligence which allow derivation of quotients to describe verbal and performance abilities or which contain both verbal and performance tests.

The *Wechsler Preschool and Primary Scale of Intelligence* (WPPSI) (Wechsler 1967) is designed to evaluate intelligence in children four to six and one-half years old. Although the test may be used with children as young as four, it may be too difficult for four year olds with intelligence quotients below 75. The WPPSI consists of a performance scale of five tests and a verbal scale of six tests.

The five WPPSI performance subtests are animal house, picture completion, mazes, geometric design, and block design. Animal house requires the child to match a colored peg to an animal following a visually presented code and requires visual association. Picture completion requires the child to tell or point to the missing part of a picture and evaluates visual closure and the ability of the child to discriminate between essential and nonessential detail. Planning ability and ocular motor control are assessed on the mazes test which requires that the child find her way out of a maze using a pencil. In the geometric design subtest, the child copies geometric forms with a pencil which reflects her motor planning and visual motor integration skills. The block design subtest requires the child to reproduce red and white block patterns and assesses her ability to analyze and form abstract designs.

The WPPSI performance subtests have verbal instructions that accompany visual-motor demonstrations. No verbal responses are required on any of the subtests. However, on picture completion, if the child points to the correct response but provides an inaccurate verbal response, he fails the item. It is difficult to administer the performance scale to the nonverbal child because of the linguistically taxing directions. Consequently, the language-impaired child may have some difficulty understanding the tasks. It is possible to administer the test to deaf children if they have the sign vocabulary to understand the instructions.

The verbal scale of the *Wechsler Preschool and Primary Scale of Intelligence* includes five subtests: information, vocabulary, arithmetic, similarities, and comprehension. There also is an optional or alternative sentences subtest which is not included in the scoring. The information subtest requires the child to answer questions such as "How many eyes do you have?" The child defines words on the vocabulary subtest. Frequently, language-impaired children receive only partial credit on this subtest because of expressive problems. Language-impaired children also may demonstrate auditory discrimination problems on the subtest and confuse test stimuli with similar sounding words. For example, they may confuse "block" with "box" and "pool" with "pull." The arithmetic subtest requires the child to respond to numerosity and to quantity terms; to count blocks, and to compute simple oral addition and subtraction problems. It is not unusual for a language-impaired child to perform more successfully on this subtest than other verbal subtests of the scale. In fact, a language-impaired child may fail initial items of the other verbal subtests but perform successfully on several arithmetic problems.

The similarities subtest is composed of pseudoanalogies in the form of oral sentence completion and includes stimuli such as "Cake and pie are both good to _____." It evaluates the ability to generalize and reason abstractly. Occasionally a language-impaired child will obtain a superficially high score on the test due to remediation procedures which have stressed categorization.

The comprehension subtest is one of the most difficult tests for the language-impaired child. Stimuli include question forms such as "What is the thing to do when _____?", "Why shouldn't _____?", and "Why do _____?" On all other verbal subtests single-word reponses are sufficient. However, on this subtest, which assesses the ability to use practical judgments in everyday social situations, a longer and more detailed response is required. Consequently, this subtest frequently will yield the lowest performance on the battery.

The sentences subtest requires the child to repeat sentences and assesses attention and immediate auditory memory. Responses from children with poor articulation may be difficult to score and may be less reliable. However, the sentence subtest score is not used for computing an intelligence quotient.

The raw score on each subtest is converted to a scaled score. The total scaled score for the performance subtests, verbal subtests, and full scale then are converted to intelligence quotients with a mean of 100 and a standard deviation of 15. The WPPSI was standardized on 1,200 children aged four years to six years and six months. One hundred boys and 100 girls were included at each of the six-month age levels. The sample was stratified with respect to geographic regions, urban-rural residence, race, and father's occupation. Reliability coefficients range from 0.71 to 0.94.

The WPPSI provides several types of information particularly pertinent to the differential diagnosis of language-impaired children. First, since the test contains both verbal and performance scales, reduced functioning on verbal items without a corresponding decrement on performance subtests compared to the standardized population helps to substantiate a finding of language impairment. Typically, a difference in performance and verbal intelligence quotients of 15 points or more is considered significant. An example profile for a language-impaired child is provided in Figure 12-1. It can be seen that the verbal quotient is significantly lower than the performance quotient. A significant reduction in functioning on both scales and therefore low performance and verbal intelligence quotients in comparison to the standardization population might be indicative of mental deficiency. It is also pertinent to note that if a remedial program for the child with language deficits is effective, it should be expected that the gap between verbal and performance scores would decrease with age.

A second type of information that can be obtained from the profile are estimates of differential performance on the skills tested by the subtests. For example, a language-impaired child may show relatively less impairment on the vocabulary and arithmetic subtests of the verbal scale if these skills have been the focus of an educational remedial program.

A third type of information obtained from the verbal subtests relates to

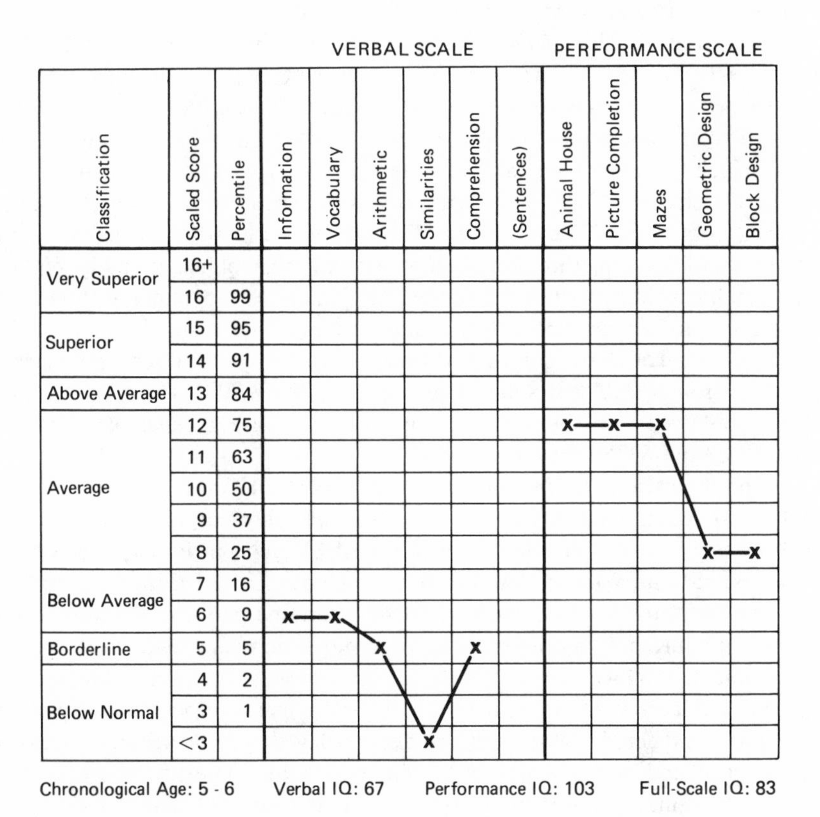

Figure 12-1 Wechsler Preschool and Primary Scale of Intelligence Profile Typical of Language-Delayed Child.

(Reproduced from the Wechsler Preschool and Primary Scale of Intelligence. Copyright 1963, 1967 by the Psychological Corporation. Reproduced by special permission.)

specific responses of the child to test stimuli. For example, a 5½-year-old boy with a verbal quotient of 74 and a performance quotient of 110 was asked "What shines in the sky at night?" on the information subtest of the WPPSI and responded "flashlight." Quite obviously, he did not have a complete understanding of the question and was responding only to the key words, "shine" and "night."

In summary, the WPPSI provides useful adjunct information for determining language impairment. It allows derivation of a performance intelligence quotient which may be used as an estimate of intellectual capability; a verbal intelligence quotient, which may serve as an indicant of language ability; and an overall or full-scale intelligence quotient. Moreover, functioning on individual subtests may help to substantiate findings of tests of specific language ability, and individual responses to items may serve as examples of particular language deficits demonstrated by the child.

The *Wechsler Intelligence Test for Children* (WISC) (Wechsler 1949) is similar in form and content to the WPPSI. In fact, the majority of the WPPSI subtests are modifications of WISC subtests. Three subtests unique to the WPPSI are sentences, animal house and geometric design which replaced subtests of the WISC which could not be easily adapted for young children. The WISC was revised (Wechsler 1974), and the revision is designed to assess intelligence in children from 6 to 16 years of age. The revised WISC performance scale has picture completion, picture arrangement, block design, object assembly, coding, and a supplementary mazes subtests. The verbal scale includes information, similarities, arithmetic, vocabulary, comprehension and a supplementary digit span subtests. The derivation of performance, verbal, and full-scale intelligence quotients from scaled scores is the same as with the WPPSI. The types of information obtained for the language-impaired child are comparable to those obtained on the WPPSI for younger children.

The *Wechsler Adult Intelligence Scale* (Wechsler 1955) is designed to assess intellectual functioning in patients 15 years old and older and norms are provided from 15 to 75 years and older. The test is similar in format and content to the WPPSI and WISC scales. The WAIS includes six verbal subtests and five performance subtests which can be used to determine performance, verbal, and full-scale intelligence quotients using procedures comparable to those of the WPPSI and the WISC. The test is useful for appraising acquired language disorders in adults. For example, for the left-hemisphere-damaged aphasic patient, it would be expected that a signifiant discrepancy should be apparent between performance and verbal scores. A patient with senile dementia, on the other hand, will demonstrate reduced verbal and performance scores with better performance overall on the verbal subtests.

In summary, the Wechsler scales encompass the age range from 4 to more than 75 years of age. The large range of the tests when considered together, the inclusion of both verbal and performance scales, and the high reliability of the scales have made them popular instruments for assessment of intellectual functioning. They are of particular value for evaluating the communicatively impaired patient because they provide estimates of both performance and verbal abilities. However, it should be noted that the instructions for the Wechsler performance scales are more linguistically taxing than earlier discussed performance measures.

A second major test of intelligence covering a large age range is the *Stanford-Binet Intelligence Scale* (Terman and Merrill 1960). The test is an outgrowth of the pioneering work of Alfred Binet in France on intelligence testing. The test was revised by Terman in 1915 and again by Terman and Merrill in 1937 and 1960 (Terman and Merrill 1960). The test was restandardized in 1972 (Thorndike 1972). The Stanford-Binet, L-M, is composed of a series of age-graded tasks. Six tests are administered at each six-month interval from two to five years of age; at yearly intervals from five to fourteen years; and at four levels of adult performance. The exception is at the "average adult" level where there are eight, rather than six, tests. The total number of successes, when added to a basal, defined as correct performance on all tests at an age level, is used to determine a mental age. The mental age is used to derive an intelligence quotient with a mean of 100 and a standard deviation of 16.

Most of the items on the test require comprehension of verbal instructions and/or verbal responses. Only approximately 20 percent of the items are performance tasks, and many of these are at the three- and five-year levels. A large number of the tasks involve verbal judgment and reasoning.

The most frequent use of the Stanford-Binet is with children under the age of seven. Since the test is primarily verbal, when used with the communicatively impaired child, it must be supplemented with a performance measure such as the *Arthur Adaptation of the Leiter International Scale of Intelligence* previously discussed.

Although the Wechsler Scales and Stanford-Binet are the most frequently used intelligence tests, other instruments have been developed which are designed to assess children of a limited age range. For example, *The Pictorial Test of Intelligence* (French 1964) was designed to assess general intelligence in normal and handicapped children between three and eight years of age. It contains seven subtests with tasks presented to determine verbal comprehension, perceptual organization, and the ability to manipulate spatial and numerical symbols. Questions are presented orally by the examiner. The child responds by choosing one of four drawings from a large picture card either by pointing or, in the case of the severely motorically impaired child, by staring at the corner of the response card containing his choice. There are no time limits which would penalize the physically handicapped child. Results of the test are compared to norms from a standardization population of 1,830 children from five to eight years of age. A mental age, deviation intelligence quotient, and percentile can be determined from results of the test.

In summary, tests of general intelligence typically include verbal and performance tasks. When compared to performance scales, they require greater language skills in terms of understanding instructions and/or responding to task items. They may be of significant value in providing information about the language problems of the testee in addition to their more important and ascribed purpose of determining intellectual functioning.

A case example may serve to illustrate the importance of intelligence testing to the appraisal of the communicatively handicapped child. S. G. was referred to the speech and hearing center with a diagnosis of mental retardation by a psychologist based on a Stanford-Binet, Form L-M, intelligence quotient of 50; a diagnosis of autism by a psychiatrist; and a diagnosis of possible hearing loss by a pediatrician. S. G.'s mother believed that the child's problems stemmed from her own illnesses while S. G. was in early infancy. Administration of the *Leiter International Performance Scale* yielded an intelligence quotient of 142. Additional testing revealed auditory acuity within normal limits and the presence of a severe deficit in the ability to derive meaning from auditory stimuli. An intensive remedial language program was instituted, and at age six the Stanford-Binet was readministered and resulted in an intelligence quotient of 115. At age 9, S. G. was administered the *Wechsler Intelligence Scale for Children* (Revised) and received a performance score of 140 and a verbal score of 125. At age 16, following long-term language remediation, she was extremely advanced academically and obtained scores of 140+ on both scales of the WISC-R. She continued to have some difficulty in interpersonal communication, however, because she interpreted all statements literally. This example serves to point out the importance of utilizing performance measures to determine intellectual capacity in the communicatively impaired patient and the value of tests of this type for monitoring the progress of remedial language programs.

ASSESSMENT OF EMOTIONAL STATUS

Determining how a child feels about himself, his family, and his environment provides diagnostic information since it places the communication deficit in the context of the child's personality. Assessments of this type are not routinely performed because the majority of communication impaired patients do not have emotional disturbances of sufficient severity to merit structured evaluation.

When a personality disorder is suspected, information obtained from the case history, measurements of adaptive behaviors, and behavioral observations will usually reveal the emotional status of the patient. Structured projective techniques also may be used, but determining the emotional make-up of the patient with these instruments is a difficult task because of questionable reliability and validity of these tests. Johnson and Myklebust (1967) point out that "Though progress is being made, there can be little question that most appraisals of the emotional status of children must be made experientially; that is, on the basis of clinical judgment. Even when projective tests of personality are used, much is dependent on the diagnostician's insights and judgments because of the subjective nature of the tests."

The most fruitful tool for assessing the emotional status of communication-impaired patients are drawings such as in the *House-Tree-Person Test* (Buck 1970). The *House-Tree-Person Test* is ". . . designed to aid the clinician in obtaining information concerning an individual's sensitivity, maturity, flexibility, efficiency, degree of personality integration and interaction with the environment, specifically and generally." The test requires the patient to make a free-hand pencil drawing of a house, a tree, and a person. Each of the drawings is considered a self-portrait. The patient next is asked to answer specific questions about the drawings. This allows an opportunity for description and interpretation. She also may be asked to draw the pictures again with crayons. By means of a qualitative analysis of the drawings and descriptions, the psychologist interprets how the child perceives her home, her environment and herself.

When drawings are used to obtain information about the child, they are seldom useful until the child is approximately five years old and has the maturity to draw recognizable objects. They may be more difficult to use with communication-handicapped children because their descriptions and interpretations may be simplified and incomplete. Even when the comments of the child are not available, the drawings may provide considerable information for the psychologist skilled at interpreting responses. For example, Figure 12-2 is a self-drawing of a five-year-old language-impaired girl. One interpretation of this drawing is that the child perceives herself as clumsy and unwanted and her world as hostile. Drawings by adults also can be very revealing. Figure 12-3 contains two drawings by a 21-year-old man with a severe hearing loss and a diagnosis of autism. The drawings are portrayals of his home (an institution). The first drawing suggests that the man sees his world as one of closed doors, windows that are opaque, and people that are almost completely out of view. The second picture portrays this man's environment as filled with medical and other paraphenalia, rather than animate objects. When this patient was asked to draw a picture of himself, he drew a baby without hands surrounded by a baby bottle, nipple, and safety pins which clearly can be interpreted to mean that he felt helpless.

As the child becomes more verbal, apperception tests can be used to explore emotional status. The *Children's Apperception Test* (Bellak 1954) was designed to ". . . facilitate understanding of a child's relationship to important figures and drives." The test is recommended for children between three and ten years of age although it seldom can be used with language-delayed children less than five years of age. The child is given ten pictures of animals engaged in humanlike behaviors and asked to tell a story about each. The pictures are designed to depict animals in situations and experiences common to all children.

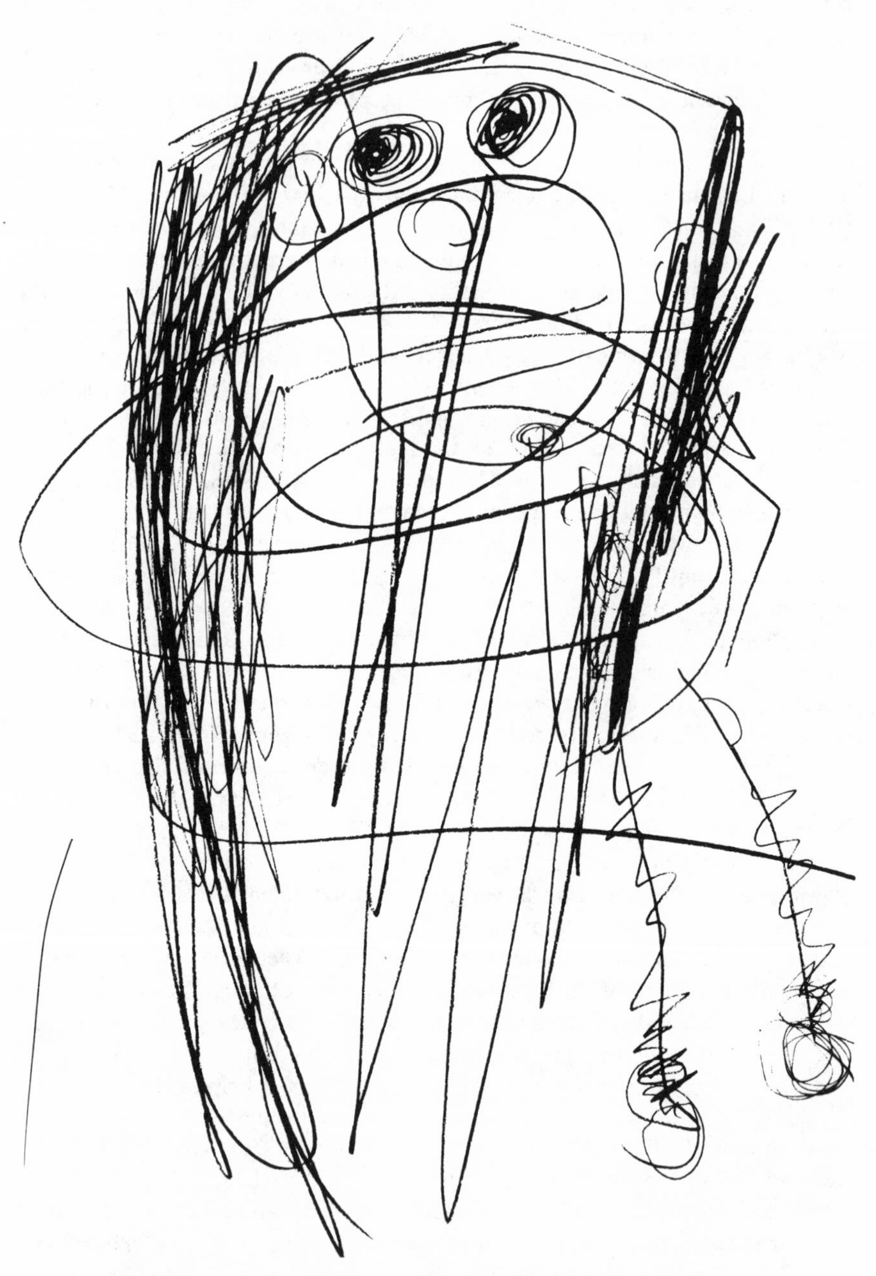

Figure 12-2 Self-portrait of five-year-old girl with language delay.

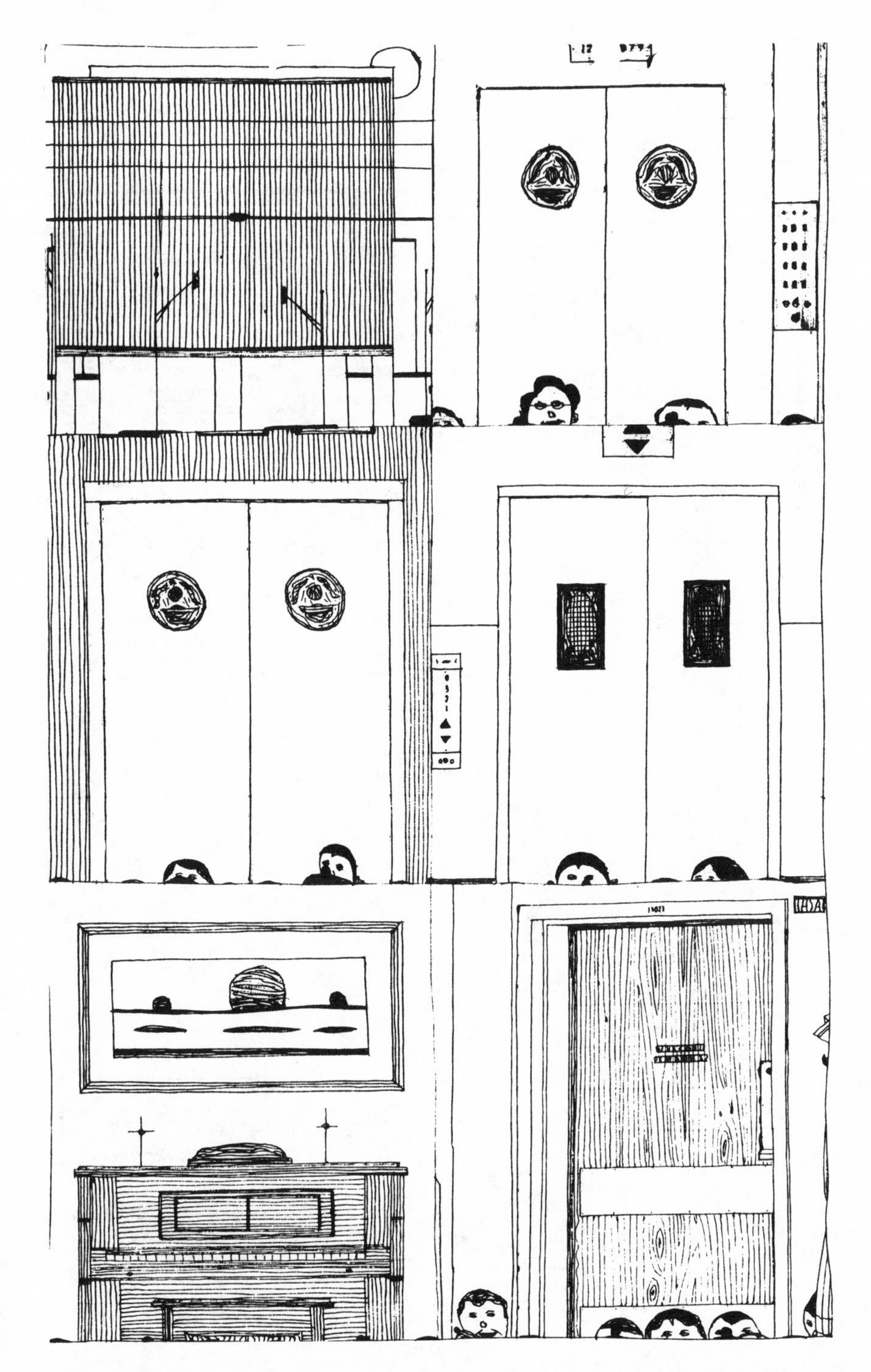

Figure 12-3 Two pictures of "home" (a state institution) drawn by a 21-year-old male with a diagnosis of severe hearing loss and autism. (continued)

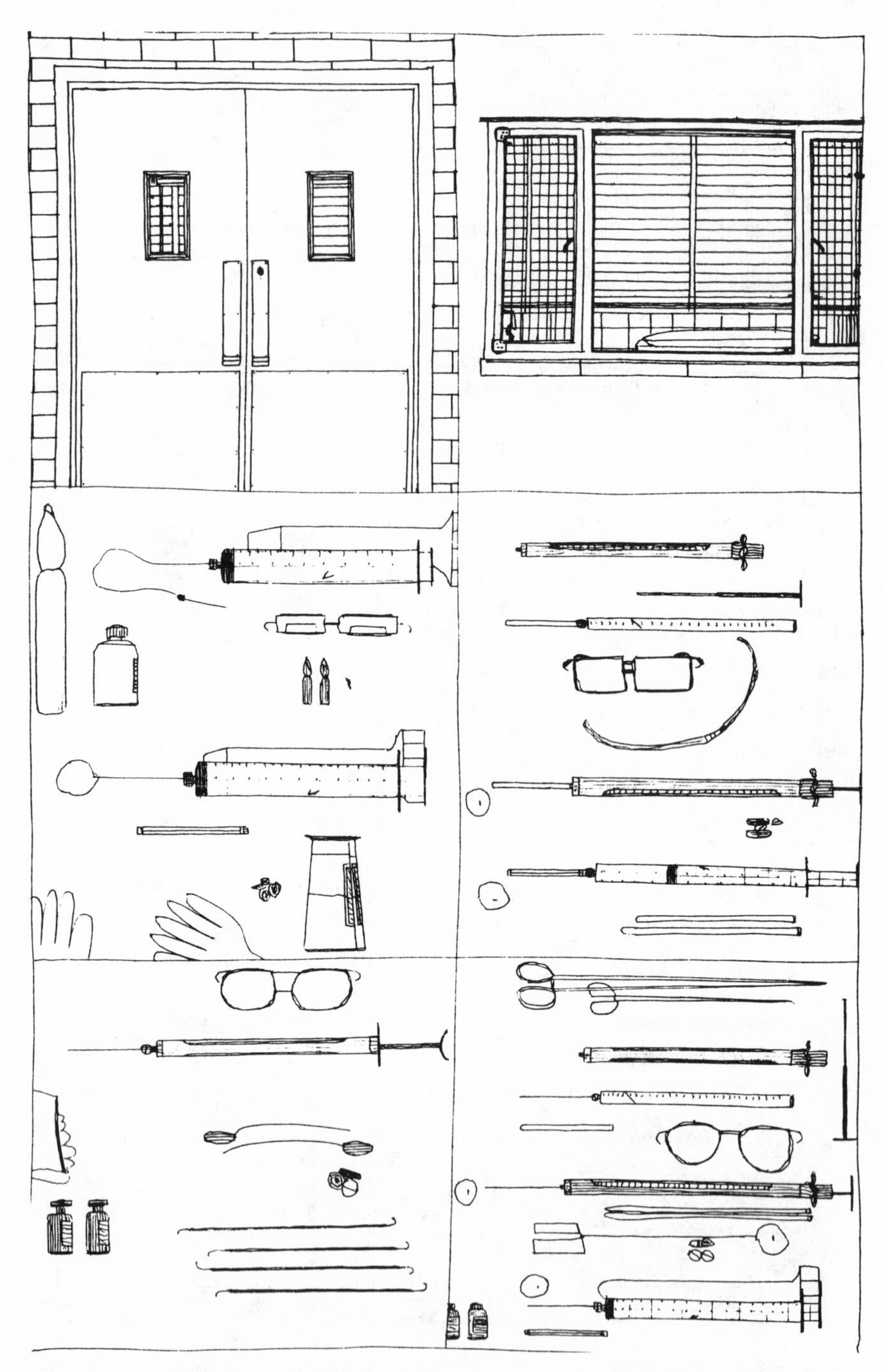

Figure 12-3 Two pictures of "home" (a state institution) drawn by a 21-year-old male with a diagnosis of severe hearing loss and autism.

What the child says about the pictures gives the clinician insights about how the child feels about himself, his family, his home, his environment, and how he handles problems. There also are ten supplemental pictures that show specific situations, such as physical disability, that are not universal to all children but which should apply to many children.

A number of other techniques are available such as sentence-completion tasks, story telling, descriptions of ink blots, and play with dolls and objects. There also are tests such as the *Bender Visual Motor Gestalt Test* (Bender 1946). This test is designed to assess neurological integrity, perceptual maturity, and emotional adjustment based upon the copying of nine figures by the patient. An overall score is determined by assessment of the integration, rotation, distortion of shape, and perseveration of the figures using an objective scoring system developed by Koppitz (1975). The drawings can be used as a projective technique, and Koppitz provides thirteen emotional indicators for interpreting the figures. For example, large drawings and confused order would be interpreted as indicative of a child who is "acting out."

The important thing to remember about tests of emotional status is that they are clinical techniques and not psychometric instruments. Consequently, the ability of the psychologist to interpret the responses and behaviors of the patient are probably more important than the technique used to elicit the responses.

SUMMARY

Tests of intellectual capacity and scholastic aptitude are the province of the psychologist but provide important information about the patient to the speech-language pathologist. Performance scales are designed to estimate intellectual capacity in children and adults with communicative impairment. Tests of general intelligence contain performance and verbal tasks and provide information about intellectual functioning and language abilities. Consequently, they are important for establishing diagnoses of mental retardation and estimating the severity of language impairment in patients with normal cognitive abilities. Psychological tests also are used to determine the emotional status of the child or adult in order to place the communication problem in perspective, but these techniques are highly subjective and their value is limited by the experience and interpretive abilities of the diagnostician.

Following this section (Table 12-1) is a summary of the intelligence tests discussed with test types and age ranges on which they were standardized as well as age ranges on which they would be appropriate for communicatively impaired and nonverbal-deaf patients.

Table 12-1 Summary of tests of intelligence

Test	*Type*	*Standardization Ages*	*Preferred Ages Communicative Disorders*	*Preferred Ages Nonverbal-Deaf*
Merrill-Palmer Scale of Mental Tests	Performance with some verbal items	1.5-6.4	2-4	2-4 omit verbal items
Leiter International Performance Scale	Performance	2.0-17.9	3-10	3-12
Arthur Adaptation of Leiter Performance Scale	Performance	3.0-7.9	3.0-7.9	3.0-7.9
Stanford-Binet, L-M	Global (Highly verbal)	2-18	3-10	Not recommended
Wechsler Preschool and Primary Scale of Intelligence	Performance	4-6.5	4-6.5	5-6.5
	Verbal	4-6.5	5-6.5	Not recommended
Wechsler Intelligence Scale for Children	Performance	5-15	7-15	8-15
	Verbal	5-15	7-15	9-15
Wechsler Intelligence Scale for Children (Revised)	Performance	6.5-16.5	7-16.5	8-16.5
	Verbal	6.5-16.5	7-16.5	9-16.5
Hiskey-Nebraska Test of Learning Aptitude	Performance	2.5-17.5	4-8	4-10
Wechsler Adult Intelligence Scale	Performance	15-75+	16+	16+
	Verbal	15-75+	16+	16+
Raven Progressive Matrices	Performance	6-69	9-65	9-65
Pictorial Test of Intelligence	Verbal Reception Motor Response	3-8	4-8	4-8

REFERENCES

Arthur, G., *The Arthur Adaptation of the Leiter International Performance Scale.* Washington, D.C.: The Psychological Service Center Press, (1952).

Bellak, L., *The Thematic Apperception Test and The Children's Apperception Test in Clinical Use.* New York: Grune and Stratton, (1954).

Bender, L., *Bender Visual Motor Gestalt Test.* New York: American Orthopsychiatric Association, (1946).

Bloom, L., and M. Lahey, *Language Development and Language Disorders.* New York: John Wiley, (1978).

Buck, J., *The House-Tree-Person Technique: Revised Manual.* Los Angeles: Western Psychological Services, (1970).

French, J., *Manual: Pictorial Test of Intelligence.* New York: Houghton Mifflin, (1964).

Hiskey, M., *Manual: Hiskey-Nebraska Test of Learning Aptitude.* Lincoln, Nebraska: Union College Press, (1966).

Horrocks, J., *Assessment of Behavior.* Columbus, Ohio: Chas. E. Merrill, (1964).

Johnson, D., and H. Myklebust, *Learning Disabilities: Educational Principles and Practices.* New York: Grune and Stratton, (1967).

Koppitz, E., *The Bender Gestalt Test for Young Children, Vol. II.* New York: Grune and Stratton, (1975).

Leiter, R., *General Instructions for the International Performance Scale.* Chicago: Stoelting Company, (1969).

Machover, K., *Personality Projection in the Drawing of the Human Figure.* Springfield, Ill.: Charles C Thomas, (1948).

Nunnally, J., *Introduction to Psychological Measurement.* New York: Mc Graw-Hill, (1970).

Raven, J., *Guide to the Standard Progressive Matrices: Sets A, B, C, D, E.* London: H.K. Lewis, (1960).

Raven, J., *Guide to Using the Coloured Progressive Matrices, Sets A, B, Ab.* London: H.K. Lewis, (1963).

Raven, J., *Advanced Progressive Matrices: Sets I and II.* London: H.K. Lewis, (1965).

Stutsman, R., *Guide for Administering the Merrill-Palmer Scale of Mental Tests.* New York: Harcourt Brace Jovanovich, (1948).

Terman, L., and M. Merrill, *Stanford-Binet Intelligence Scale.* Boston: Houghton Mifflin, (1960).

Thorndike, R., *Stanford-Binet Intelligence Scale: 1972 Norms Tables.* Boston: Houghton Mifflin, (1972).

Wechsler, D., *Manual: Wechsler Intelligence Scale for Children.* New York: The Psychological Corporation, (1949).

Wechsler, D., *Manual for the Wechsler Adult Intelligence Scale.* New York: The Psychological Corporation, (1955).

Wechsler, D., *Manual: Wechsler Preschool and Primary Scale of Intelligence.* New York: The Psychological Corporation, (1967).

Wechsler, D., *Manual: Wechsler Intelligence Scale for Children, Revised.* New York: The Psychological Corporation, (1974).

Clinical Reporting and Record Keeping

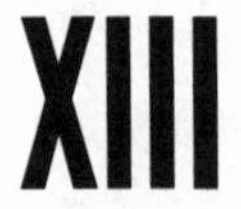

An expert gives an objective opinion, he gives his own.

Desai

The clinical report in the field of speech pathology and audiology has grown up in this age of accountability. It is no longer adequate or acceptable, if it ever was, for the report of a half-year's therapy contact with a child to be reduced to an informationally empty statement such as: "Johnny is doing well, is more cooperative than at first, and will be continued in therapy." Even if we assume that we know what he is "doing well" at, there are no behavioral descriptions and no measurements on which to base clinical judgments. Accountability implies measurement—measurement as base-line performance and as an increment of progress toward an agreed-upon and stated goal. Accountability demands that the purchaser of services be able to decide whether the benefits to be derived outweight the investments of time, inconvenience, and money. The documentaton of speech and language skill was the concern of the bulk of the preceeding chapters. The interpretation and communication of the significance of these performance skills is both the basis and the reason for the clinical report. We will discuss three types of clinical reports, according to the purposes for which they are written: the diagnostic, or initial evaluation report; the periodic or terminal clinical summary, and the daily contact report. These reports differ in form but not in purpose—they are each constructed to communicate necessary clinical information.

WHAT A REPORT IS—AND WHAT IT IS NOT

A report is an answer to a stated or implied question; therefore, the writer's first task is to determine what question is to be answered, and to whom the answer is directed. The question may be whether or not a communication problem exists; or if there is agreement that a problem exists, the question may be "what can be done about it?" Clinical settings are also an important consideration. As Taylor (1977) has pointed out, not only will form and style differ among similar clinical settings, but specific settings may require specialized types of reporting. For example, a speech consultation in a medical setting usually is brief. The need for clarity and brevity exists in every setting but may be of paramount importance here. The medical speech consultation report does not include the extensive case history information typically found in other parts of the hospital record, and most test details and specifics are not included although they are maintained for your records. Your consultation report for most medical-setting purposes may include only what would have been summary, conclusions, and recommendations of the report you write in another setting. In most medical settings you are asked to supply a short description of the communication problem presented—and what can be done about it.

However, our purpose here is not to outline standards of form for all clinical settings. Purposes as well as local preferences dictate a variety of forms and procedures in report writing. What the variety has in common is that all reports should be designed to communicate the nature of the problem, if one exists, and to outline a plan of care for its remediation. Nation and Aram (1977) outline the diagnostician's task in these words (p. 332):

> The diagnostician asks himself four interrelated yes/no questions. Can the client change his disordered behavior? Is therapeutic intervention necessary to do so? Are referrals necessary? Is service available? Depending on his answers to these questions, he proceeds to think through the various management alternatives appropriate to the disorder, its causes, and the personal characteristics of the client. He develops a definitive plan of action to offer to the client during the interpretive conference.

and (p. 328), "The information of prime importance to impart is who is going to do what, when, and where."[1]

[1] From James E. Nation and Dorothy M. Aram, *Diagnosis of Speech and Language Disorders* (St. Louis: The C. V. Mosby Co., 1977), pp. 328, 332.

What a report is not is an excuse to pontificate, confabulate, or obfuscate. In other words, one should avoid the unnecessary use of words, such as is contained in the last sentence because they are less likely to transmit the answer you wish to communicate than if you choose less exotic words. The language used in a report should not be pompous or dogmatic, it should not be chatty or informal, and the information contained should not be confused or obscured by the inclusion of irrelevant statements.

WRITING STYLE

There are a number of publications concerned with writing style in the speech and hearing literature. Notable among them are articles by Jerger (1962), Moore (1966), and Pannbacker (1975). These three have been singled out from the larger number of well-written and informative articles because of the free use of examples of bad writing style which they include to help make their points clear. There is general agreement as to what constitutes good writing style (see also: Good 1970; Knepflar 1976; Sanders 1972; Wolfe 1967) and few points of disagreement.

Use of Pronouns. One such point of apparent disagreement is in the use of personal pronouns.. Jerger (1962) advocates their use–but not overuse–on the assumption that personal pronouns will make the report sound more natural.

> Nothing livens up dull material like personal references. Use them often. Especially, use personal pronouns like I, me, we, you, she, they, etc. Don't use them to excess–the excessive repetition of anything makes dull reading–but don't be afraid to use them when they are clearly necessary in order to say a thing naturally. (Jerger 1962)

Emerick and Hatton (1974), on the other hand, think that first-and second-person pronouns should be avoided. Johnson and others (1963) stated that the tone of the report should be impersonal, and personal pronouns should be used only to make a statement clearer. English and Lillywhite (1963) advocate the use of personal pronouns only when the writer wishes to emphasize that an opinion or a feeling is being expressed for which she has no immediate objective, supportive evidence. A probable consensus among experienced report writers would be to maintain an impersonal and relatively formal tone in reporting clinical information, but not to abrogate personal responsibility, especially in expressing an opinion. In other words, use personal references when necessary. More important than the use of personal pronouns, as such, is the issue of clarity. Jerger (1962) reminds us that in scientific reporting the object is to convey to the reader what you did, why you did it, and what you found.

A comprehensive list of *dos* and *don'ts* specifically applicable to clinical reports would be difficult to write partly because it almost certainly would include many personal preferences and therefore be more biased than stylistic. Moore (1969) liberally quoted from Strunk and White's (1959) *The Elements of Style* in listing a set of rules to be followed in writing clearly and concisely. She listed three primary "symptoms" in determining when writing was defective. According to Moore (1969, p. 535), report writing is defective when it is (1) unintelligible–the report is not clear, (2) conspicuous–the reader pays more attention to how the report is written than to the content, or (3) confusing–if the reader is confused the writer may well have been confused. Clear thinking cannot be illustrated by fuzzy writing.

Most of the Strunk and White's rules are straightforward. For example, "Use definite, specific, concrete language. Prefer the specific to the general, the definite to the vague, the concrete to the abstract." This effectively translates as "say what you mean and mean what you say."

Avoid Jargon. A number of authors (for example, Taylor 1977; Knepflar 1976; Fisher 1969; Wolfle 1967) express the admonition to avoid jargon. One of Moore's quoted examples (p. 536) expressed this "conspicuous writing" symptom as:

> The patient exhibited apparent partial paralysis of motor units of the superior sinistral fibres of the genioglossus resulting in insufficient lingual approximation of the palatoalveolar region. A condition of insufficient frenulum development was noted, producing not only sigmatic distortion but also obvious ankyloglossia.

Translation: "The patient was tongue-tied and dysarthric." Similarly, a report of "dactyl speech" is not as informative as "finger spelling." Commenting on this same point, Pannbacker (1975) has urged that "only terms in common use by professionals should be used." The difficulty results from the fact that:

> . . . . . (professional workers) all have their jargons; fads abound; authors strain for effects; long words replace short ones, and ignorance, carelessness, a false idea of what constitutes proper style, overuse of the passive voice, and kindred sins all make unnecessary trouble for the readers. (Wolfle 1967, p. 55)

Use of Qualifiers. One of those kindred sins is the overuse of qualifiers. One Strunk and White rule (quoted by Moore 1969) was to avoid the use of qualifiers–words like "rather," "very," "little," "pretty" ". . . are leeches that infest the pond of prose, sucking the blood of words." An earlier rule we quoted was to use definite, concrete, specific language. Qualifiers insert a lack of precision and an indefinite tone to otherwise acceptable descriptions. Less experienced report writers are especially prone to hide behind nebulous descriptors–"a little restless," "somewhat delayed," "seems to be," "appears to have," as if they could abrogate the responsibility of their professional judgment by being less precise. A report *is* a professional opinion and only that. As we discussed at the beginning of this text, there is no ethical requirement that the clinician always be right—only that she make her best professional judgment based on appropriate tests and observations.

A valid point can be made that not all of our observations and test results can be precisely calibrated or determined. There is a place for "in my opinion" or "it appears to me" statements. Therefore the suggestion may be made that after you write a report, go back through and scratch off all the qualifier words. Go through again and put back only those which must be included. When we discuss the form or the outline for reports, it will be apparent that sections concerning the history of the problem, the data concerning measurement of the speech and language problem, and your interpretation of the significance of the data and recommendations for amelioration of the problem will contain different types of information.

In the case history report section, the qualifiers that state "Mrs. Jones reported that . . ." or "According to . . ." are appropriate because they remind the reader that the information or judgment is second-hand. When you report performance data gathered from speech-language testing and observations, the report is to be as calibrated and precise as you can make it, and qualifiers are to be avoided. When you interpret the results, the reader should already be aware that what he is reading is a qualification in that it is not necessarily *the* truth but *your* truth.

One of the more succinct summary sets of report guidelines is that offered by Jerger (1962, p. 104):

1. Write short sentences. Use a new sentence for each new thought.
2. Avoid artificiality and pompous embellishment. Write it the way you would say it.
3. Use active verb construction whenever possible. Avoid the passive voice.
4. Use personal pronouns when it is natural to do so.

FORM AND CONTENT OF THE REPORT

A variety of forms are in use as outlines or guidelines for clinical reporting. That is to say that there are many acceptable forms and that any form which is functionally adequate to the communicative task is acceptable. For that reason, the example form for an Examination Report and for a clinical summary or Progress Report included in this chapter are only examples. The form, as such, is of lesser importance than the content to be included, but the use of such an outline form is useful, especially for less experienced report writers, as a reminder of what information should be included. Figure 13-1 is an example format for an initial or diagnostic report outline.

(Date report typed)

TO: Referring source
Address, including
zip code

RE: Client's name, File Number
PARENTS: (If child)
Address, zip code
BIRTHDATE: AGE:
DIAGNOSTIC CATEGORY:
DATE OF EVALUATION:

HISTORY:

Pertinent birth and early developmental histories; all medical information; Parental description of early speech and language development

SIGNIFICANT FINDINGS:

Observations and test findings

SUMMARY:

Brief summary of test results

RECOMMENDATIONS:

Disposition--reevaluation, therapy, parental counseling, referral, and so on

Reported by:

Name, degree, certification
Speech Pathologist

Assisted by: Student clinician(s) name

Copies to: (if any)

Figure 13-1

Examination Report

Patient Identification. The identifying information obviously includes the patient's name and address, and if the patient is a child, the parents' name should also be included. The inclusion of birthdate rather than age may be a bias, but it is preferred because the precision of a birth date may help prevent confusion at a later time.

A file number system is probably in use at every clinical facility. This number system may be a simple numerical listing or a code (Mueller and Peters 1976) which identifies a patient, the presenting problem, and the clinical setting. The advantages of including a file number on a report are obvious. In the same way as a file number uniquely identifies an individual patient, every report and each bit of test or informational data preserved *must* be dated. An undated report is useless. In essence, the importance of the identification heading is that it uniquely identifies a specific set of test results and interpretations for a particular patient at a specified time and place.

Complaint. At the writer's (or the clinic's) option, a statement that "Susie was referred by Dr. Glotz, her pediatrician, with a concern of delayed language development," may be placed here. One alternative to this separate heading, is the inclusion of the referral reason within the background or history section.

History. The critical guideline for what is to be included is the word *pertinent.* In the interpretation of test results which indicate a speech and language delay, for example, either normal or deviant developmental milestones could be significant. On the other hand, if the patient and problem in question were a 48-year-old adult who had suffered a stroke, early developmental history would probably not be important, although status prior to the cerebral damage is important in terms of expected or acceptable recovery performance. Again the key word is pertinent. The diagnostician in his detective role, as discussed in Chapter II, is expected to include here the information which *could be* significant to the problem or problems presented and to the remediation plan proposed.

Examination Results. Knepflar (1976) has suggested separate sections with headings for case history, hearing, speech mechanism, articulation, voice, language, fluency and rate, psychological factors, clinical impressions, and recommendations. Let us assume agreement with Knepflar on the advisability of separating case history, clinical impressions, and recommendations. In Chapter II we discussed the importance of separating information which we gathered by direct observation from what was reported to us—and is therefore objective, rather than subjective. When writing reports, it is important to maintain that distinction. It is also important to separate test results from interpretation. In contrast it is not important whether the form used maintains separate headings for speech mechanism, hearing, articulation, voice, and so on. In other words, you should certainly include a statement relative to the patient's hearing acuity, because it could be pertinent to any speech and language disorder, but you may or may not wish to set it off under a separate heading.

There is less agreement among report writers about the inclusion of a statement of fluency or one on adequacy of voice when fluency or voice are not considered part of the presenting problem. There should be no difference of opinion among professionals as to whether voice and rate, for example, should be at least informally evaluated—the difference of opinion is whether "normal" bears reporting. It at least takes little time and space to report that "voice and fluency were within normal limits," and it alerts the reader to the fact that your evaluation was concerned with the total communication picture. In that sense, it may be a worthwhile habit for the diagnostician to develop.

As we commented earlier, the purpose of the outline for formulation of your report is to cue the reader to the information found in different sections. Obviously, it also should remind the writer what is included where. The data collected and their significance are a function of the measurement device used. For example, you may well report that, "Henry obtained a vocabulary recognition age-score of 6-3 (C.A. 5-7) on the *Peabody Picture Vocabulary Test.*" This system immediately does two things: It shows where the data came from, and it provides a comparison by your inclusion of the child's chronological age. In the summary or impressions section you would report the vocabulary recognition score was within normal limits for his age. It is important to report how you measured or judged a performance. If you report that the child obtained a language age score of 6-5 (C.A. 6-5) on the *Utah Test for Language Development* and was therefore normal in his expressive language skills, you at least give the knowledgeable reader a chance to disagree. The Utah test, as we discussed in Chapter V, is more developmental in nature than specific to syntax, grammar, and so on, as a measurement of language. In that sense you would not have the same theoretical basis for your judgment that expressive language skills were within normal limits, that you would have from a structural description such as obtained from the *Developmental Sentence Scoring* procedure. One more example may help to emphasize this point. If four-year-old Johnny's articulation skill was determined from your administration of the *Templin-Darley Screening Test of Articulation* (described in Chapter III), your report would indicate number of correct productions and the relevance of that number.

> John correctly produced 30 of the 50 articulation screening items on the *Templin-Darley Tests of Articulation.* The average performance for a boy of this age is approximately 35 correct, but 23 correct productions is considered 'adequate'. Errors in articulation were primarily on /s/ and /l/ sounds in two- and three-element blends but which John correctly produced in other contexts. Articulation skill is judged as within normal limits for his age.

If you used a single-phoneme test, as was discussed in Chapter III, your judgment of adequate or inadequate would be based on which phonemes were in error and which set of age-of-acquisition norms you chose for comparison.

The point to be emphasized is that your examination data are to be reported as specific to a test, with necessary descriptive or normative comparisons, and that test results are separated from the interpretive summary. Your data, with the necessary comparisons and qualifications, are shown as examination results. Your interpretation of the significance of the total results, included in the clinical impressions or summary section, is then your professional judgment. It should be possible for another professional reader to accept your data and make a different interpretation of their overall significance.

Diagnostic Summary–or Clinical Impressions. As the writer of the diagnostic examination report, you are being asked to express your professional opinion. This is the answer to the question we began with. It is appropriate in this section of your report to summarize the pertinent results and make an interpretation. Earlier we talked about the use of personal opinions and personal pronouns (English and Lillywhite 1963; Jerger 1962) in making it clear to the reader that what is being expressed as an opinion may go beyond the available data. In other words, this is *your* truth.

Recommendations. Your professional opinion also extends into the recommendations section which some forms separate from summary–and some do not. Again we may say that the separation and designation of sections of a report with specific headings is of lesser importance than the fact that the information is there and can be readily located for the readers' purposes. That last sentence is a recognition of the fact that not all of your report may be read by the one to whom it is addressed–or may not be read with the same care. Your recommendations for case management should include a specifically stated plan of care. The most important statements you write may be those which summarize the problem as you see it and recommend what can be done about it. In other words, who will do what, to whom, where, and when–as well as the expected outcome.

Progress Report

A progress report, or therapy summary, by definition, is an answer to a different question. The purpose of the initial or diagnostic evaluation is to provide the data base or description of what the problem was like when first identified–at least in your shop. If the initial evaluation was your baseline data, the progress report is a measurement of change as a function of treatment. The progress report outline shown as Figure 13-2 is obviously only an example. Identifying information as previously described is a constant on all reports. In addition

PROGRESS REPORT

Name:	Clinic No:
Address:	Diagnostic Category:
	Period Covered: (Quarter, Year)
Phone No:	Date of Report: (Date report typed)
School Status:	
Birthdate: Age:	
Clinic Schedule:	Hours Individual (I) Therapy:
Sessions per week:	Hours Group (G) Therapy:
Length of session:	Cumulative Hours of I Therapy:
Number of Clinic Visits:	Cumulative Hours of G Therapy:

STATUS AT BEGINNING OF PERIOD:

(Short, abstract of information taken from first contact with Clinic--such as diagnostic, reevaluation, hearing report--description of previous therapy--description of all behaviors (speech, language, attentiveness, motivation) at the beginning of this reporting period.)

SUMMARY OF THERAPY:

(The summary is to include goals, procedures, results and/or evaluations of the case. Also to be included are description of response to therapy, impressions of performance, problems in therapy.)

RECOMMENDATIONS:

(Be specific so next clinician will have an idea where to start next quarter. Even though you or your supervisor feel the client should continue but for some reason they can't, won't, put it in report here. This paragraph is used for scheduling information and what they will do or are going to do is needed -- not what you think they should do.)

(Supervisor will sign here)
Supervised by: (Type name, degree)
Speech Pathologist

(Sign name)
(Type name) Student Clinician

Figure 13-2

the identification of how long and with what frequency therapy has been scheduled is helpful for a number of comparative and bookkeeping purposes. One obvious example is for the ease of collecting length-of-stay data for audit purposes. That is, how many hours of therapy are usually required in your clinical setting for any particular diagnostic category (an aphasic adult, a cerebral-palsied child, a teenager who stutters, and so on) to reach maximum potential? Of course not every patient will present the same problems, and not every client responds equally well to the remediation regime, but your range and median hours when compared to that of other clinicians and clinics can tell you something about the relative effectiveness of your therapeutic process. We mentioned the idea of accountability at the beginning of this chapter. It will be discussed more fully in the section concerned with the daily reporting of clinical activities.

Status at Beginning of Period. By analogy to the examination report, this section of the progress report represents the baseline for the reporting period. Information from the previous description (or descriptions) is briefly abstracted to show the entering baseline performance the speech-language performance at the beginning of the current period for comparative purposes, and any important considerations that influenced change or lack of change.

Summary of Therapy. Essentially, a summary of therapy amounts to a statement of what was done or attempted, why and how, and to what effect. Many training programs will require students to write out a specific set of goals and procedures before therapy begins. The difference between the clinician-in-training and the experienced clinician in this respect may be the degree to which the goals and procedures are written out, not the degree to which plans are formulated. For the purposes of the progress report, the critical information is once again a description of current speech and language performance. The more precise your descriptions, the more readily you can determine changes toward the goal originally set, or as modified, in your plan of care statement. For example, if one of your goals for a child was the inclusion of past-tense morphemes in her speech, your summary may report that "Susie was correct on 80 percent of her regular verb, past-tense endings and 75 percent of the irregular verb endings in structured response situations." This section is a summary or abstract in the truest sense of the word. All of the details of your day-to-day contact are not included for obvious reasons. It is, however, important to include sufficient description of the *how* and *why* of your intervention procedure to allow either a continuation of successful procedures or a modification of goals and procedures, if expected progress was not realized. Descriptive statements of this type will allow a comparative audit of procedures at a later time.

Recommendations. The primary requirement in writing recommendations is to be specific. Recommendations are the nearest thing to prescriptions that speech-language clinicians write. Tell the reader what, in your opinion, is to be done as continuation or modification from what was done in the current therapy period, for what continued or changed purposes, with what frequency, where, and by whom.

One word has been occuring with some degree of frequency throughout this chapter. That word is *opinion.* One chord that was struck in Chapter I, and repeated in a number of other locations, was the idea of fallibility. The diagnostic instruments and observations we have discussed may not have appraised everything that is important for the formulation of our interaction. If for no other reason than the recognition that this, like other people-oriented professions, is not an exact science, the "in-my-opinion" statement is an acceptable fence-riding hedge. That statement is the basis for our caveat that the report writer must label and separate statements of fact, reports and conjecture, and interpretation. Just as another speech-language pathologist may find it possible to make a different interpretation from your reported data, it may also be possible for him to arrive at a different set of recommendations.

Daily or Therapy Contact Reports

At the beginning of this chapter we commented on accountability in our evaluation and therapy reporting. Over the last few years much more attention has been paid to report writing, both as periodic summaries and daily contact notes. To a large degree this greater concern and greater precision has been required because of third-party accounting. Medicare, Medicaid, and the federal mandates contained in Public Law 94-142 are examples of this third-party interest. In addition to the inevitability of death and taxes, there are two inevitable accompaniments to the occurrence of state and federal support for speech-language and hearing services. One is the proliferation of regulatory guidelines, and the second is the acrostic use of initials to identify what otherwise might have been descriptive phrases. Examples in point for our reporting purposes are PCAs, IEPs, POMR and SOAP.

PCAs. PCAs or Patient Care Audits are only peripherally part of our current report writing concern. Patient Care Audits are part of a larger issue identified as quality assurance. An assurance that the services we provide are qualitatively adequate is not only a logical concern, for the provider as well as for the purchaser of services, it is also the implicit reason for all of the recording and reporting of clinical contact. Patient Care Audits are frequently retrospective in the sense that they may be concerned with whether or not we have routinely included in our clinical folders all of the information we have decided is minimal. For example, the members of a clinical group may have decided that all folders for clients seen on an initial speech-language evaluation must include:

a. a complete case history form
b. a pure-tone hearing screening

c. a vocabulary assessment
d. an articulation test
e. a measure of receptive and expressive language skill, and
f. an examination of the oral mechanism

Because we did not specify a number of variables such as age of subjects, or degree of cooperation, it would not be logical to assume that 100 percent of the folders to be reviewed for these data will include all of what we decided were minimum requirements. For example, it may be fair to assume that 100 percent of the folders would have a case history interview but that some of the clients were young children on whom we could not get a hearing screening test or a vocabulary test, and the like. It would be usual to set our performance criteria at something less than 100 percent but more than 75 percent, if it is considered "minimal."

We may select 90 percent, or 85 percent, or some other reasonable degree of compliance. Our retrospective review may include all of the cases of this type seen in the previous six months, or the last 50 cases of this category, or some other representative number. Those folders are pulled from the file and checked to see if they include evidence of the criteria we had chosen. Folders which do not contain all of the listed measures are reviewed by a professional member of the clinic group to see why the noted deficiencies occurred. This information, along with the tally of the percentage of folders that did contain each of the specified measures, is then presented to the entire clinic group for discussion. The identification of deficiencies in the folders or the reports is not to fix blame on individuals but to decide if changes in clinic procedures are necessary to insure that all the necessary data are collected and reported. It is also possible, as a result of the discussion, that some measures earlier specified as minimal may be deleted from the "minimal" list. The next audit on the same category, at some specified future time, would tell whether the changed procedures had accomplished the desired data.

Patient Care Audits may be on diagnostic categories, as the previous example; they may be on procedures of therapy or testing and test selection; or they may be outcome audits. An outcome audit is concerned with the effectiveness of the intervention regime. It has to do with total hours of therapy contact and whether the client had reached her maximum potential when dismissed. In the strictest sense, the outcome audit is the real measure of quality of services provided. Drucker (1974), in a text concerned with business management, defines two words that are frequently confused and which are pertinent to our discussion of quality of services. The words are *efficiency* and *effectiveness.* Efficiency is defined as doing well those procedures which we selected; effectiveness is selecting the most appropriate procedures. It is possible to be efficient in procedures which may not be the most effective in outcome. Delivery of quality services–outcomes audits–are concerned with the efficiency of effective procedures.

IEPs. Individualized Educational Plans (IEPs) are mandated by Public Law 94-142–The Education of all Handicapped Children Act of 1975–which demands an appropriate free public education for all handicapped children from three to twenty-one years of age.* The law states that IEPs are to be developed by the parent, the classroom teacher, and a representative of the local educational agency. To insure the completeness and the appropriateness of the specialized intervention plan, representatives of professional specialties involved in this educational plan may also be included. The IEPs as developed, and as periodically reviewed, must include:

a. a statement of the present levels of educational performance of each such child;
b. a statement of annual goals, including short-term instructional objectives;
c. a statement of the specific educational services to be provided to each child and the extent to which such child will be able to participate in regular educational programs;
d. the projected date of initiation and anticipated duration of such services, and;
e. appropriate objective criteria and evaluation procedures and schedules for determining, on at least an annual basis, whether instructional objectives are achieved.

In other words, for the purposes of this discussion, our analysis of what the child requires in terms of his speech-language-hearing needs is assembled with his other total educational requirements. The IEP inclusions listed obviously require descriptive statements of the problems presented, concise plans for remediation, and goals and objectives which are sufficiently objective to allow measurement. Once again, statements of the problem, descriptive data, interpretations and recommendations must be separable.

POMR–SOAP. Just as IEPs are usually associated with school programs, POMR and SOAP (Bouchard and Shane 1977) most often are associated with hospital-based programs. POMR stands for Problem Oriented Medical Records. This record-keeping system was not developed specifically for speech-language pathology, but like the IEP format can be used effectively by speech-language pathologists. The data base is the core of information which is collected for description of the patient. It includes such things as the development of the problem, the present complaint, the life situation insofar as it bears on the problem or the remediation of identified problems, and the results of evaluations from speech pathology and others concerned with the "total" patient. Problems are identified, listed, and numbered on a "problem list" at the front of the patient folder. This list serves as a table of contents and

*The inclusion of children under five and over 18 is not required if it is inconsistent with the state law and practice.

includes the initial plans for patient care as well as a rationale for new testing when appropriate, plans for therapy, and patient education. For example, with a stroke patient, problems identified may include self-help and self-care skills (or activities for daily living), muscle reeducation and locomotion, language and communication, and education of the patient and family as to what to expect in terms of recovery. Problem notes are placed in the daily record and identified with appropriate problem numbers.

The patient information is placed under four columns in the record, and this is where SOAP comes in. SOAP stands for Subjective, Objective, Assessment, and Plans. The four headings are defined by Bouchard and Shane (1977) as:

Subjective –information supplied by the client and his family including the complaint and the symptoms from their point of view,

Objective –those observations made by the clinician from his viewpoint as well as all objective information received from referral sources,

Assessment–evaluation of the problems presented based on subjective and objective findings–i.e., the diagnosis, and

Plans –plans for further testing, for therapeutic intervention, and for patient education for the numerically identified problems each member of the therapeutic regime is concerned with.

This discussion holds no brief for any particular type of daily record keeping. Obviously some have more relevance for specific settings than others. What is important is the daily, brief, descriptive notation of what happened, when, and to what avail. Daily notes must be recorded in ink and signed by the clinician as part of the Medicare regulations. Medicaid is administered by states so regulations are more variable. One other comment may be appropriate to underline the importance of daily therapy records. They can be considered legal documents and are subject to review and audit, especially for the Special Education Act and Medicare purposes. It probably goes without saying that the certified clinician-in-charge (Case Manager) writes and signs the daily therapy notes rather than the student-trainee in clinician training programs.

SUMMARY

We have discussed both form and substance of report writing. Listings of do's and don'ts have been provided in a number of published sources for the writing of reports. What they have in common is the insistence on clarity and the requirement that a report communicate information from the writer to the reader. The importance of concise, informative, and descriptive reports cannot be overemphasized. In a legal sense, if the therapeutic contact was not documented and recorded, for all practical purposes it did not occur. A report is a communication which also has relevance beyond the immediate information to be conveyed. Knepflar (1976) expressed it this way:

> The need for effective report writing (is important) to all professionals in our field. How do physicians, dentists, psychologists, social workers, educators, and other professionals judge our capabilities, whether we represent a hospital, a community agency, a public school system, or a college or university? The answer to that question is: through our ability to communicate concisely and effectively, in language that can be easily understood. More often than not, this communication is written rather than oral. (p. xii)

We have discussed three types of clinical reports: initial or diagnostic descriptions, periodic or so-called progress reports of ongoing clinical contact, and special purpose reports including daily record keeping. Outlines for the diagnostic report and for the progress report were included as examples. There is no single acceptable format for writing reports. What is important is that information be included which adequately describes the problem and what will be (or has been) done about it. The interpretation of subjective and objective findings is a professional judgment—and the interpretation of significance and recommendations for what is to be done are statements of the writer's professional opinion. That fact does not make the judgment inherently good, bad, or otherwise. It only means that the writer must be certain that baseline data and interpretations of those data are separable.

REFERENCES

Andrews, J. K., Operationally written therapy goals in supervised clinical practicum. *Asha,* 13, 385-387 (1971).

Bouchard, M. M., and H. C. Shane, Use of the problem-oriented medical record in the speech and hearing profession. (Special Report) *Asha,* 19, 157-159 (1977).

Caccamo, J. M., Accountability—a matter of ethics? *Asha,* 15, 411-412 (1973).

Chapey, R., Consumer satisfaction in speech-language pathology. *Asha,* 19, 829-833 (1977).

Drucker, P. F., *Management: Tasks, Responsibilities, Practices.* New York: Harper & Row, (1974).

Eisenstadt, A. A., Weakness in clinical procedures—a parental evaluation. *Asha,* 14, 7-9 (1972).

Emerick, L., and J. Hatten, *Diagnosis and Evaluation in Speech Pathology.* Englewood Cliffs, N.J.: Prentice-Hall, Inc., (1974).

English, R., and H. Lilywhite, A semantic approach to clinical reporting in speech pathology. *Asha,* 5, 647-650 (1963).

Fisher, L. I., Reporting: In the schools to the community, in *Clinical Speech in the Schools,* ed. R. J. Van Hattum. Springfield, Ill.: Charles C Thomas, (1969).

Good, R., The written language of rehabilitation medicine: Meanings and usages. *Arch. Phys. Med. Rehabil.,* 51, 296-36 (1970).

Jerger, J., Scientific writing can be readable. *Asha,* 4, 101-104 (1962).

Johnson, W., F. L. Darley, and D. C. Spriestersbach, *Diagnostic Methods in Speech Pathology.* New York: Harper & Row, (1963).

Knepflar, K. J., *Report Writing in the Field of Communication Disorders.* Danville, Ill.: The Interstate Printers and Publishers, (1976).

Moore, M., Pathological writing. *Asha,* 11, 535-538 (1969).

Mowrer, D., Accountability and speech therapy. *Asha,* 14, 115 (1972).

Mueller, P. B., and T. J. Peters, A clinical record-keeping system. *Asha,* 18, 352-353 (1976).

Nation, J. E., and D. M. Aram, *Diagnosis of Speech and Language Disorders.* St. Louis, Mo.: C. V. Mosby Co., (1977).

Pannbacker, M., Diagnostic report writing. *J. Speech Hearing Dis.,* 40, 367-379 (1975).

Sanders, L., *Procedure Guides for Evaluation of Speech and Language Disorders in Children.* Danville, Ill.: Interstate Press, (1972).

Strunk, W. Jr., and E. B. White, *The Elements of Style.* New York: Macmillan, (1959).

Taylor, M. F., Report writing in the medical setting: some special considerations. *J. Speech Hearing Dis.,* 42, 581-582 (1977).

Wolfle, D., Bad writing. *Science, N.Y.,* 155, 37 (1967).

AUTHOR INDEX

Y

Z

SUBJECT INDEX

A

B

C